AF878966

Pharmacology of Diabetes

Diabetes Forum Series, Volume 3

Pharmacology of Diabetes

Present Practice and Future Perspectives

Editors: C. E. Mogensen, E. Standl

Walter de Gruyter
Berlin · New York 1991

Deutsche Bibliothek Cataloging-in-Publication-Data

Pharmacology of diabetes : present practice and future perspectives / ed.: C. E. Mogensen ; E. Standl. – Berlin ; New York : de Gruyter, 1991
ISBN 3-11-012636-2
NE: Mogensen, Carl E. [Hrsg.]

Library of Congress Cataloging-in-Publication Data

Pharmacology of diabetes : present practice and future perspectives / editors, C. E. Mogensen, E. Standl.
Includes index.
ISBN 0-89925-742-9
1. Diabetes—Chemotherapy. I. Mogensen, Carl Erik. II. Standl, E. (Eberhard)
[DNLM: 1. Diabetes Mellitus—drug therapy. 2. Hypoglycemic Agents—therapeutic use. 3. Insulin—therapeutic use. Wk 825 P536]
RC661.A1P43 1990
616.4'62061—dc20
DNLM/DLC
for Library of Congress 90-14121
CIP

© Copyright 1990 by Walter de Gruyter & Co., Berlin 30. All rights reserved, including those of translation into foreign languages. No part of this book may be reproduced in any form – by photoprint, microfilm or any other means nor transmitted nor translated into a machine language without written permission from the publisher.

Medical science is constantly developing. Research and clinical experience expand our knowledge, especially with regard to treatment and medication.

For dosages and applications mentioned in this work, the reader may rely on the authors, editors and publisher having taken great pains to ensure that these indications reflect the standard of knowledge at the timc this work was completed.

Nevertheless, all users are requested to check the package leaflet of the medication, in order to determine for themselves whether the recommendations given for the dosages or the likely contraindications differ from those given in this book. This is especially true for medication which is seldom used or has recently been put on the market and for medication whose application has been restricted by the German Ministry of Health.

The quotation of registered names, trade names, trade marks, etc. in this copy does not imply, even in the absence of a specific statement that such names are exempt from laws and regulations protecting trade marks, etc. and therefore free for general use.

Typesetting: Arthur Collignon GmbH, Berlin. – Printing: Gerike GmbH, Berlin. – Binding: Lüderitz & Bauer GmbH, Berlin. – Printed in Germany.

Editors

Prof. Dr. C. E. Mogensen
Medical Department M
Second University Clinic
of Internal Medicine
(Diabetes and Endocrinology)
Kommunehospitalet
DK-8000 Aarhus C
Denmark

Prof. Dr. E. Standl
III. Med. Abteilung
des Städtischen Akad.
Lehrkrankenhauses
München-Schwabing
Kölner Platz 1
D-8000 München 40
West Germany

List of first-mentioned contributors

C. Bain, M. D.
East Birmingham Hospital
Bordesley Green East
Birmingham B 9 5ST
England

H. Beck-Nielsen, M. D.
Medical Department M
Odense Sygehus
DK-5000 Odense
Denmark

K. J. Berg, M. D.
Medicinsk afdeling
Rikshospitalet
Pilestredet 32
0027 Oslo 1
Norway

D. J. Betteridge, M. D.
University College London
The Rayne Institute
University Street
GB-London WC1E6JJ
England

J. S. Christiansen, M. D.
Medical Department M
Diabetes and Endocrinology
Kommunehospitalet
DK-8000 Aarhus C
Denmark

M. P. Cohen, M. D.
University City – Science Center
Institute of Metabolic Research
3508 Market Street, Suite 420
Philadelphia/Pensylvania 19104
USA

J. A. Colwell, M. D.
Department of Medicine
Medical University of South
Carolina
171 Ashley Avenue
Charleston, South Carolina
29425 – 2220
USA

J. Giardino, M. D.
Diabetes Research Center of
Medicine of Yeshiva University
1300 Morris Park Avenue
Bronx, N. Y. 10461
USA

D. A. Greene, M. D.
The University of Michigan
Medical Center
Department of Internal Medicine
5570 MSRB II, Box 0678
Ann Arbor, Michigan 48109–0678
USA

T. Jensen, M. D.
Research Fellow
Steno Memorial Hospital
DK-2820 Gentofte
Denmark

E. M. Kohner, M. D.
Hammersmith Hospital
Du Cane Road
GB-London W12 OHS
England

A. Kribben, M. D.
Zentrum für Innere Medizin
Universitätsklinikum Essen
Hufelandstr. 55
D-4300 Essen 1
West Germany

J. G. Larkin, M. D.
Department of Medicine
Gardiner Institute
University of Glasgow
GB-Glasgow G11 6NT
Scotland

H. Lithell, M. D.
Department of Geriatrics
Uppsala University
Box 12042
S-750 12 Uppsala
Sweden

N. Lotz, M. D.
III. Med. Abt.
d. Städt. Krankenhauses
München-Schwabing
Kölner Platz 1
D-8000 München 40
West Germany

C. E. Mogensen, M. D.
Medical Department M
Kommunehospitalet
DK-8000 Aarhus
Denmark

L. Mølsted-Pedersen, M. D.
Department of Gynecology and
Obstetrics
Rigshospitalet
Blegdamsvej 9
DK-2100 København 0
Denmark

G. Schernthaner, M. D.
I. Med. Abteilung
der Krankenanstalt Rudolfstiftung
Juchgasse 25
A-1030 Wien
Austria

E. Standl, M. D.
III. Med. Abt.
d. Städt. Krankenhauses
München-Schwabing
Kölner Platz 1
D-8000 München 40
West Germany

M. Toeller, M. D.
Diabetesforschungsinstitut der
Universität Düsseldorf
Auf'm Hennekamp 65
D-4000 Düsseldorf
West Germany

J. P. Vora, M. D.
Department of Medicine
University of Wales
Health Park
GB-Cardiff CF4 4XN
Wales

A. W. Zorgniotti, M. D.
33 East 74th Street
New York
N. Y. 10021
USA

Contents

Introduction

Treatment of diabetes has become an increasing challenge to the clinicians in recent years. A rapid development has taken place within a number of pharmacological areas both with respect to insulin-dependent and non-insulin-dependent diabetes and also within the prevention and treatment of complications of both types of patients. Within diabetes treatment problems can usually be divided into two phases, namely the acute or short-term treatment of patients aiming at well-being and perfect physical abilities for professional and leisure activities, mainly related to good metabolic control. The long-term perspective of treatment is the prevention of complications of the microvascular and the macrovascular system. Insulin treatment has changed considerably during recent years with the introduction of multiple insulin injection programmes with pens and intensified self-monitoring. This development has also had a considerable effect on other short-term treatment areas, namely prevention and treatment of infections and also treatment related to pregnancy where short-term metabolic control is very critical. Also, other acute metabolic aberrations may be ameliorated by new treatment modalities, for instance lipid lowering agents or agents modifying glucose absorption or possibly appetite regulation. Regarding type II diabetes new perspectives are also on the horizon, although the classical treatment with sulphonyluria and biguanides, along with diet remains the cornerstone of treatment of this type of diabetes.

An important area is obviously prevention of treatment of complications and considerable development has taken place in the last few decades. The development of diabetic complications is undoubtful a multifactorial process, and therefore it is not surprising that researchers attack the problem from many different angles, all discussed in the present volume which tries to cover almost all aspects of the pharmacological treatment of diabetes. Attempts have also been made to introduce a real cure for diabetes, both in insulin-dependent and non-insulin-dependent diabetes, but still we are only on the track on such radical achievements. Pharmacological treatment also involves problems related to diabetogenic drugs and this important field is also discussed in the present volume.

The book is meant as a working guide for the practical diabetologists active in all parts of the health care system and, along with the previous volume in this series and a future one "Concepts of the Ideal Diabetes Clinic", the Diabetes Forum Series should indeed cover most parts of diabetes management, not only from a treatment point of view, but also from the point of diagnosis and etiology of the disease.

The editors have had the pleasure to cooperate with many colleagues and specialists within the field and it is really impressive to see how many new aspects are related to diabetes. However, the physicians have to treat the individual patients. It is essential, therefore, that up-to-date knowledge is available on the desk where this volume is meant to be placed. We look forward to comments and proposals with regard to the present volume in this series.

Finally, the editors would like to express their sincere thanks to Bayer AG for a very fine and effective cooperation. We would also like to acknowledge the excellent and kind cooperation with the publisher, Walter de Gruyter & Co. in Berlin.

Munich and Aarhus
August 1990 *Eberhard Standl and Carl Erik Mogensen*

Immunomodulation in the initial phase of type I diabetes mellitus: a critical analysis

G. Schernthaner

Introduction

There is now overwhelming evidence that insulin dependent (type I) diabetes is an immunological disease [1 – 5]. What initiates the disorder – a viral infection or an autoimmune stimulus – is not known, but that the subsequent gradual destruction of β-cells is immune-mediated can no longer be in doubt [1 – 6]. This knowledge has emerged over the past 15 years from research [2 – 10], indicating (a) a genetically determined predisposition to type I diabetes, associated with HLA DR genes, which is almost a prerequisite for development of disease; (b) immunoglobulins (islet-cell antibodies) are present in almost all newly-diagnosed cases and (c) more recently, high levels of activated T-lymphocytes have been found in new cases, but not in patients with longstanding disease. The concept that type I diabetes is an autoimmune disease is supported by two recent observations: The recurrence of insulitis and disease in transplanted pancreata of monozygotic twins [11] and the successful immunotherapy of newly-diagnosed cases with cyclosporine-A [12].

Rationale of immune intervention in type I diabetes

Conventionally treated type I diabetes is still associated with considerable excess mortality and morbidity [13]. However, impressive improvements in the prognosis of type I diabetes have been achieved during the last few decades. The increase of 15 – 30 years of life expectancy of type I diabetic patients can most likely be explained by a 30% decline of the incidence of diabetic nephropathy [14]. Nevertheless, about 35% of the newly diagnosed type I diabetic patients will still develop diabetic nephropathy. We have to realize that the widely used secondary therapy with functional insulin substitution, patient education and blood glucose self-control 4 – 5 times daily seems to be insufficient to prevent late diabetic complications in all cases [15 – 17]. Secondary therapy is still associated with impaired quality of life, vascular complications, a high mortality rate and decreased life expectancy. Many long-term cases need tertiary forms of treatment, such as photocoagulation, vitrectomy or kidney transplantation. Although prolongation of life expectancy and improvement in the quality of life is possible even at that stage, a primary therapy with the hope of a "cure" would obviously be most desirable. An important factor in consideration of immunotherapy trials is the seriousness of type I diabetes, which does not appear to have changed dramatically. Previously published data [18], as well as the most recent update by Danish colleagues indicate a 40% 30 year mortality [19]. In addition to such mortality figures, the morbidity from retinopathy, nephropathy and other vascular complications is distressing.

Strategies and types of immune intervention in type I diabetes

The previously described observations transformed our ideas of the pathogenesis of the disease and led to attempts to curtail the process of β-cell destruction by immunosuppression. Different therapeutic approaches have already been described in patients with newly diagnosed type I diabetes [4], including preliminary attempts at both immunosuppression [12] and immunomodulation [20]. Immunomodulation can reduce or enhance a particular activity of the immune system at a given time or stage of a disease, while immunosuppression changes the overall activity of the immune system. Immunomodulatory drugs or procedures can either modify the immunoregula-

Table 1 The potential therapeutic strategies of type I diabetes at onset of the disease

Insulin to maintain normoglycaemia
Glucocorticoids
Interferon (s)
Immunoregulants (dapsone, levamisole)
Plasmapheresis
Thymic hormones
Anti-thymocyte-globulin
Intravenous gamma-globulin
Nicotinamide
Antimetabolites (azathioprine, cyclosporine-A)
Anti-lymphocyte serum
Total lymphoid irradiation
Monoclonal antibodies against cell subsets
Monoclonal antibodies against idiotypes
Anti-lymphokines
Suppressor factors

tory balance or they can effect a lymphocyte subpopulation at the effector-cell level. In contrast, immunosuppression basically operates by blocking the proliferation of immune cells. Thus, it is possible that the effects are due mainly to the proliferative stage of lymphocyte subpopulations at the time of treatment. The potential therapeutic strategies of type I diabetes at the onset of the disease are summarized in Table 1.

Immunomodulatory drugs and procedures

Plasmapheresis

Plasmapheresis was one of the earliest immunomodulatory procedures used in type I diabetes mellitus. The action of plasmapheresis is based on two separate mechanisms: (a) the depletion of the patient's plasma leads to reduction of autoantibodies and antigen-antibody complexes and (b) the donor plasma may add components which are lacking in the patient's plasma, i. e. anti-idiotypic antibodies. Some studies have been carried out with plasmapheresis in human type I diabetes [21 – 24]. Ludvigsson et al. [21, 22] were unable to show a significant effect of plasmapheresis on islet-cell antibodies, complement dependent antibody-mediated-cytotoxicity, or on complement-dependent, antibody-mediated cytotoxicity against RINm5F cells [23]. In contrast, positive effects were observed even after 18 months on basal and stimulated C-peptide secretion, the duration of total remission and metabolic control. In another small pilot study [24] plasmapheresis was used in combination with azathioprine, prednisolone and anti-lymphocyte globulin administration. All three patients in this study came off insulin for a period between 6 and 12 months, but relapsed later on.

Levamisole

Levamisole is a synthetic derivate of tetramisole and one of the first chemically derived immunostimulants. Several mechanisms of action of levamisole have been proposed [25]. It acts directly on lymphocytes, macrophages, granulocytes to modify their mobility, secretion an proliferation. The principal mechanism of action appears to be facilitation of monocyte chemotaxis. It can be immunostimulatory or immunosuppressive in its effect depending on the dose and time of administration. When levamisole is administrated clinically, it acts on the cellular limb of the immune response and does not affect antibody production. Levamisole can restore impaired cell-mediated immune responses to normal, but it will not hyperstimulate a normal immune system. The most interesting action of levamisole is mediated by the induction of a serum factor with a thymopoetin-like activity which is thymus independent, as shown in athymic mice. Consequently, several T-lymphocyte functions (mitogen- and antigen-induced proliferation, suppressor activity, lymphokine production, etc) as well as phagocytic functions are restored. Up to how, the therapeutical experience with levamisole is restricted to 3 type I diabetic patients [26], who received the drug for variable amounts of time. After six months, none of the patients showed any improvement concerning the stimulated C-peptide secretion.

Thymic Hormones

The central role of the thymus gland in the development and maintenance of the immune system has been recognized for many years. Several peptides have been isolated from thymic tissues and were found to circulate in the peripheral blood, establishing the role of the thymus as a endocrine gland. A number of hormones have been identified including thymosin fraction 5, thymosin $\alpha 1$, thymopoietin, thymulin and thymic humoral factor, among others. Several thymic polypeptides are now available and have been used for therapy in several immune- or autoimmune-mediated diseases [27]. In human diabetes, only thymostimulin (TP1), either alone or in association with azathioprine, has been used. Recent experience in 35 newly diagnosed patients shows some effect on induction and maintenance of remission [28], although the observed findings were not very different from figures obtained in historical control patients.

Theophylline

Theophylline acts mainly on T-suppressor cells. This is of some interest for patients with type I diabetes, since lymphocytes from patients with this disease have shown a loss of theophylline sensitivity in vitro [29], identified as an inhibition of E-rosette formation and a proliferative response to mitogens (ConA, PHA). Therefore, theophylline administration might restore impaired suppressor-cell function in diabetes. The therapeutic use of theophylline (800 mg/day for 1 month) has been evaluated in a small single-blind controlled study [30]. The findings observed are rather disappointing, since only a temporary partial remission (less than 0.2 U insulin requirement/kg/day) was achieved in 4 out of 5 patients, whereas in the placebo group two out of 4 patients also fulfilled these criteria.

Interferon

Interferon is a natural and broad spectrum antiviral glycoprotein that is species specific and produced by virtually all nucleated animal cells. Although it is usually referred to as a single molecule, three different types of interferon have been identified, i. e., α-, β-, and γ-interferon. There a 14 subtypes of α-interferon produced mainly by mononuclear leukocytes; β-interferon is made by fibroblasts in connective tissue, and γ-interferon is produced by T-cells. Interferon is normally produced after a virus infection by infected cells and it protects other cells from infection. Thus, interferon is a potent natural antiviral substance. Interferon activates both NK cells and macrophages [31], but in type I diabetes these effects have to be considered with caution since both cell types are likely to be involved in the process of β-cell destruction. In two newly diagnosed diabetic children adminstration of interferon failed to have any beneficial effect on metabolic control [32]. Likewise, in a single-blind controlled study in 43 patients, no difference was found between patients treated with α-interferon or placebo [33]. The control group as well as the placebo group showed a partial remission rate in 42% of the subjects studied. No difference in stimulated C-peptide levels and insulin requirements during the 12 months follow-up was observed. It is expected that the results of α-interferon treatment might be more promising in diabetic patients with a confirmed virus infection rather than in unselected cases.

Intravenous gamma-globulin

The effect of intravenous gamma-globulin can be explained by different actions. The gamma-globulin fraction may contain antiidiotypic antibodies which bind to autoantibodies and autoreactive B-cells inhibiting their activity. Furthermore, a decrease in the CD4/CD8 lymphocyte ratio and in particular, a reduction of B-helper cells were observed in patients with idiopathic thrombozytopenic purpura during treatment [34]. The experience in type I diabetes is limited to a small study performed in six children newly diagnosed with the disease, whereby 0.4 g/kg/day was infused over a period of five days [35]. In 2 of the 6 children a clinical remission was observed, one for a short period only and the other for 12 months. Several controlled studies using gamma-globulin and immunosuppressants in combination are running to clarify whether intravenous gamma-globulin administration is beneficial in the treatment of early type I diabetic cases.

Nicotinamide

Experimental animal studies have demonstrated, that nicotinamide can significantly diminish the diabetogenic effect of alloxan and streptozotozin [36]. Recent studies have shown that nicotinamide increases the β-cell NAD content by inhibiting poly-(ADP-ribose) synthetase, and favours insulin synthesis [37]. Up to now, two studies using nicotinamide have been performed in human diabetes mellitus [38, 39]. The effect of high dosage nicotinamide (3 g/day) has been analysed in seven patients with type I diabetes in comparison with nine placebo-treated patients [38]. Of the seven patients treated with nicotinamide 5 had gone into total remission after six months and three after 12 months. Of the nine placebo patients the figures were two and zero, respectively. In the second study only low dosages of nicotinamide (200 mg/day) were used [39] and also showed some beneficial effects. After six and twelve months a significant increase of C-peptide was observed in 22 patients on nicotinamide treatment in comparison with 13 control patients.

Ciamexone

Ciamexone acts mainly on B-lymphocytes by reducing antibody production, cell proliferation and suppressing antibody-dependent cellular cytotoxicity. Ciamexone was used in an open pilot study in 11 newly diagnosed type I diabetic subjects [40]. In that study 8 out of 11 patients under ciamexone treatement had a complete or partial remission as compared to only 3 out of 9 control patients. Based on these preliminary data, the German/Austrian Ciamexone Study Group was established. One hundred sixty-nine patients were treated either with ciamexone or placebo; after 6 months of treatment clinical remission was observed in 17.1% in ciamexone treated patients, but in only 1.9% in the placebo group. It must be noted that the clinical remission rate of 17.1% in the ciamexone-treated group is very similar to the clinical remission rate in the placebo group of the controlled cyclosporine-A studies [41]. Furthermore, a significant increase of C-peptide secretion could not be observed in the controlled ciamexone trial [41] in contrast to the randomized placebo-controlled Canadian-European cyclosporine-A study [42].

Anti-thymocyte-globulin

The action of the anti-thymocyte-globulin (ATG) treatment is the in-vivo destruction of mature T-cells and their precursors. Thus, the targets of this treatment with ATG are immune T-regulatory and effector T-cells, whereas

B-lymphocyte activity should not be affected. In one pilot study [43], 6 patients were treated with ATG (7 – 15 mg/day over a period of 1 – 4 weeks) in combination with prednisone (1 mg/kg/day). A decrease in the CD4/CD8 lymphocyte ratio and in improved metabolic control were observed and compared to patients receiving prednisolone only or the control group (insulin only). Two out of the 6 patients had a complete remission of the disease for more than 8 months. In the second study [44] the combined effect of ATG and prednisone was tested in 4 children with recent-onset type I diabetes. No clinical improvement could be detected after 6 months of treatment.

Immunosuppressive drugs

Azathioprine in type I diabetes

Azathioprine, a well known and widely used compound, is a cell-cycle-active antiproliferative agent effective in preventing the induction of primary immune responses, at both humoral and cellular levels [45]. Azathioprine produces a greater effect on autoantibody than on antibody production. It has a different effect on T-cell-dependent, compared with T-cell-independent, antibody responses. Up to now, three controlled studies [46 – 48] with azathioprine have been performed in type I diabetes; in one of the three studies the combined use of azathioprine and glucocorticoids [48] was tested. In the first trial azathioprine was administered alone to patients with recent-onset type I diabetes [46]. At 12 months, when azathioprine was discontinued, 7 of the 13 azathioprine group patients were in clinical remission, whereas only one such remission occurred in the placebo-treated group. Five of the patients in remission at one year relapsed during the first year after discontinuation of azathioprine treatment. A relationship of β-cell function and clinical remission was indicated by the finding that plasma-C-peptide levels were elevated on the group of azathioprine-treated patients who were non-insulin receiving at 1 year. This beneficial effect of azathioprine monotherapy was not confirmed in a randomized double-blind controlled trial using single treatment with azathioprine in 49 diabetic children in Australia [47]. None of the patients (mean age: 11 years; age range. 2 – 20 years) entered "clinical remission" and there was no significant difference in the rates of "partial remission" in the two treatment groups. At 6 months, 10 placebo- and 7 azathioprine-treated patients were in partial remission, and at 12 months the corresponding numbers were 4 and 4. Plasma C-peptide concentrations did not change significantly in the placebo group, but significantly rose between 0 and 3 months in the azathioprine-treated group. Thus, using a treatment regimen with azathioprine similar to that effective in adult patients, there was only a modest and transient effect on the basal C-peptide levels in plasma, whereas no difference between the treatment groups in terms of meal-stimulated β-cell function or clinical remission rates was noted [47].

Controlled trial with azathioprine and glucocorticoids

Forty-six patients with a mean age of 12 years (range 4–32 years) were entered [48] within two weeks of beginning insulin treatment, and were assigned to groups receiving either corticosteroids for 10 weeks together with azathioprine for 1 year, or no immunosuppressive therapy. The dose of azathioprine was initially 2 mg/kg body weight and was adjusted to maintain leucocyte counts of 3000–5000 cells/ml^3. Methylprednisolone was given intravenously in a dose of 30 mg/kg on alternate days for 4 dosages at entry, with oral prednisone 2 mg/kg/day. The dose of prednisone was reduced every 2 weeks with discontinutaion after 10 weeks. In the immunosuppressed group 10 patients discontinued insulin for periods of more than 1 week through the year of study, and 3 maintained normal-range blood glucose and HbA_{1C} levels without insulin therapy until more than one year after diagnosis. In contrast, only 2 patients in the control group became temporarily independent of insulin treatment during the year. The levels of standard-meal stimulated C-peptide at 1 year was significantly higher in the azathioprine-group than in the control group.

Immunosuppression with cyclosporine-A

Since the discovery of azathioprine in 1961 and the introduction of heterologous antilymphocyte serum in 1967, very little innovation has occurred in the area of immunosuppression. During the previous several decades, cytotoxic drugs have been used to induce immune tolerance by destroying replicating cells. The cytotoxic drugs are divided into cell-cycle drugs that destroy rapidly multiplying cells and the non-cycle drugs that are injurious to all cells and usually result in a depletion of small lymphocytes. The most dramatic discovery has been the introduction of cyclosporine. This is the first immunosuppressive agent that allows selective alteration of the immune system and is unlike all other available immunosuppressants. The mechanism of the action of cyclosporine in both in vitro and in vivo studies relates to its inhibition of lymphokine production by impairing interleukin-2 production by both quiescent and activated helper T-cells. This blockade of T-cell help required for B-cell activation, cytolytic T-cell generation, and further expansion of helper/inducer T-cell subpopulations underscores the potent mechanism of action of cyclosporine. There is also a simultaneous expansion of suppressor T-cell populations. Cyclosporine-A does not interrupt primary antibody responses unless introduced during the early steps of B-cell activation. The advantages of cyclosporine-A are well known from world-wide experience in the field of organ transplantation: the high immunosuppressive potency, the selectivity for T-lymphocytes, the lack of bone marrow toxicity, the possibilities of drug monitoring by radioimmunologic measurement of blood levels, as well as the fact that the effect of cyclosporine-A on the immune system is rapidly reversible. Cyclosporine depresses both cell-mediated immunity and antibody formation but its immunosuppressive effect is more powerful on cell-mediated than on humoral immunity [49]. Cyclosporine-A blocks the synthesis, as well as the release of interleukin 1 and interleukin 2, leading to modulation and suppression of the ongoing autoimmune process [50]. However, it is important to realize that this type of immunosuppression is totally unspecific.

Uncontrolled trials with cyclosporine-A in type I diabetes

In November 1982 a pilot-clinical trial of the effects of the administration of cyclosporine-A to volunteer subjects with recent onset type I diabetes mellitus was initiated in London, Ontario, Canada. The first results of the pilot studies were published in 1984 [12]. One group of patients received cyclosporine-A within 6 weeks after manifestation of disease, which means that immunotherapy started no later than 6 weeks after onset of insulin treatment. The daily insulin requirement decreased progressively in the majority of the patients, and an increasing number of patients maintained glycemic control in the absence of exogenous insulin. When this status had been maintained for at least two weeks, the subjects were designated "non-insulin-requiring". Approximately half (16 out of 30) of these patients attained a non-insulin requiring ("NIR") status. By contrast, only 2 of 11 subjects with diabetes between 2 and 11 months duration received positive benefit from this therapeutic intervention. From that point on, recruitment of further volunteers was confined to patients with disease of less than 6 weeks duration. Similar promising findings have been observed in the French pilot study [51], although the cyclosporine-A dosage was lower and onset of cyclosporine-A administration was somewhat later in the course of the disease. Four out of 12 patients went into total remission, 4 patients achieved partial remission and no effect was noted in the remaining four patients [51]. A non-insulin-requiring state was obtained in 47% in the Canadian open study [12] and in 33% in the first French open study [50]. These two studies [12, 50] had been performed in adult type I diabetic patients and the mean follow-up was 12 and 7 months respectively. Later on, the effect of cyclosporine was investigated in diabetic children in France. Forty diabetic children were followed up for a period of 6 months by one group [52] and another 40 patients for 12 months by a second group [52]. Surprisingly, the total remission rate obtained in diabetic children was even higher, namely 55% and 50% at 6 and 12 months after onset of cyclosporine treatment. The demonstrated efficacy of cyclosporine-A in the prevention of diabetes in the BB rat [54], and the promising results of pilot studies in type I diabetes in man, indicated a need for controlled clinical trials of the effects of cyclosporine-A in patients with type I diabetes of recent onset. The design of controlled studies, the entry criteria and the cyclosporine-A dosage used have been summarized previously [55].

Placebo-controlled cyclosporine-A studies

In 1984 the Canadian/European Diabetes Study group consisting of 13 diabetes treatment centers initiated a randomized double-blind placebo controlled trial designed to determine whether administration of cyclosporine-A induces remission of the disease, and if such a remission can be maintained for one year [42]. Concurrently, a comparable, but not identical study was initiated by a French multicenter group [57]. Both studies were randomized controlled trials, whereby parallel groups of patients treated with either insulin and cyclosporine-A or insulin and placebo are compared. Classical recent-onset type I diabetic patients were studied, whereby strict exclusion criteria with respect to safety were taken into consideration. In both studies, the French and the Canadian/European trial, the dose of insulin was minimized as far as was consistent with maintenance of the target control of near normoglycemia.

French multicentre double-blind cyclosporine-A study

In the French multicentre double-blind trial, 106 cases were analysed at 6 months after treatment [56]. Incidence of remission was increased 5-fold in the cyclosporine-A-treated patients as compared with the placebo group. 24% of cyclosporine-A-treated, but only about 5% of placebo-treated patients went into total remission. Further analysis showed a significant correlation between the average cyclosporine-A trough levels in the first three months and the incidence of complete remission at nine months. In patients whose cyclosporine-A blood trough levels in the first three months were 300 ng/ml or higher, the complete remission rate at 6 months was 37,5% and the complete and partial remission rate combined was 65%. By contrast those with lower blood trough levels had about the same rate of remission as the placebo group at six months. The French group reported no serious nephrotoxicity. Plasma creatinine rose above normal in 26% of cyclosporine-A treated subjects but never exceeded 160µmol/l.

Canadian-European controlled cyclosporine-A study

Nine Canadian and five European centres participated in the Canadian-European trial [42]. Out of the 187 patients, more than 40 newly diagnosed patients have been treated in Vienna [57] and almost the same number in Copenhagen. In the Canadian/European trial, patients were entered within 6 weeks after diagnosis and within 14 weeks after onset of classical symptoms. Administration of cyclosporine-A was initiated with 10 mg/kg/day and dosage was adjusted to maintain whole blood concentrations of 400 – 600 ng/ml at onset of the study and later on, of 300 – 400 ng/ml as determined by radioimmunoassay. Fig. 1 shows the effect of cyclosporine on remission rates in the Canadian/European multicenter trial. At three months of follow-up approximately 25% of both groups were in total remission. The total remission rate continued to rise in the cyclosporine-treated group significantly higher and peak later than in the placebo group. The total remission rate was

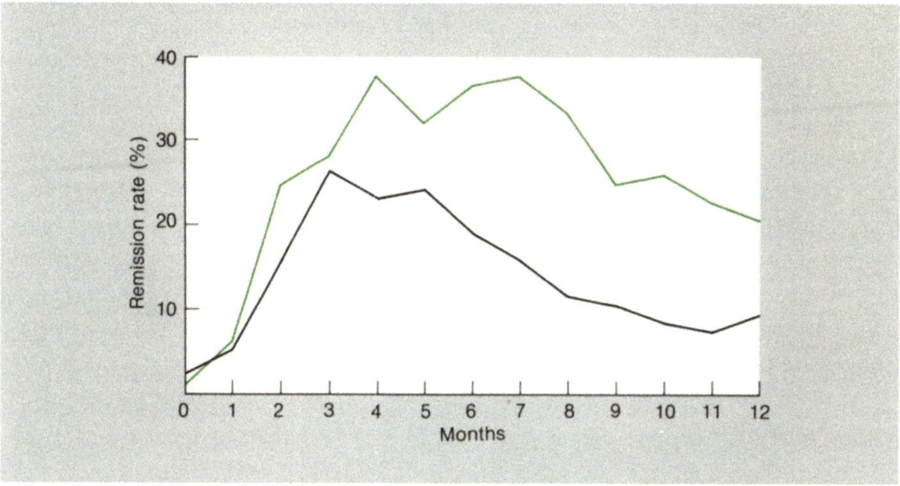

Fig. 1 Effect of cyclosporine-A (green) or placebo (black) on remission rates in the Canadian/European multicentre trial [42].

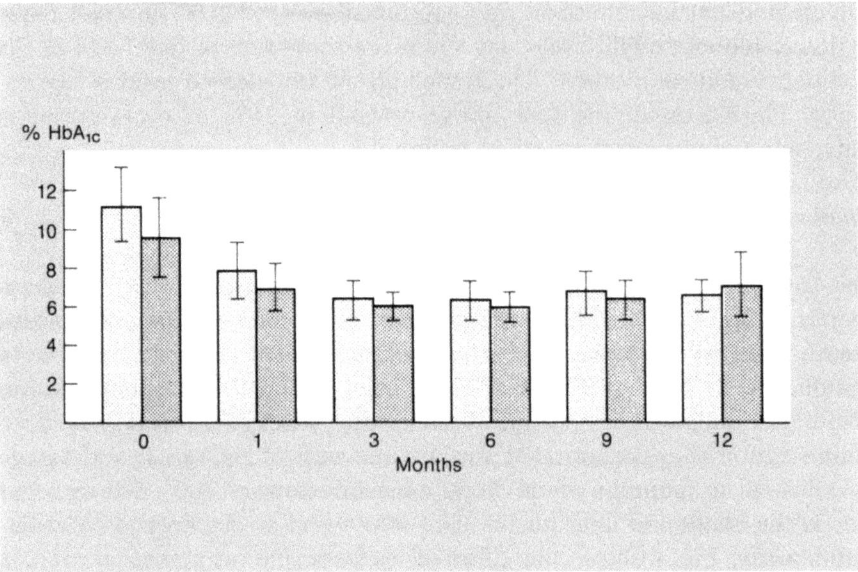

Fig. 2. Haemoglobin A_{1C} values of type I diabetic patients during the first 12 months of the disease treated in Vienna [58] with either cyclosporine-A (green) or placebo (grey).

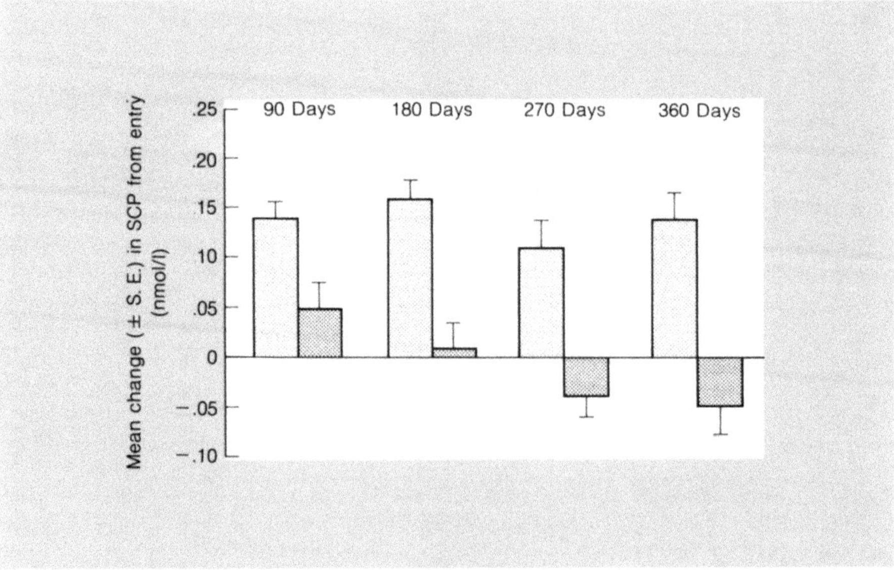

Fig. 3. Changes in the response of plasma C-peptide to glucagon [42] from baseline in groups treated either with cyclosporine-A (green) or placebo (grey).

maintained for several months in the cyclosporine-treated type I diabetic patients. Thereafter, the total remission rate decreased in both groups at follow up between 8 and 12 months. After 6 months of follow-up, total remission rate was 38.7% in cyclosporine-treated patients, but only 19.1% in the placebo group. After 12 months 24% of cyclosporine-treated patients, but only 9.8% of placebo-treated patients were still in total remission. The observed loss of remissions in the interval 6–12 months is troublesome in regard to potential for the clinical benefit.

The total remission rate was even higher in the patients treated with cyclosporine-A in the Vienna diabetes centre [57], which can be explained most likely by the very short duration of disease before starting cyclosporine treatment. Fig. 2 illustrates the haemoglobin A1C values of the type I diabetic patients treated with either cyclosporine-A or placebo in Vienna [57]. Both treatment groups demonstrated high HbA_{1C} values at manifestation of disease and a similar significant decrease in the upper range of normal at 12 months after onset of the study. Fig. 3 shows the changes in the responses of plasma C-peptide to glucagon from baseline in the two treatment groups. Changes in the cyclosporine-treated group were significantly different from those in the placebo-treated groups at all times. The C-peptide response of the placebo group decreased significantly from 3 to 12 months, whereas that of the cyclosporine group was maintained through the second half of the year, suggesting that progressive deterioration of β-cell function did not occur within that time. The maintenance of relatively high levels of C-peptide in the blood of cyclosporine-treated patients and their greater rate of remission are consistent with the importance of those factors in determining the insulin requirement. At the present time, we have no conclusive explanation for the loss of remissions during the second half of the year. Whether relapses result from inadequate immunosuppression, non-compliance with other modes of treatment, or are unavoidable is not known.

The effect of duration of diabetes and cyclosporine on remission is shown in Table 2. Interestingly, a relatively short duration of diabetes – meaning entry less than 6 weeks after onset of symptoms with less than 2 weeks of insulin therapy – was associated with greater efficacy of cyclosporine. Total remission rate was 55% after 6 months of cyclosporine treatment in the patients with short duration of disease compared to 13% of placebo treated patients. After one year of treatment the total remission rate was 32% in the cyclosporine-treated patients with short-term disease in comparison with less than 3% in placebo-treated patients. In contrast, total remission rate was relatively low and very similar in cyclosporine- and placebo-treated patients with longer-duration of disease. The relatively low rate of spontaneous total

Table 2 Effect of duration of diabetes and cyclosporine-A on remission in the Canadian/European multicentre Trial [42]

Outcome	6 mo		12 mo	
	Short*	Long	Short*	Long
NIR or CP ≥ 0.6 nM				
Cyclosporine	71.1 (38)	38.2 (55)	39.5 (38)	28.3 (53)
Placebo	31.6 (38)	30.4 (56)	16.2 (37)	23.6 (55)
P	.001	.39	.02	.58
P diff†	.02		.15	
NIR				
Cyclosporine	55.3 (38)	27.3 (55)	31.6 (38)	18.9 (53)
Placebo	13.2 (38)	23.2 (56)	2.7 (37)	14.5 (55)
P	.001	.62	.001	.55
P diff†	.003		.06	

Values are percentages, with number of subjects in parentheses. The minor discrepancies between numbers of subjects in the 2 response groups are accounted for by data falling outside predetermined time windows. NIR, non-insulin-requiring; CP, C-peptide.
* ≤ 6 wk symptoms and ≤ 2 wk insulin before entry.
† Difference in treatment effect between short-duration and long-duration subsets.

remission in short-duration diabetes mellitus in comparison with longer-duration disease in the placebo group is consistent with a more agressive process in short-duration diabetes.

Combined treatment with cyclosporine-A and glucocorticoids

The combined use of cyclosporine-A and methylprednisolone (1.25 g infused over 72 hours) was analysed in 38 patients with recent onset type I diabetes in order to test whether the additional administration of glucocorticoids could induce an earlier and higher occurrence rate of remission [57]. Seventeen of 38 patients received cyclosporine-A in an initial dose of 10 mg/kg/day and the remaining 21 patients a dose of 7.5 mg/kg/day. The control group was treated with cyclosporine-A (7.5 mg/kg/day) alone. No difference was noted in the clinical remission rate or in the C-peptide increase versus baseline among the 3 treatment groups. Further studies are necessary to clarify whether the combined administration of cyclosporine-A and glucocorticoids is superior to cyclosporine-A therapy alone or not.

Side effects of cyclosporine-A treatment

Hypertrichosis was the most frequent clinical side effect, seen in 45% of the cyclosporine-A group in the French trial [56]. Hypertension was noted in 3 placebo and 9 cyclosporine-A patients. The proportion of patients who had one or more infections was 61% in the cyclosporine group and 48% in the placebo group, not reaching a statistically significant difference. No severe infections were observed in either group. The side effects of cyclosporine treatment in the Canadian-European study [42] were very similar to those reported in the French trial. The most important side effect was chronic nephrotoxicity. The creatinine clearance rate fell by 21% from baseline by 6 months and by 25% from baseline by 12 months in the cyclosporine-treated group. The rise in mean diastolic blood pressure in the cyclosporine-treated group was modest and was not significantly different at 12 months from the placebo group [42]. In view of the risk of structural damage to the kidney, biopsies from 15 patients treated for more than 12 months were evaluated and classified by two independent pathologists. Histopathological changes associated with administration of cyclosporine were rated on 4 scales concerning tubulus atrophy, interstitial fibrosis and arteriolopathy. The majority of the patients had a relatively low histologic score [42]. Remarkably, the histologic score showed a close relationship with the cyclosporine treatment score. Histologic changes were minimal in the set of biopsies from patients in whom the mean cyclosporine trough blood level was less than 400 ng/ml. In light of these results, our study group has adopted an upper limit of 400 ng/ml whole blood for the 12-h trough level of cyclosporine in continuing studies. In a recently published uncontrolled cyclosporine study performed in diabetic children in France [53], a high remission rate of 67% at 4 months and of 50% at 12 months was observed even when low non-toxic cyclosporine-A dosages were used. The blood trough levels in this study ranged between 150 and 350 ng/ml. Nephrotoxic side effects were almost absent in the kidney biopsies of the diabetic children, who were treated with low cyclosporine dosages for a period of one year [52]. The lack of nephrotoxicity might be explained by the fact that cyclosporine blood trough levels were less than 400 ng/ml.

Critical analysis of cyclosporine-A studies in type I diabetes

What have we learned from the pilot and controlled cyclosporine-A studies in recent onset type I diabetes patients? Total remission was seen in 20% to 50% of cyclosporine-A-treated patients at 12 months follow up, but in only

Table 3 Pros and cons of cyclosporine-A treatment in type I diabetes mellitus

Pros	Cons
• Diminuation of β-cell destruction • Improvement of quality of life • Decrease/delay of late complications • Primary therapy (cure) • Development of new therapeutic concepts	• Onset of intervention too late? (80% of β-cells destroyed) • Non-responders (30–70%) • Lifelong therapy • Induction of lymphoma • β-cell Toxicity • Nephrotoxicity

3–10% of placebo-treated patients. The difference between cyclosporine-A and placebo-treated patients is statistically highly significant in both controlled studies. These findings strongly support the concept that type I diabetes is indeed a member of the family of autoimmune diseases. A higher response rate was seen when the duration of diabetes prior to treatment with cyclosporine-A was short. The chronic nephrotoxicity of cyclosporine-A demonstrate by kidney biopsies in transplanted patients and in subjects with other autoimmune diseases must, however, limit efforts to halt the β-cell destructive process by use of cyclosporine-A in diabetes.

Table 3 lists the pros and cons of cyclosporine-A treatment in type I diabetic patients. A diminuation of β-cell destruction, an improvement of quality of life and hopefully a decrease or postponement of late complications form the rationale for immune intervention in the early phase of type I diabetes. Moreover, it is hoped that further improvements in such forms of primary therapy might be curative at least in a representative number of cases. It is clear that cyclosporine-A treatment at the present time is still an experimental therapeutic intervention and should not be used outside controlled studies. The development of new therapeutic concepts with the goal of primary therapy is a further point within the pros for immune intervention in type I diabetic patients. The available experience with immunosuppression indicates that the intervention comes too late in many cases, since 70–80% of the β-cell mass seems already to be destroyed at onset of the immune intervention. Thus, very early immunosuppression is necessary. Efficacy of cyclosporine-A is minimal when patients have symptoms for more than two weeks prior to administration of cyclosporine-A. These findings suggest that the destructive process of β-cells show very rapid and progressive course during the very last few weeks before manifestation of the disease, although the immunologic prediabetic phase may have been present for many months or years before clinical manifestation. Whether or not viral infections [5] are involved in this final precipitation of the disease must be clarified in further studies. A relatively high non-responding rate and the necessity for a lifelong treatment have to be viewed as disadvantages. Increased risk of development of lymphomas has also been discussed, although the risk seems to be very low for cyclosporine-A monotherapy according to the experience of cyclosporine-A treatment in about 1000 cases with other autoimmune diseases [20]. A toxic effect of cyclosporine-A on Langerhans' islets has been suggested in some animal studies [20], but this notion is contradicted by the persistance of clinical remission in type I diabetic patients and by the absence of hyperglycaemia in patients receiving cyclosporine-A alone for therapy of autoimmune diseases. Chronic cyclosporine-A therapy in patients with multiple sclerosis during 2 years did not affect glucose homeostasis or islet β-cell function [61]. The unsolved problem of cyclosporine-A treatment is the chronic nephrotoxicity [62] of this otherwise extremely useful drug. Finally, in the Canadian open study [12] and in the controlled cyclosporine-A trials [42, 56] most patients relapsed within a few weeks after discontinuation of cyclosporine-A, indicating the need for a long-term immunomodulatory therapy.

Immunotherapeutic intervention in the prediabetic phase?

Experimental animal studies, in particular in the BB Wister rat and NOD mouse, have indicated that immunotherapy started before clinical diabetes may prevent the onset of the disease. Current knowledge of the pathogenesis of type I diabetes suggests that the onset of the disease occurs close to the time when immunological markers appear. Thus, an immunotherapeutic intervention should theoretically take place at this time or in any case before the disease becomes clinically manifest. However, with the present available methods, we cannot precisely predict whether the disease will develop. Since we do not know enough of the natural history of the disease in the prediabetic period, it is not ethically justifiable to treat normoglycaemic subjects with immunosuppression. However, a mild form of immunointervention, i. e. immunostimulation could be tested in nondiabetic patients with longstanding islet cell antibody persistence and decreasing insulin secretion capacity. Preliminary uncontrolled studies with nicotinamide by Elliot in New Zealand have shown, that none of 63 prediabetic children has progressed to overt type I diabetes so far.

Prospects and future of immune intervention in type I diabetes

We end with the outstanding problems with immunotherapy of type I diabetes as well as the aims of future work. We are not yet ready for specific immune intervention in type I diabetes, because the sequence of the immune-mediated destruction of β-cells is largely unknown. The heterogeneity of the disease itself [63] could hinder identification of clear selection criteria for patients who will show total remission in 80 to 90%. Effective therapy will probably have to be initiated in the very early stages of the disease, most likely in the late period of the prediabetic phase. The side effects and in particular the long-term risks must be evaluated further. It is not yet known whether remission in diabetes can be maintained with low cyclosporine-A dosages as successfully achieved in long-term transplant recipients. We are still at the beginning of a new and until now experimental therapeutic strategy. We must realize that the presently available immunotherapeutic agents are rather unspecific and are used at the end of a long-lasting β-cell destroying process.

New immunotherapeutic strategies should be tested first in experimental animal models of type I diabetes, i. e. in the BB-rat, the NOD-mouse or in the low-dose streptozotocin-mouse-model. Studies in experimental animals have shown that the autoimmune β-cell destructive mechanisms are a multifactorial and complex process, indicating that basically very different immune intervention strategies could be effective. In fact, administration of silica prevents diabetes in the BB-rat [64]. A preventive effect on the development of diabetes in the NOD-mice has been shown, when either silica [65], anti-Lyt2-antibody [65] or monoclonal anti-L3T4 antibody [66] had been administered. Recent studies have shown that L3T4 and Lyt-2 T-cells are both involved in the generation of low-dose streptozotocin-induced diabetes [67]. Antibodies to immune response gene products have a suppressive effect [68] on the development of diabetes in this experimentally-induced diabetes type. A recent study [69] indicates that antiinterleukin 2 receptor antibody suppresses murine diabetic insulitis and lupus nephritis. Short-term treatment with a combination of a monoclonal antiinterleukin 2 receptor antibody and a subtherapeutic dose of cyclosporine-A cures frequently manifested diabetes in BB-rats [70].

In summary, very different immuno-therapeutic strategies, such as inhibition of macrophages [64, 65], suppression of helper/inducer $CD4^+$-cell function [66, 67], inhibition of cytotoxic/suppressor $CD8^+$-cell function [65, 67] and administration of antibodies directed against class II-MHC genes [68] or interleukin 2 receptors [70], showed significant positive effects in the experimental animal models of type I diabetes. Based on these findings it cannot be excluded that combined immune intervention strategies – effective at different targets of the autoimmunologic process – are necessary for a complete blockade of the β-cell destructive process. Further carefully controlled trials are necessary to show whether nontoxic monoclonal antibodies could be used in the first phase of the disease. In addition, we need further studies to clarify whether an initial combined treatment with cortisone and a relatively low dose of cyclosporine-A might be beneficial. In evaluating new or potent therapies, one must never overlook the most important principle in medicine: Primum nil nocere.

References

[1] Schernthaner G. Neue Aspekte in der Pathogenese und im Krankheitsverlauf des Typ-I Diabetes mellitus. Wiener Klinische Wochenschrift 1980; 92 (Suppl. 115): 1–36.

[2] Bottazzo GF, Dean BM, McNally JM et al. In situ characterization of autoimmune phenomena and expression of HLA molecules in the pancreas in diabetic insulitis. N Engl J Med 1985; 313: 353–60.

[3] Rossini AA, Mordes JP, Like AA. Immunology of insulin dependent diabetes mellitus. Annu Rev Immunol 1985; 3: 289–320.

[4] Kolb H, Schernthaner G, Gries FA. Diabetes and Immunology: Pathogenesis and Immunotherapy. Bern–Stuttgart–Vienna: Hans Huber Publishers, 1983; 1–144.

[5] Schernthaner G, Banatvala JE, Scherbaum W et al. Coxsackie-B-virus specific IgM responses, complement-fixing islet-cell antibodies, HLA DR antigens, and C-peptide secretion in insulin-dependent diabetes mellitus. Lancet 1985; 2: 630–632.

[6] Banatvala JE, Bryant J, Schernthaner G et al. Coxsakie B, mumps, rubella and cytomegalovirus specific IgM responses in patients with juvenile-onset insulin-dependent diabetes mellitus in Britain, Austria and Australia. Lancet 1985; 1: 1409–1412.

[7] Mandrup-Poulsen T, Bendtzen K, Nerup J et al. Mechanisms of pancreatic islet cell destruction. Allergy 1985; 41: 249–259.

[8] Luger A, Schernthaner G, Urbanska A et al. Cytokine production in patients with newly diagnosed insulindependent (type-I) diabetes mellitus. European Journal of Clinical Investigation 1988; 18: 233–236.

[9] Eisenbarth GS. Type I diabetes mellitus: a chronic autoimmune disease. Diabetes 1986; 314: 1360–1367.

[10] Tarn AC, Thomas JM, Dean BM et al. Predicting insulin-dependent diabetes. Lancet 1988; I: 845–850.

[11] Sibley RK, Sutherland DER, Goetz FC et al. Recurrent diabetes mellitus in the pancreatic iso-and allograft period: a light and electron-microscopic and immunohistochemical analysis of four cases. Lab Invest 1985; 53: 132–144.

[12] Stiller CR, Dupre J, Gent M et al. Effects of cyclosporine immunosuppression in insulin-dependent diabetes mellitus of recent onset. Science 1984; 223: 1362–1367.

[13] Green A, Borch-Johnsen K, Kragh Andersen P et al. Relativ mortality of Type I (insulin-dependent) diabetes in Denmark: 1933–1981. Diabetologia 1985; 28: 39–342.

[14] Kofoed-Enevoldsen A, Borch-Johnsen K, Kreiner S et al. Declining invidence of persistent proteinuria in type I (insulin-dependent) diabetic patients in Denmark. Diabetes 1987; 36: 205–209.

[15] Schade DS, Santiago JV, Skyler JS et al. Intensive Insulin Therapy. Amsterdam: Excerpta Medica, 1983.

[16] Stephenson JM, Schernthaner G. Dawn phenomenon and somogyi effect in insulin-de-

pendent diabetes mellitus: Clinical relevance and intraindividual comparison during conventional and basal-bolus insulin therapies. Diabetes Care 1989; 12, 245–251.
[17] Mühlhauser I, Jörgens V, Berger M et al. Bicentric evaluation of a diabetes teaching and treatment programme for type-I (insulin-dependent) diabetic patients: Improvement of metabolic control and other parameters of diabetes care for up to 22 months. Diabetologia 1983; 25, 470–476.
[18] Deckert T, Poulsen JE, Larsen M. Prognosis of diabetics with diabetes onset before the age of thirty-one. Diabetologia 1978; 14: 363–377.
[19] Borch-Johnsen K. The prognosis of insulin-dependent diabetes mellitus – an epidemiological approach (thesis). Dan Med Bull 1989 (in press).
[20] Andreani D, Kolb H, Pozzilli P. Immunotherapy of type I diabetes. Chichester Sussex: John Wiley & Sons Ltd., 1989; 1–251.
[21] Ludvigsson J, Heding L, Lieden G et al. Plasmapheresis in the initial treatment of insulin-dependent diabetes mellitus in children. Br Med J 1983; 286: 176–179.
[22] Marner B, Lernmark A, Ludvigsson J et al. Islet cell antibodies in insulin-dependent (type 1) diabetic children treated with plasmapheresis. Diabetes Res 1985; 2: 231–236.
[23] Rabinovitch A, MacKay P, Ludvigsson J et al. A prospective analysis of islet-cell cytotoxic antibodies in insulin-dependent diabetic children. Transient effects of plasmapheresis. Diabetes 1984; 33: 224–228.
[24] Leslie RD, Pyke DA, Denman AM. Immunosuppressive therapy in diabetes. Lancet 1985; I: 516.
[25] Symoens J, Rosenthal M. Levamisole in the modulation of the immune response: the current experimental and clinical state. J Reticuloendothel Soc 1977; 21: 175.
[26] Cobb WE, Molitch M, Reichlin S. Levamisoe in insulin-dependent diabetes mellitus. N Engl J Med 1980; 303: 1065–1066.
[27] Sundal E. Thymopentin in experimental and clinical medicine. Surv Immunol Res 1985; 4: 1–154.
[28] Moncada E, Subira ML, Barberia JJ et al. Effect of thymic hormone and azathioprine administration on remission rate and insular function of 35 recent diagnosed type I (insulin-dependent) diabetic patients. A one year follow-up study. Diabetologia 1987; 30: Abstr. 599 A.
[29] Crosti F, Secchi A, Ferrero E et al. Impairment of lymphocyte-suppressive system in recent onset insulin-dependent diabetes mellitus. Correlation with metabolic control. Diabetes 1986; 35: 1053–1057.
[30] Secchi A, Pontiroli AE, Falqui L et al. Prednisone, indomethacin or theophylline administration and the remission phase in recent onset Type I insulin-dependent diabetic patients. Transplant Proc 1986; 18: 1540–1542.
[31] Ennis FA, Meager A, Bear AS et al. Interferon induction and increased natural killer cell activity in influenza infections in man. Lancet 1981; I: 891–893.
[32] Rand KH, Rosenbloom AL, MacLaren NK et al. Human leukocyte interferon treatment of two children with insulin dependent diabetes. Diabetologia 1981; 21: 116–119.
[33] Koivisto VA, Aro A, Cantell K et al. Remission in newly diagnosed type 1 (insulin-dependent) diabetes: influence of interferon as an adjunct to insulin therapy. Diabetologia 1984; 27: 193–197.
[34] Stiehm ER, Ashida E, Sik Kim K et al. Intravenous immunoglobulins as therapeutic agents. Ann Int med 1987; 107: 367–382.
[35] Heinze E, Thon A, Vetter U et al. Gamma-Globulin therapy in 6 newly diagnosed diabetic children. Acta Pediatr Scand 1985; 74: 605–606.
[36] Lazarus SS, Shapiro SH. Influence of nicotinamide and pyridine nucleotides on streptozotocin and alloxan induced pancreatic B-cell cytotoxicity. Diabetes 1973; 22: 499–506.
[37] Okamoto H. The role of poly (ADP-ribose) synthetase in the development of insulin-dependent diabetes and islet B-cell regeneration. Biomed Biochim Acta 1985; 44: 15–20.

[38] Vague PH, Vialettes B, Lassemann-Vague V et al. Nicotinamide may extend remission phase in insulin-dependent diabetes. Lancet 1987; 1: 619.
[39] Pozzilli P, Visalli N, Ghirlanda G et al. Nicotinamide therapy in patients with newly-diagnosed type 1 (insulin-dependent) diabetes. Diabetologia 1988; 31: 533 A.
[40] Usadel KH, Teuber J, Schmeidl R et al. Management of type 1 diabetes with ciamexone. Lancet 1986; 2: 567.
[41] Usadel KH. Immunotherapy of type I diabetes with ciamexone a multicenter double-blind trial. 1st International Symposium on Immunotherapy of type I diabetes, Rome, 1989.
[42] The Canadian/European Randomized Control Trial Group. Cyclosporin-induced remission of IDDM after early intervention: association of 1 yr of cyclosporin treatment with enhanced insulin secretion. Diabetes 1988; 37: 1574–1582.
[43] Eisenbarth GS, Srikanta S, Jackson R et al. Anti-thymocyte globulin and prednisone immunotherapy of recent onset type 1 diabetes mellitus. Diab Res 1985; 2: 271–276.
[44] Silverstein J, Riley W, Barret D et al. Immunosuppressive therapy for newly diagnosed insulin-dependent diabetes mellitus with antithymocyte globulin and prednisone. Pediatr Res 1983; 71: Abstr. 295.
[45] Schwartz R. Immunosuppressive Drugs II. Fed. Proc 1967; 26: 914–17.
[46] Harrison LC, Colman PG, Dean B et al. Increase in remission rate in newly diagnosed type 1 diabetic subjects treated with azathioprine. Diabetes 1985; 34: 1306–1308.
[47] Cook JJ, Hudson I, Harrison LC et al. A double-blind controlled trial of azathioprine in children with newly diagnosed type 1 diabetes. Diabetes 1989; 38: 779–783.
[48] Silverstein J, MacLaren N, Riley W et al. Immunosuppression with azathioprine and prednisone in recent onset IDDM. N Engl J Med 1988; 319: 599–604.
[49] Borel JF, Feurer C, Magnee C et al. Effects of the new antilymphocytic peptide cyclosporin A in animals. Immunology 1977; 32: 1017.
[50] Cohen DJ, Loertscher R, Rubin MF et al. Cyclosporine: a new immunosuppressive agent for organ transplantation. Ann Intern Med 1984; 101: 667.
[51] Assan R, Bach JF, DuRostu H et al. Metabolic and immunological effect of cyclosporine in recently diagnosed type I diabetes mellitus. Lancet 1985; 1: 67–71.
[52] Levy-Marchal C, Czernichow P. Effect of different dosages of cyclosporin A (Cs A) on the early phase of overt insulin-dependent diabetes mellitus (IDDM) in children. Transplant Proc 1986; 18: 1543–1544.
[53] Bougneres PF, Carel JC, Castano L et al. Factors associated with early remission of type I diabetes in children treated with cyclosporine. N Engl J Med 1988; 318: 663–70.
[54] Laupacis A, Stiller CR, Gardell C. Cyclosporin prevents diabetes in BB Wistar rats. Lancet 1983; I: 10–12.
[55] Graffenried B. Cyclosporin in insulin-dependent diabetes mellitus: design of controlled studies. In: Schindler R, ed. Cyclosporin in Autoimmune Diseases. Berlin, Heidelberg, New York, Tokio: Springer-Verlag, 1985; 128–129.
[56] Feutren G, Papoz L, Assan R et al. Cyclosporin increases the rate and length of remission in insulin-dependent diabetes mellitus of recent onset. Lancet 1986; 2: 119–124.
[57] Majon JL, Arkison P, Dawson KG et al. Methylprednisolone combined with cyclosporine in remission induction in Typ 1 diabetes. Autoimmunity 1989; (in press).
[58] Schernthaner G, Aschauer-Treiber G, Gaube S et al. Ergebnisse der Cyclosporin-A Therapie in der Frühphase des Typ-I Diabetes mellitus. Wr. Klin. Wschr. 1988; 100: 454–459.
[59] Mihatsch MJ, Bach JF, Coovadia HM et al. Cyclosporin-Associated Nephropathy in Patients with Autoimmune Diseases. Klin. Wochenschrift 1988; 66: 43–47.
[60] Helmchen U, Schmidt WE, Siegel EG et al. Morphological and functional changes of pancreatic B cells in cyclosporin A-treated rats. Diabetologia 1984; 27: 416–18.
[61] Robertson RP, Franklin G, Nelson L. Intravenous glucose tolerance and pancreatic islet β-cell function in patients with multiple sclerosis during 2-yr treatment with cyclosporin. Diabetes 1989; 38: 58–64.
[62] Myers BD. Cyclosporine nephrotoxicity. Kidney Int. 1986; 30: 964–74.

[63] Schernthaner G. The relation between clinical, immunological and genetic factors in insulin-dependent diabetes mellitus. In: Köbberling J, Tattersall RB. Genetics of diabetes mellitus. Proceedings of the 2nd International Conference. London – New York – Toronto – Sidney – San Francisco: Academic Press, 1982; 99 – 114.
[64] Oschilewski U, Kiesel U, Kolb H. Administration of silica prevents diabetes in BB rats. Diabetes 1985; 34: 197 – 199.
[65] Charlton B, Bacelj A, Mandel TE. Administration of silica particels or anti-Lyt2 antibody prevents β-cell destruction in NOD mice given cyclophosphamide. Diabetes 1988; 37: 930 – 935.
[66] Koike T, Hoh Y, Ishi T et al. Preventive effect of monoclonal anti-L3T4 antibody on development of diabetes in NOD mice. Diabetes 1987; 36: 539 – 541.
[67] Kantwerk G, Cobbold S, Waldmann H et al. L3T4 and Lyt-2 T cells are both involved in the generation of low-dose streptozotozin-induced diabetes in mice. Clin Exp Immunol 1987; 70: 585 – 592.
[68] Kiesel U, Kolb H. Suppressive effect of antibodies to immune response gene products on the development of low-dose streptozotozin-induced diabetes. Diabetes 1983; 32: 869 – 871.
[69] Kelley VE, Gaulton GN, Hattori M et al. Anti-interleukin 2 receptor antibody suppresses murine diabetic insulitis and lupus nephritis. J Immunol 1988; 140: 59 – 61.
[70] Hahn JH, Lucke S, Klöting I et al. Curing BB rats of freshly manifested diabetes by short-term treatment and a combination of a monoclonal anti-interleukin 2 receptor antibody and a subtherapeutic dose of cyclosporin A. Eur J Immunol 1987; 17: 1075 – 1078.

Pharmacokinetic aspects of insulin therapy – with special reference to pumps and pens versus conventional insulin treatment

J. S. Christiansen, T. Lauritzen

Introduction

In recent years the treatment of insulin-dependent diabetes has been based on the concept that metabolic control should be maintained as close to normal as possible [1]. It has ben argued that this offers the best hope of preventing, delaying, arresting, or even reversing progression of microvascular complications in diabetic patients, thus improving their prospects of prolonged well being and survival. This concept is supported by the experimental findings that long-term strict metabolic control in rats [2] and dogs [3] can delay the development of microvascular complications, and that reversal of diabetic glomerulopathy in rats has been documented after islet transplantation [4]. Furthermore, reprospective surveys in humans have shown that diabetic patients treated with trice daily insulin developed microaneurysms at a slower rate than those treated with one injection per day [5].

The concept of a relationship between metabolic control and the development of microvascular diseae is crucial to the understanding of clinical management of diabetes. It is, however, not within the scope of the present book to discuss this in any detail. We will therefore restrict ourselves to discussing the pharmacological aspects of insulin as a therapeutic tool to obtain normo- or near-normo-glycaemia.

Within the past two decades short-term normalization of blood glucose has become possible using an artificial pancreas, which delivers intravenous insulin based on feed-back measurement of blood glucose (closed loop) [6]. Despite intensive research, the closed loop system has so far not been further developed to such a degree, that it can be used clinically. The main reasons for this rather disappointing fact are problems relating to the life time of the glucose sensor. Therefore, closed loop insulin infusion can presently be used only for short-term investigation. It is on the other hand obvious that closed loop insulin infusion systems will have an immediate clinical application as soon as reliable glucose sensors are developed — even if these glucose sensors have a relatively short (2—3 days) life span.

More than 10 years ago, it became evident that near-normalization of blood glucose was also possible using a pre-planned intravenous insulin infusion without feed-back (open loop system) [7, 8]. Long-term studies using the intravenous route are, however, very difficult because of risks such as microembolism and septicemia. For that reason the open loop intravenous insulin infusion systems have not gained widespread use. The next discovery was the near-normalization of blood glucose was also possible with a continuous subcutaneous insulin infusion (CSII) without feed-back from a glucose sensor [9]. The CSII pumps have — in contrast to the closed loop and open loop intravenous infusion system — proven to be useful in certain clinical settings. A number of long-term clinical trials have been conducted using such pumps, thereby increasing our knowledge of the influence of long-term changes in metabolic control upon certain pathophysiological variables and microvascular manifestations in IDDM [10—13].

Simultaneously, the idea of improved metabolic control by means of multiple insulin injection regimens was further explored [14], and the feasibility of this multiple injection therapy (MIT) regimen was later facilitated by the introduction of various pen-devices for repeated injections of insulin.

An obvious difference between conventional insulin treatment (CIT) with twice daily injections, and MIT or insulin infusion treatment (whether by artificial beta-cell, preplanned intravenous insulin infusions, or CSII) lies in the different insulin preparations employed. CIT is based on the use of intermediate or long-acting insulin combined with short-acting insulin, whereas infusion systems and MIT mainly or exclusively use short-acting insulin. In evaluating the different treatment regimens we must therefore look upon the pharmacokinetic characteristics of these different insulin preparations.

Pharmaceutical preparations of insulin

In 1923, Banting stated, "In our view a prolongation of the period of action is most desirable, and whether this is to be obtained by slowing the rate of absorption or by more frequent injections is a matter for further study" [15].

Hagedorn was the first to report on a pharmaceutical modification of soluble insulin designed to have a slower rate of absorption [16]. This preparation was produced by adding protein from fish sperm to a neutral solution of soluble insulin — thus creating protamin insulin, which was later refined to the neutral protamin Hagedorn insulin or NPH insulin [17]. Sixteen years later another Danish investigator, Hallas Møller, reported an alternative method of slowing the rate of insulin absorption by adding a suspension of zinc to a neutral solution of soluble insulin [18]. This process lead to the development of the "lente" insulin.

These preparations, together with subsequently developed modifications were widely accepted in clinical use, and many insulin formulations with different timing characteristics are now available.

The preparations currently available fall into 3 main groups i. e. 1) short-acting (soluble), 2) intermediating-acting (e. g. NPH and "lente" insulin) and 3) long-acting insulin (e. g. zinc protamin insulin).

Within the next few years, however, a number of newer insulin preparations – e. g. very rapid or very slow absorptive insulin analogues, insulin for nasal administration and perhaps even oral insulin preparations – will undoubtedly be developed and offered for clinical use (see chapter "Future aspects of insulin treatment").

Variability in insulin absorption

Unfortunately, absorption of the insulin preparations so far known is extremely variable [19 – 21]. The variation in insulin absorption between patients can be expressed as the coefficient of variation (CV) of the time required for 50% of the insulin to disappear from the injections site. This CV is approximately 50% for intermediate-acting insulin [20].

Absorption of a given insulin preparation also varies greatly within the same patient [20, 21]. An example of this is given in the left part of Fig. 1, which shows the absorption curves of NPH insulin during 12 consecutive days in one patient. The patient CV for the time required for 50% of the injected insulin to disappear is approximately 25% [20].

A number of known factors contribute more or less to the variability in insulin absorption (Table 1). It has long been known, that the region of injection has significant impact on the absorption rate in general, showing a faster absorption form the abdominal wall than from the upper arm, which again has a faster absorption than injections performed in the thigh [19, 22]. Recent investigations have shown that a number of lean diabetics using vertical injection technique will often accidentally inject themselves intramuscularly due to a very thin subcutaneous tissue layer [23]. This problem is probably of increasing clinical importance, as vertical injection often has been recommended in connection with the use of insulin-pens. It is also well-known that absorption from areas in which lipohypertrophies have developed due to frequent insulin injections is significantly slower as compared to absorption

Table 1 Factors influencing insulin absorption

Factors influencing absorption	Comment	References
Insulin formulation	Fast, intermediate and slow acting	[19, 39]
Patients; between and within	Large spontaneous variation	[19–21]
Concentration, volume and insulin dose	Slow absorption with increasing dose, increasing concentration and decreasing volume	[19, 40–42]
Method of administration	Fast absorption with multiple small depots and jet injection	[39, 43]
Region of injection	Faster absorption from abdomen than arm or leg	[19, 22]
Lipohypertrophies	Slower absorption from lipohypertrophies	[24]
Body weight	1. No relation to skin fold thickness 2. Faster absorption in lean patients	[19] [24]
Exercise	Increased absorption from exercising limb	[44–46]
Smoking	Decreased absorption during and after smoking	[47]
Temperature	Cooling and heating of injection site results in slower, or faster absorption	[45, 48]
Local massage	Faster absorption when massage is applied to the injection site	[48]
Neuropathy	Increased absorption in patients with decreased vibration sense	[19]
Serum bicarbonate	Increased absorption in patients with low bicarbonate	[24]
Beef, pork or human insulin	Faster absorption of pork than beef insulin. No significant difference between pork and human insulin	[49–51]
Insulin degradation	Only in rare patients with insulin needs in excess of 120 IU/day	[39]

from otherwise normal subcutaneous tissue [24]. Factors such as exercise, smoking, body temperature, local massage, and fluctuations in plasma pH all have minor influence on absorption – probably due to changes in regional blood flow. A number of these factors are shown in Table 1. Altogether the clinical impact of these factors are relatively small when compared to the large intraindividual variation in absorption using intermediate action insulin. The factors shown in the table are probably not of major importance in patients treated with MIT or CSII. With these treatment modalities, long-term near-normal blood glucose levels can be maintained during daily life [13, 14], probably due to the small insulin depot in the subcutaneous tissue (see below).

Subcutaneous degradation of insulin is of no clinical importance in the majority of patients. In patients with insulin needs in excess of 120 IU/day it might, however, explain brittleness [25–27]. High amounts of circulating insulin antibodies can in rare cases explain brittleness [28].

The impact of variation in insulin absorption upon changes in blood glucose

What effect does variation in insulin absorption have upon blood glucose regulation? Binder [19] considered that the amount of intermediate acting insulin absorbed within 24 h was only a minor determinant of variations in blood glucose. This view is perhaps not surprising if the impact of other factors with known influence on blood glucose – such as the timing of meals, amount of calories, absorption rate of carbohydrates from the intestinal tract, and the amount of exercise etc. are considered as well. Such variables will, of course, strongly influence the relationship between insulin and blood glucose within the same 24 h time period.

Of greater importance, however, is the fact that we now have solid data suggesting that the so-called "unexplained" variations in blood glucose, to some extent, are due particularly to variability in the absorption of intermediate acting insulin. The first study to further elucidate this problem was published in 1979 [21]. The 9 patients who took part in the study, were selected at random from patients admitted to a diabetes clinic for blood glucose stabilization. The insulin dosage was adjusted before the study period and remained constant throughout the study, during which the patients remained in hospital and followed a regular pattern of diet and exercise. A radio-labelled intermediate acting insulin was given as a morning dose on each of 12 consecutive days, and the absorption from each SC injection site was followed during the same period.

The amount of radio-labelled insulin injected over a 24 h period (I) was compared with the amount of insulin actually absorbed over the same 24 h period (A). A rather large spontaneous variation in the absorbed amount of insulin was seen despite constant daily insulin dosage. The A/I ratio in the patient with the smallest fluctuation varied from 0.8–1.2 and the patient with the greater fluctuation from 0.5–1.5.

Importantly, there was a significant linear correlation between the amount of insulin absorbed over 24 hours, and the corresponding 24 h mean blood glucose concentration with the mean correlation coefficient of 0.81. The right part of Fig. 1 shows this correlation for one of the patients in that study [21].

These observations were further supported by the work of Molnar et al. [29], who found a significant correlation between day to day mean serum insulin concentrations and corresponding day to day blood glucose in patients treated with intermediate acting insulin.

It can therefore be concluded that the increased understanding of the absorption characteristics of intermediate acting insulin has been of particular clinical importance, since variations in SC absorption of these insulins appeared to be inevitable, and that they offer an explanation for the apparently "inexplicable" swings in blood glucose concentrations.

Post-hypoglycaemic hyperglycaemia

Somogyi was the first to attempt to quantify the relationship between insulin dose and blood glucose changes over a 24 h period [30]. He defined the G/I ratio, which is grams of glucose utilized/units of insulin injected, and observed "that blood sugar and glycosuria in diabetic patients often show wide fluctuations, even when both carbohydrate content of the diet and the insulin dosage are unchanged". Now we know that some of the variations in blood glucose, despite an apparently constant G/I ratio, are due to the fact that the amount of injected insulin (I) is not necessarily the same as the amount of absorbed insulin on a day to day basis. As already shown in Fig. 1, the changes in mean blood glucose can easily be explained in terms of the amount of insulin absorbed. Thus, it is – although hardly surprising – a fact, that when little insulin is absorbed, blood glucose values are higher and glucose appears in the urine, as compared to the situation when more insulin is absorbed.

The observations made by Somogyi [30] have been used to form the basis of the widely held concept of post-hyperglycaemic hyperglycaemia [31]. This concept has in particular been clinically applied with respect to nocturnal hyperglycaemia. It can be seen from Fig 2, that variations in the absorption of intermediate-acting insulin may be an important part of the explanation for this phenomenon. In this figure, blood glucose excursions in the same 9 patients are shown following nocturnal hyperglycaemia ($\leq$ 3 mmol). It is clearly demonstrated that post-hyperglycaemic insulin absorption is significantly decreased in the event in which hyperglycaemia developed as compared to the events when hyperglycaemia did not develop in response to hypergly-

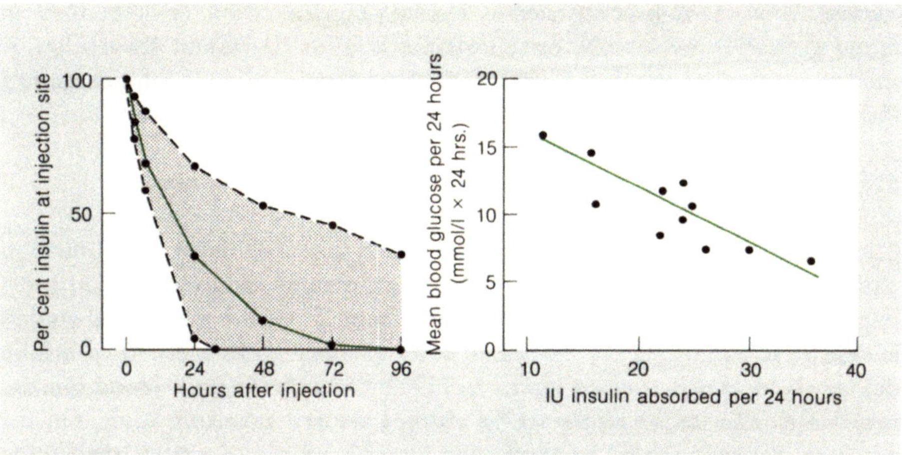

Fig. 1 Variation in insulin absorption and its impact upon blood glucose concentration.
Left part: This illustrates the median and range of the absorption curves of a morning insulin injection of 24 units of intermediate-acting insulin (NPH) during 12 consecutive days in 1 patient.
Right part: The absorbed amount of insulin in IU per 24 hours during 11 consecutive days, and corresponding mean 24 hours blood glucose concentration. These data are from the same patient as the data in the left part of this illustration. The correlation coefficient $r = -0.81$, $p < 0.01$.

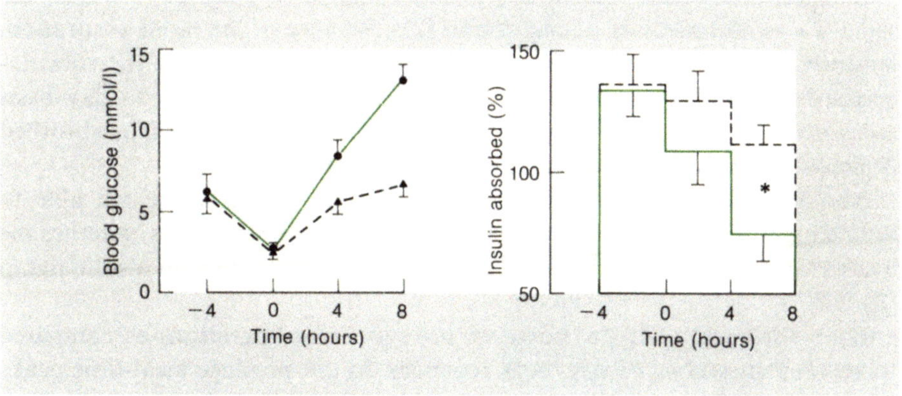

Fig. 2 Posthypoglycaemic hyperglycaemia.
Left part: All spontaneous blood glucose values ≤ 3 mmol/l over 11 consecutive days in 9 patients are superimposed at time 0. Patients were studied in the hospital on a balanced and constant insulin dose and diet and performed regular exercise. The hypoglycaemic episodes were divided into 2 groups; one which did and one which did not increase above 10 mmol/l during the first 8 hours following hypoglycaemia.
Right part: The mean amount of insulin absorbed before and after hypoglycaemia in per cent of the amount absorbed when all blood glucose values were considered. The amount of insulin absorbed in the period preceding hypoglycaemia was equally elevated in the two groups, whereas insulin absorption was significant decreased during the following 8 hours in those patients who showed the greatest rise in blood glucose (: $p < 0.05$).*

caemia. Thus post-hyperglycaemic hyperglycaemia could be explained in terms of relative insulin efficiency owing to a failure in insulin absorption. A similar conclusion emerged from the work of Gale et al. [32], who examined the same phenomenon in terms of blood plasma free insulin levels.

Clinical implications of variation in intermediate insulin absorption

Clinicians often find it difficult to understand unstable glycaemic control in patients following a described pattern of diet, insulin and exercise. The most important clinical conclusion to be drawn from the above mentioned studies is that these variations are inevitable consequences of the method of insulin delivery, and that it is often unfair to blame patients for poor blood glucose regulation. The intermediate-acting insulins are not precision tools. On the contrary, patients should be taught the variable nature of insulin absorption so that they might anticipate and understand these otherwise "unexplainable" variations in blood glucose levels.

The use of short-acting insulin in intensive insulin treatment

The absorption of subcutaneously injected soluble insulin shows almost the same CV as intermediate-acting insulin [21]. Because of the rapid absorption, however, all insulin is absorbed within 10–12 hours from the the subcutaneous depot. Therefore, no accumulation of insulin on a day to day basis takes place, and thus – on a 24 h basis – the amount of insulin absorbed is almost identical to the amount of insulin injected.

Another advantage of the short-acting insulin is that these are able to provide relatively reproducible postprandial serum insulin peaks, whether the insulin delivered is a part of the MIT regimen or comes from an insulin pump [29, 33].

Both MIT and CSII do, however, have inherent limitations as compared to an ideal situation. Firstly, both regimens do not produce meal-time peaks in plasma insulin which fully resemble those in non-diabetics. Secondly, they both deliver insulin into the systemic circulation with the inevitable consequence of systemic hyperinsulinaemia and inadequate insulin delivery to the liver. Finally, neither form of treatment completely overcomes the problem of variations in insulin absorption. Thus – as mentioned above – the coefficient of variation of infused or injected insulin remains around 30% within an individual [19, 33]. Thus, the important difference between MIT and CSII as compared to conventional insulin treatment lies in the size of the insulin depot [34]. With conventional insulin treatment, a large depot of intermediate acting insulin is present and variable absorption can produce wide swings in insulin delivery and consequently in the blood glucose levels. When using the MIT regimen, the depots are much smaller and the overall variability is thus reduced. Using CSII, the depot is extremely small – approximately 1–4 IU [33] – and a variation of 30% around this small depot will clearly have much smaller consequences for blood glucose regulation.

Bearing the limitations of MIT and CSII in mind, it is clear that near-normalization rather than complete normalization of blood glucose must be the aim of present insulin therapy.

It can be concluded that, given the insulin preparations presently available, the use of short-acting insulin whether given by MIT or CSII is a logical approach to near-normalization of blood glucose.

Practical aspects of subcutaneous insulin administration

There are two main problems with everyday subcutaneous insulin therapy. The first is to administrate insulin in such a way that peak insulin concentrations occur in connection with main meals and the second problem is to achieve stable plasma insulin levels overnight. The latter problem is of particular importance since the conventional insulin treatment as well as the MIT regimen tends to create an excess insulin level in the early part of the night and an inappropriate decline in insulin concentration before breakfast. The only treatment regimen which can presently maintain stable overnight plasma insulin levels is the CSII insulin pumps.

Conventional insulin treatment

For many years, insulin injection therapy has been conducted through once or twice daily injections. With one injection daily it is impossible to achieve a plasma insulin profile which resembles the normal profile. Patients treated with one daily injection will have relatively low prandial and postprandial plasma insulin levels, while preprandial values will be relatively high. A large number of the patients will have hyperglycaemia, especially in morning hours, due to insufficient insulin action in the late night hours. On the other hand, if the insulin dose is increased in order to create an acceptable prandial and postprandial insulin level, the risk of preprandial and nocturnal hypoglycaemia will be imminent.

A number of patients, however, will achieve acceptable blood glucose control with one insulin injection per day. This may especially be the case in patients with a relatively high residual endogenous insulin production. But, one daily injection may also be considered satisfactory in a number of other patients in whom for various reasons, the therapeutic goals must be rather modest.

A number of the disadvantages of once daily insulin injection can be overcome by giving insulin, both morning and evening, and this should be considered in most patients in which the total daily insulin dose exceeds 0.4 U/kg. In this case, insulin is best given half an hour before the main meals in the morning and in the evening – approximately 60–70% of the total dose in the morning and 30–40% in the evening. The conventional insulin therapy regimen may be further refined by giving a mixture of short-acting and NPH insulin which will be particularly useful in the morning dose.

Some patients will accept 3 injections per day, and in such cases, a satisfactory insulin profile – and blood glucose control – can be obtained by giving a mixture of NPH and short-acting insulin in the morning and an injection of short-acting insulin with the evening meal, and finally, an injection of NPH insulin around bedtime (10–11 p.m.).

The main disadvantage with the conventional insulin treatment regimen is that strict adherence to the meals – both in terms of timing and amount – is a prerequisite for the success of the regimen. This is one of the main reasons why a number of patients in recent years have found that changing to the multiple injection therapy regimen has offered them more freedom, and is thus considered an improvement in their quality of life.

Multiple injection therapy regimen (insulin pens)

The introduction of a number of different syringes for repeated subcutaneous administration of insulin – so-called insulin pens – has made multiple insulin injection therapy much more attractive to many IDDM patients.

The principal is that a more or less basal insulin level during the night and part of the day will be achieved through an injection of NPH, or even longer-acting insulin at bedtime and that the rest of the insulin administration takes place as soluble insulin administration in connection with main meals 3 or 4 times a day. This treatment regimen often creates satisfactory prandial and postprandial insulin peaks, but, it unfortunately does not always solve the problem of stable insulin concentration during the night.

It has been shown, without any reasonable doubt, that highly motivated patients on the MIT regimen can obtain very satisfactory glycaemic control – almost equal to the control obtained by insulin pumps [35]. Studies in larger unselected groups of patients have shown, however, that the introduction of insulin pens normally will induce only minor, if any, improvement in the metabolic control. One explanation for this apparent discrepancy might be that the patients really enjoy the "freedom" of the MIT regimen with respect to meals, and therefore do not adhere to a strict diabetic diet. Importantly, most patients do find that the MIT regimen is preferable to the traditional insulin treatment, and in most clinics the acceptability of MIT by means of insulin pens has been more than 90%.

From a practical point of view, one could start giving the patients 30% of the total insulin dose as NPH insulin at bed time (10–11 p.m.), 30% before breakfast, 20% before lunch, and 20% before dinner. The first thing to establish is whether the night dose is correct, and for that reason it will be advisable to perform blood glocuse measurements during the night, e.g. at 3 a.m.

It is presently being debated whether the MIT regimen results in an increase in the number of hypoglycaemic attacks. This, however, will of course depend on the therapeutic goal set for each patient, which of course must be highly individual.

Continuous subcutaneous insulin infusion (insulin pumps)

Treatment with insulin pumps using the subcutaneous route (CSII) has been applied as a research tool, but also in routine treatment since the original work by Pickup [36].

The advantage of CSII treatment is that it is superior to all other currently available regimens with respect to near-normalisation of blook glucose. One of the reasons for this success in maintaining glucose homeostasis is undoubtedly the fact that insulin pumps can achieve and maintain a stable insulin level during the night and can, in some cases even be programmed in such a way that an increase in plasma insulin can be obtained in the early morning hours.

From a practical point of view, approximately 50% of the total daily insulin dose is given as a constant 24 h infusion, while the second half of the daily insulin dose is given in connection with meals and snacks – again observing the fact that the breakfast is normally quite "expensive" due to relative insulin resistance in the morning hours.

The drawback of a CSII treatment – apart from the physical inconvenience caused by the pump – is the risk of severe ketoacidosis. Clinical experience has shown that ketoacidosis develops *extremely fast* in CSII treated patients. This is of course due to the fact, that the size of the insulin depot in the subcutaneous tissue is very small (1–4 units), and therefore severe insulin deficiency develops with a few hours if insulin infusion stops. The causes of irregularities in insulin infusion are often related to catheters [37]. And for that reason it is recommended that catheters should not be used for more than 3 days.

Because of the risk of severe ketoacidosis, CSII treatment can only be recommended in highly motivated, well trained and very disciplined patients, who should be instructed to perform at least one daily check of blood glucose for safety reasons, and who should have access to immediate advice from a specialist unit on a 24 h basis.

Treatment of diabetic ketoacidosis

Diabetic ketoacidosis is, unfortunately, still a frequent complication to IDDM – despite intensive patient education including prophylactic measures. The condition is in principal simple to treat, but it is nevertheless associated with a mortality of 5% or more – depending upon the degree of acidosis, the age of the patient and the availability of specialized care.

Most centres have now adopted various modifications of the so-called "low-dose" insulin regimen for the treatment of diabetic ketoacidosis introduced by Alberti [38].

The following brief recommendations apply to adults without cardiac insufficiency.

Insulin

Insulin should be administered promptly – either as a continuous infusion of soluble insulin – 6–8 IU/h diluted in saline, or as repeated i. m. injections – normally starting with 10 IU i. m. (+10 IU i. v.) and continuing with 10 IU/90 min.

Once blood glucose has fallen below 13 mmol/l, insulin administration should be reduced to 4 UH/h (i. v. infusion) or 6 IU/90 min. (i. m. injection).

Fluid replacement

Isotonic saline (0.9%) should be infused with an initial infusion rate of 1 l/h the first hour, ½ l/h the next 4–6 hours and thereafter gradually decreasing infusion rates – giving a total of 6–10 l during the first 24 hours. Isotonic glucose (5.5%) should be infused once blood glucose is below 13 mmol/l in order to maintain levels below 6–12 mmol/l as long as acidosis is present.

Potassium

Potassium levels will fall at once when the replacement and insulin therapy begin. It is therefore wise to begin potassium replacement as soon as fluid replacement commences. The following protocol is commonly used for infusion of potassium chloride.

Start with 20 mmol/h.

When serum potassium values become available:
if potassium > 6 mmol/l stop;
if potassium > 5 mmol/l give 10 mmol/h
if potassium < 4 mmol/l give 30 mmol/h
if potassium < 3 mmol/l give 40 mmol/h

Bicarbonate

Sodium bicarbonate is still a controversial issue. Most centres recommend cautious use of alkali because of the risk of rebound alkalosis and sodium overload associated with brain oedema.

A practical approach is to use alkali only if arterial pH is below 7. In this case, an infusioin of 100 mmol sodium bicarbonate should be given over 40–60 min. Arterial pH should then be rechecked and further sodium bicarbonate given only if pH still is below 7.

Insulin administration during surgery

For adult patients without cardiac insufficiency, the following approach may be convenient in connection with pre-planned surgery:

Give 40–50% of the usual total daily insulins dose as intermediary (NPH) insulin in the morning.

Simultaneously, an intravenous infusion of isotonic glucose (5.5%) should be given at an infusion rate of 80–120 ml/h.

Alternatively, no subcutaneous insulin is given in the morning. Instead, an intravenous infusion of glucose (10%) added 15–20 IU soluble insulin per litre and 20 meq potassium chloride per litre is commenced in the morning with an infusion rate of 50–120 ml/h.

Future aspects of insulin treatment

Before the end of this century, a number of new insulin treatment modalities will undoubtedly be offered for clinical use. First of all, the new DNA technology has made it possible to construct monomeric insulin analogues with either very fast or very slow absorption profiles. The introduction of the very fast absorptive insulin will make it possible to further normalize prandial and postprandial insulin profiles, while the introduction of very slow absorptive insulin preparations might make it possible to create a stable basal insulin level. It is, however, a prerequisite for the slow absorptive insulins that they prove to have considerably smaller variations in absorption from the subcutaneous depot as compared to currently available intermediate and long acting insulin.

In order to avoid the inconvenience of injection therapy, insulin preparations for nasal application are presently under development and may be a clinical option within few years.

The problem of peripheral hyperinsulinaemia and the relative insulin insufficiency in the portal circulation might be solved if insulin preparations for oral ingestion are successfully developed.

Finally, the next years will undoubtedly offer smaller, more reliable, more convenient and safer insulin pumps. Hopefully, we will also see the construction of a subcutaneous needle type glucose sensor with a stable lifetime more than 24 h which then could be used in a glucose controlled (closed loop) insulin infusion system.

References

[1] Cahill GF, Etzwiler DD, Freinkal N. "Control" and diabetes. N Engl J Med 1976; 294: 1004–1005.

[2] Rasch, R. Prevention of diabetic glomerulopathy in streptozotocin diabetic rats insulin treatment. Diabetologia 1979; 17: 243–248.

[3] Engerman R, Bloodworth JMB Jr, Nelson S. Relationship of microvascular disease in diabetes to metabolic control. Diabetes 1977; 26: 760–769.

[4] Mauer SM, Steffes MW, Sutherland DER et al. Studies on the rate of regression of glomerular lesions in diabetic rats treated with islet transplantation. Diabetes 1975; 24: 280–284.

[5] Eschwege E, Job D, Guyot-Argenton C et al. Delayed progression of diabetic retinopathy by divided insulin administration: A further follow-up. Diabetologia 1979; 16: 13–5.

[6] Albisser, AM, Leibel BS, Ewarts TG et al. Clinical control of diabetes by the artificial pancreas. Diabetes 1974; 23: 396–404.

[7] Slama G, Hautcouverture M, Assan R et al. One to five days of continuous insulin infusion on seven diabetic patients. Diabetes 1974; 23: 732–738.

[8] Deckert T, Lørup B. Regulation of brittle diabetes by a preplanned infusion programme. Diabetologia 1976; 12: 573–579.

[9] Pickup JC, Keen H, Parsons JA et al. Continuous subcutaneous insulin infusion: an approach to achieving normoglycaemia. Br Med J 1978; 1: 204–207.

[10] Lauritzen T, Frost-Larsen K, Svendsen PAa et al. The effect of six months strict metabolic control on eye and kidney function in insulin-dependent diabetics with background retinopathy. A randomized, prospective study. Lancet 1982; I. 121–123.

[11] Lauritzen T, Frost-Larsen K, Larsen H-W et al. Steno Study Group. The effect of one year near-normal blood glucose levels on retinopathy in insulin-dependent diabetics. Lancet 1983; I: 200–204.
[12] Tamborlane, WV, Puklin JE, Bergman M et al. Long-term improvement of metabolic control with the insulin pump does not reverse diabetic microangiopathy. Diabetes Care 1982; 5: suppl. 1: 58–64.
[13] Dahl-Jørgensen K. Near normoglycemia and late diabetic complications. The Oslo study. Acta Endocrinol (Copenh) 1987; 115: suppl. 284: 1–38.
[14] Schiffrin A, Belmonte M. Multiple daily self-glucose monitoring: its essential role in long-term glucose control in insulin-dependent diabetic patients treated with pump and multiple subcutaneous injections. Diabetes Care 1982; 5: 479–484.
[15] Banting FG, Campbell WR, Fletcher AD. Further clinical experience insulin (pancreatic extracts) in the treatment of diabetes mellitus. Br Med J 1923: I: 8–12.
[16] Hagedorn HC, Jensen BN, Karup NB et al. Protamine insulinate. JAMA 1936; 106: 177–180.
[17] Krayenbühl C, Rosenberg T. Crystalline protamine insulin. Rep Steno Hospital (Copenh) 1946; 1: 60–73.
[18] Hallas-Møller K, Jersild M, Petersen K et al. Zinc insulin preparations for single daily injections. JAMA 1952; 150: 1667–1671.
[19] Binder C. Absorption of injected insulin: a clinical-pharmacoalogical study. Acta Pharmacol et Toxicol (Copenh) 1969; 27: suppl. 2: 1–84.
[20] Kølendorf K, Aaby P, Westergaard S et al. Absorption, effectiveness and side effects of highly purified porcine NPH-insulin preparations (Leo®. Eur J Clin Pharmacol 1978; 14: 117–124.
[21] Lauritzen T, Faber OK, Binder C. Variations in ^{125}I-insulin absorption and blood glucose concentration. Diabetologia 1979; 17: 291–295.
[22] Koivisto VA, Felig P. Alternations in insulin absorption and blood glucose control associated with varying insulin injection sites in diabetic patients. Ann Intern Med 1980; 92: 59–61.
[23] Fried A, Linde B. Where do lean diabetics inject their insulin? A study using computed tomography. Br Med J 1986; 292: 1638.
[24] Kølendorf K, Bojsen J, Deckert T. Clinical factors influencing the absorption of ^{125}I-NPH-insulin in diabetic patients. Horm Metab Res 1983; 15: 274–278.
[25] Deckert T, Hansen B, Lauritzen T et al. Subcutaneous degradation of insulin. Diabetologia 1981; 21: 161–162.
[26] Galloway JA, Spradlin CT, Nelson RL et al. Factors influencing the absorption, serum insulin concentration, and blood glucose responses after injections of regular insulin and various insulin mixtures. Diabetes Care 1981; 4: 366–376.
[27] Dandona P, Foster M, Healey F et al. Low-dose insulin infusion in diabetic patients with high insulin requirements. Lancet 1978; II: 283–285.
[28] Kurtz AB, Nabarro JDN. Circulation insulin-binding antibodies. Diabetologia 1980; 19: 319–334.
[29] Molnar GD, Taylor WF, Langworthy AL. Plasma immunoreactive insulin patterns in insulin-treated diabetics. Mayo Clin Proc 1972; 47: 709–717.
[30] Somogyi M. Exacerbation of diabetes by excess insulin action. Am J Med 1959; 26: 169–191.
[31] Marks V. Drug-induced hypoglycaemia. In: Marks V, Rose FC eds. Hypoglycaemia, second edition. London: Billing and Sons Limited 1981; 357–386.
[32] Gale EAM, Kurtz AB, Tattersall RB. In search of the Somogyi effect. Lancet 1980; II. 279–282.
[33] Lauritzen T, Pramming S, Deckert T et al. Pharmacokinetics of continuous subcutaneous insulin infusion. Diabetologia 1983; 24: 326–329.
[34] Blinder C, Lauritzen T, Pramming S et al. Pharmacokinetics of insulin. In: Mngola EN, eds. Diabetes 1982. Amsterdam–Oxford–Princeton: Excerpta Medica 1983; 277–279.

[35] Schiffrin A, Belmonte M. Combined continuous subcutaneous insulin infusion and multiple subcutaneous injection in type I diabetic patients. Diabetes Care 1981; 4: 595–600.
[36] Pickup JC, Keen H, White MC et al. Long-term continuous subcutaneous insulin infusion in diabetics at home. Lancet 1979; II: 870–873.
[37] Christiansen JS, Sonnenberg GS, Kverneland A et al. Clinical outcome of using insulin at 40 UI/ml and 100 IU/ml in pump treatment. Acta Med Scand 1987; 222: 65–70.
[38] Alberti KGMM. Diabetic emergencies. Br Med Bull 1989; 45: 242–263.
[39] Lauritzen T. Pharmacokinetic and clinical aspects of intensified subcutaneous insulin therapy (Thesis). Dan Med Bull 1985; 32: 104–118.
[40] Lauritzen T, Pramming S, Gale EAM et al. Absorption of isophane (NPH) insulin and its clinical implications. Br Med J 1982; 285: 159–162.
[41] Lauritzen T, Thorsteinson B, Pramming S et al. Subcutaneous absorption of U-40 and U-100 insulin. Horm Metab Res 1984; 16: 611–612.
[42] Hildebrandt P, Sestoft L, Nielsen SL. The absorption of subcutaneously injected short-acting soluble insulin: influence of injection technics and concentration. Diabetes Care 1983; 6: 459–462.
[43] Taylor R, Home PD, Alberti KGMM. Plasma free insulin profiles after administration of insulin by jet and conventional syringe injection. Diabetes Care 1981; 4: 377–379.
[44] Koivisto VA, Feling P. Effects of leg exercise on insulin absorption in diabetic patients. N Engl J Med 1978; 298: 79–83.
[45] Kølendorf K, Bojsen J, Nielsen SL. Adipose tissue blood flow and insulin disappearance from subcutaneous tissue. Clin Pharmacol Ther 1979; 25: 598–604.
[46] Ferrannine E, Lind B, Faber OK. Effect of bicycle exercise on insulin absorption and subcutaneous blood flow in normal subjects. Clin Physiol 1982; 2: 59–70.
[47] Klemp P, Staberg B, Madsbad S et al. Smoking reduced insulin absorption from subcutaneous tissue. Br Med J 1982; 284: 237.
[48] Berger M, Cüppers HJ, Hegner H et al. Absorption kinetics and biologic effects of subcutaneously injected insulin preparations. Diabetes Care 1982; 5: 77–91.
[49] Faber OK, Lauritzen T, Binder C et al. Comparison of absorption and clinical effect of insulin Monotard® and Insulin Novo Lente®. Ugeskr Læg 1975; 137: 2510–2514.
[50] Sestoft L, Vølund Aa, Gammeltoft S et al. The biological properties of human insulin. Acta Med Scand 1982; 212: 21–28.

Future trends in insulin therapy: clinical implications of novel insulin analogues and nasal administration of insulin

J. P. Vora, D. R. Owens

Introduction

The outstanding medical achievement of the discovery and administration of insulin had a dramatic impact on the survival of insulin-dependent diabetics (IDDs) [1]. Insulin-dependent diabetes mellitus, previously an acute fatal disease, became a chronic disorder of long-term macro-and micro-vascular complications, resulting in increased mortality and morbidity in IDDs [2, 3]. There is increasingly convincing evidence that the development of the micro-vascular complications is related to the degree and duration of the metabolic derangement of diabetes mellitus [4 – 7]. The present day clinician is, therefore, committed to strive for the best glycaemic control feasible, without placing the patient at undue risk from hypoglycaemia [8].

The design and degree of success of a given insulin therapy regimen depends on the stringency of its goals. As the current aim is to achieve normoglycaemia, insulin substitution must mimick normal physiology [9 – 11]. Physiological endogenous insulin secretion in normals can be separated into absorptive and post-absorptive phases [12 – 15]. The absorptive phase consists of meal-related increases in insulin secretion, which are primarily responsible for tissue uptake and storage of nutrients. This increase is followed by a rapid decline in insulin secretion to basal rates between meals and during nighttime. The post-absorptive phase regulates hepatic glucose production and amino-acid and fatty-acid release from muscle and adipose tissue. The plasma insulin profile of normal subjects closely follows plasma glucose levels and the fineness of beta-cell regulation is exemplified by the control of plasma glucose within narrow margins [12 – 15].

Deficiencies of the commonly utilised conventional subcutaneous insulin regimen of twice daily injections of admixtures of short- and intermediate-acting insulin preparations were illustrated by the introduction of closed- and open-loop devices for insulin administration [16 – 18]. These devices achieved an improvement in glycaemic control, compared with conventional insulin therapy, by differentiating between between meal related and basal insulin requirements [16–18]. The result was the development of a multiplicity of insulin formulations, regimens and delivery systems, in an attempt to fulfill meal related (bolus) and basal insulin requirements [19]. Continuous subcutaneous insulin infusion, using portable pumps with adjustable rates, undoubtedly improved glycaemic control [17, 18]. Comparable glycaemic control can, however, be obtained using intensive 'conventional' insulin therapy (multiple injection therapy) involving multiple pre-prandial bolus injections of soluble insulin and once-daily intermediate- or long-acting insulin preparations (bolus/basal regimens) [17, 19, 20]. One of the therapeutic challenges of such subcutaneous insulin regimens is the achievement of rapid increments in plasma insulin levels to coincide with meal ingestion, in order to control post-prandial hyperglycaemia.

Short-acting insulins

Meal ingestion in normal subjects results in a rapid rise in plasma insulin levels, reaching a peak within 30–60 min and declining rapidly to basal levels by 120–180 min [9, 10, 13–15]. By contrast, peak plasma insulin levels are attained at 90–150 min following the subcutaneous administation of soluble insulin [19, 21–23]. Thereafter, plasma insulin concentrations decline gradually but remain inappropriately elevated for an extended period of approximately 120 min [19, 21–23]. The relatively slow rise in plasma insulin levels following subcutaneous injection of soluble insulin leads to an initial phase of hypoinsulinaemia, particularly affecting the portal circulation with inadequate suppression of hepatic glucose production, resulting in post-prandial hyperglycaemia [24]. The delayed exaggerated plasma insulin levels may cause late hypoglycaemia, necessitating between meal-time snacks. The hypoglycaemic effect of the administered soluble insulin may be extended further by the presence of circulating insulin-binding antibodies [25]. In an attempt to reduce the effect of the initial delay in the absorption of subcutaneously administered soluble insulin on post-prandial hyperglycaemia, soluble insulin is injected between 30–60 min prior to meal ingestion [26, 27]. Despite this inconvenient practice, the risk of delayed hypoglycaemia due to the inappropriately elevated plasma insulin levels remains. Attempts at increasing the initial rate of absorption of soluble insulin and produce more physiological plasma insulin profiles have included the use of jet injection devices [28, 29], sprinkler needles [30], massage of the injection site [31] and pharmacological manipulations using potent vasodilators [32, 33]. These manœuvres have, however, produced only modest enhancement of the absorption of soluble insulin.

The slow initial rise in plasma insulin levels after subcutaneous injection of soluble insulin results from a phase of low but increasing rate of insulin absorption, the so-called lag-phase [30, 34–36]. The rate of absorption of soluble insulin gradually increases until a maximum rate is attained at approximately 120 min after injection [35]. Although the pharmacokinetics of soluble insulin absorption have been extensively studied [21–23], the precise mechanisms of the absorption process have remained obscure until recently. A major determinant of the rate of soluble insulin absorption is the local blood flow at the injection site [34, 36]. A curvilinear relationship between the rate of soluble insulin absorption and subcutaneous blood flow has been reported [26]. Thus, at low to medium subcutaneous blood flow rates, an increase in blood flow with recruitment of capillaries reduces the diffusion distances and increases the concentration gradient between the interstitial space and the intravascular compartment. Therefore, increasing blood flow within this range results in an enhancement of the soluble insulin absorption. However, at high subcutaneous blood flow rates, factors other than blood flow become rate-limiting. These factors include the rate of diffusion within the interstitial space, and therefore the particle size, and the total area and permeability of the capillary membrane.

The predominant configuration of insulin in neutral soluble insulin is a hexameric unit [37]. Current evidence suggests that following soluble insulin injection, the insulin depot undergoes substantial dilution and the removal of the zinc from the hexameric unit. Thereafter, the hexameric insulin dissociates within the subcutaneous tissue, diffuses to the capillaries and is absorbed in a predominantly dimeric or monomeric form [34, 38, 39]. The dilution of the injected insulin depot and the dissociation of the hexameric insulin unit would account for the initial delay in the absorption of soluble insulin, with the rate of dissociation of the 2 zinc-hexamer of insulin being the final determinant of the rate of absorption.

At supraphysiological concentrations (above 1 nmol/l) insulin molecules self-associate into dimers [37]. In neutral solutions, in the presence of zinc ions, three dimers form the 2 zinc-hexamer of insulin molecules [37]. Based on the factors that limit the rate of diffusion, a decrease in the size of the insulin/unit would allow for faster diffusion and absorption through the capillary membrane. Current information regarding the absorption of subcutaneously administered soluble insulin would suggest that insulin with reduced tendency to self-association would be absorbed faster than the neutral soluble human insulin preparation.

The formation of a dimer is a prerequisite for higher association of insulin molecules [40]. As the capacity of proteins to dimerize can be abolished by site-specific mutagenesis [41], the main targets in the production of insulins of reduced association state have been the residues involved in dimer formation [42–44]. The aggregation surfaces between monomers in dimerization involve the B-chain residues, principally B8, B9, B12, B13, B16 and B23 to B28 [37, 45]. Of these residues, B12, B16 and B23 to B25 are also included in the putative receptor binding region of insulin [37, 45]. Amino acid residues chosen for mutation were those involved in dimer formation but on the periphery of the putative receptor binding region. The residues principally chosen were at B9, B10, B12, B26, B27 and B28 positions [42]. Single or double substitutions were performed by oligonucleotide directed mutagenesis or by total gene synthesis [42].

The principle of amino acid substitutions of the above sites was to introduce charge repulsion or steric hinderence into the monomer to monomer interface. As the isoelectric point of insulin is approximately 5.4, addition of positive charges would tend to reduce the solubility of the resulting insulin at physiological pH (see Section 2). Therefore, negative charges, in the form of amino-acids with carboxyl groups in the side-chains were utilised. In most instances negatively charged carboxyl-group side-chains of aspartate or glutamate residues are already present in the interface. These side-chains were chosen as opposites to the inserted negative charge in the opposite monomer of the dimer [42]. Alternative approaches at reducing the self-association of insulin into hexamers have been the introduction of hydrophilic residues at the hydrophobic interfaces and the removal of metal binding sites.

The association state of the resulting analogues was evaluated by means of osmometry and size-exclusion chromatography [42–44]. Standards utilised for comparisons with the analogues were 2 zinc-human insulin and zinc-free human insulin, which have mean association states of 6 and 4.4 respectively. Of the analogues produced, one-third are essentially monomeric (for example, B9Ser → Asp and B27 Thr → Glu; termed INA AspB9, GluB27: (Fig. 1)), one-third are dimeric (B10His → Asp; termed INA AspB10) and the remaining demonstrate slightly decreased association state compared with the parent compounds at pharmaceutical concentrations of 10^{-4}–10^{-3} M (B12 Val → Ile; termed INA IleB12). Compared with human insulin, the insulin analogues possess unchanged or negative net charge at physiological pH. The in-vitro activity for the insulin analogues, measured by the free fat cell assay, varies between 0–600% compared with human insulin, whilst the in-vivo biological activity (mouse blood glucose assay) is similar to the parent compound [42, 46–48].

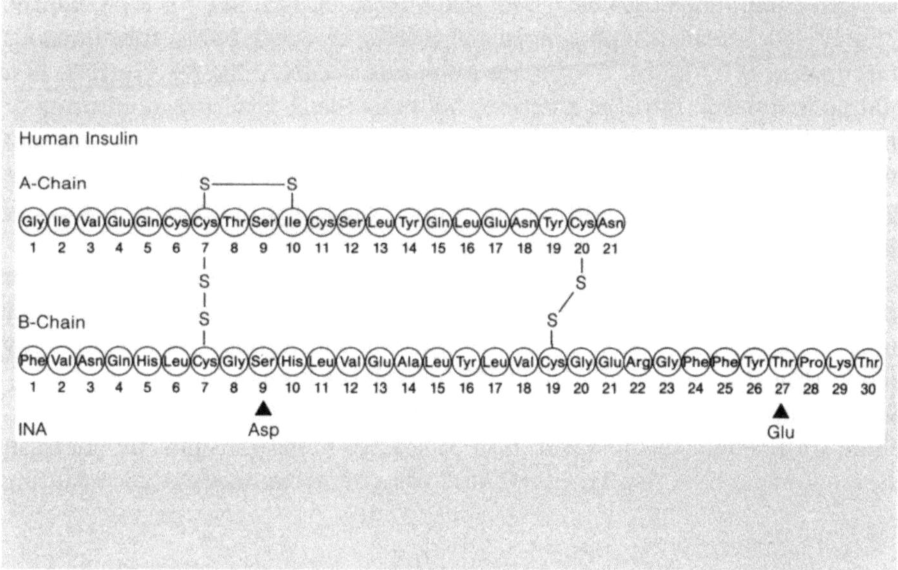

Fig. 1 The amino acid sequence of human insulin, with an example of an insulin analogue with reduced association state resulting from the substitution of the B9 serine and B27 threonine residues with aspartate and glutamate respectively.

The influence of the association state of the insulin analogues on the rate of absorption from subcutaneous injection sites has been examined in pigs [42, 44, 49]. Comparisons were performed between a series of analogues and the parent human insulin [42, 44, 49]. The disappearance of the various insulins, containing A14 mono-^{125}I -insulin tracer, after subcutaneous administration was determined by external monitoring of residual radioactivity at the injection site [34, 39]. The time to 50% initial radioactivity at the injection site (T50%) was significantly shorter for the insulin analogues with reduced association state compared with human insulin [42, 44, 49]. The T50% values for the analogues and human insulin demonstrate a strong positive correlation with the mean association state of the insulin [49]. The faster absorption of the monomeric INA AspB9, GluB27 compared with human insulin was evident in a faster rise in plasma insulin levels and quicker and shorter-lived hypoglycaemic effect [42].

Demonstration in animal studies of the faster absorption of the analogue INA AspB9, GluB27 compared with human insulin prompted clinical evaluation of this analogue, firstly in normal subjects and then in insulin-dependent diabetics. In a group of normal subjects, the rate of absorption from subcutaneous tissue and the resulting hypoglycaemic response were compared between equimolar doses of ^{125}I soluble human insulin and ^{125}I INA AspB9, GluB27 [50]. Rested supine normal subjects received bolus subcutaneous injections of 0.IU/kg of ^{125}I soluble insulin or ^{125}I INA AspB9, GluB27, in a randomised order, into the anterior abdominal wall. External monitoring of the residual radioactivity at the injection site [34], together with frequent blood sampling for plasma glucose and immunoreactive insulin and the insulin analogue, were conducted for 6 h following the adminstration of the respective insulins.

The disappearance from the subcutis of the INA AspB9, GluB27 was faster than the reference soluble human insulin, as reflected by significantly lower levels of residual radioactivity at the injection site throughout the 6 h study period (Fig. 2). The calculated T50% for soluble human insulin was 145 ± 8 min compared with 67 ± 11 min for INA AspB9, GluB27. An initial lag-phase was evident in the absorption of soluble human insulin. By contrast, the monomeric INA AspB9, GluB27 follows a monoexponential course during

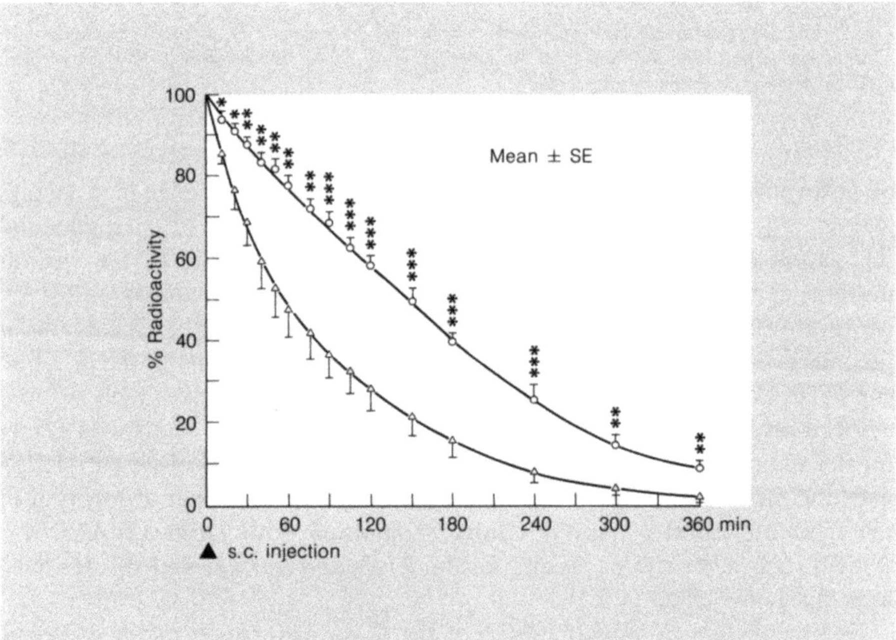

Fig. 2 Mean (± SEM) residual radioactivity at the injection site following the administration of 0.1 U/kg of 1251 labelled soluble human insulin (○———○) and 1251 labelled INA AspB9, GluB27 (△———△).

* $P < 0.05$ ** $P < 0.01$ *** $P < 0.001$

the entire absorption process, with the rate of absorption during the initial 20 min after subcutaneous injection being approximately three times faster for the analogue than soluble human insulin. Administration of the analogue resulted in a rapid rise in plasma insulin levels, to approximately seven-fold higher peak levels compared with soluble human insulin, followed by a gradual decline (Fig. 3). The nadir in plasma glucose levels was reached at

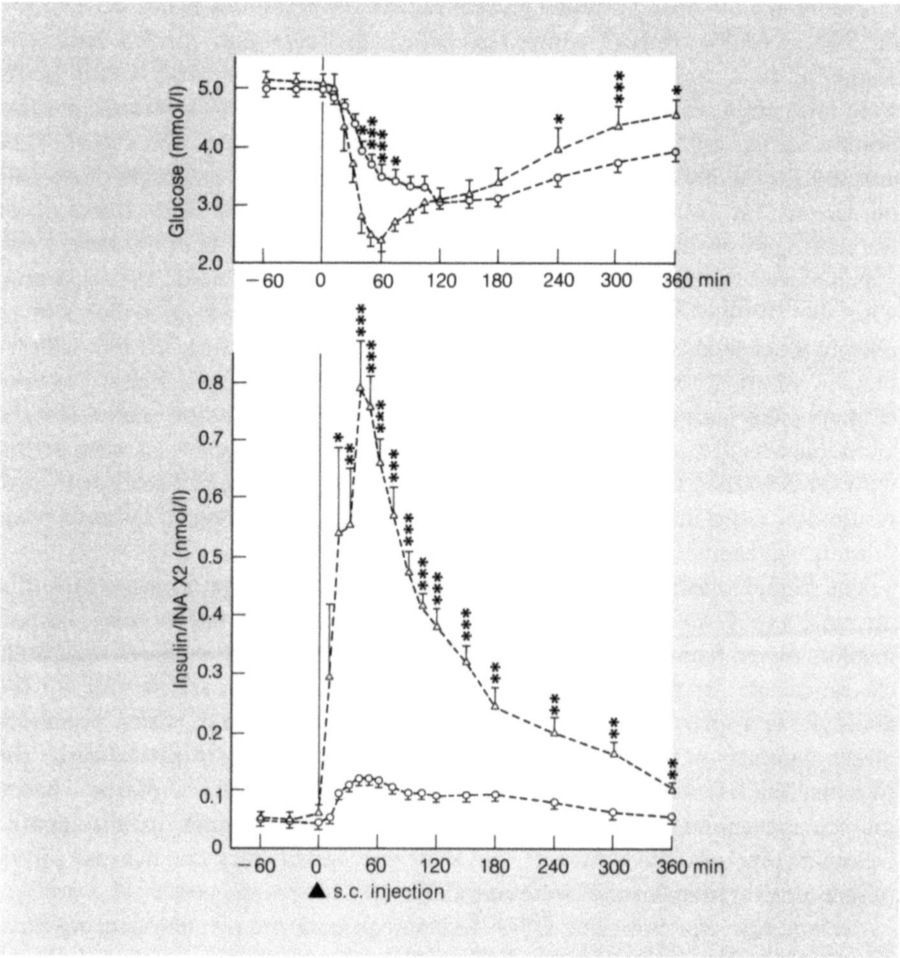

Fig. 3 Plasma glucose, insulin and insulin analogue levels (INA AspB9, GluB27) following the administration of 0.1 U/kg soluble human insulin (○– – –○) and INA AspB9, GluB27 (△– – –△).
* $P < 0.05$ ** $P < 0.01$ *** $P < 0.001$

120 min following soluble human insulin injection. By contrast, a faster and greater hypoglycaemic effect was observed following INA AspB9, GluB27 administration, with a nadir in plasma glucose levels at 60 min post-injection (Fig. 3). The recovery in plasma glucose levels was also faster following the analogue administration. Preliminary data from disappearance studies in normal subjects, using other ^{125}I labelled analogues, indicates a strong inverse relationship between the association state and the rate of absorption for the analogues [51], confirming results from the animal studies [49].

The effect on post-prandial glycaemic excurions of the faster absorption of INA AspB9, GluB27 compared with soluble human insulin has been studied in insulin-dependent diabetics [52]. Plasma glucose and insulin levels were measured following the administration of 1OU (UIOO) of soluble human insulin or INA AspB9, GluB27 immediately prior to the ingestion of a standardized 500 kcal (2.1 kJ) physiological mixed meal. Injection of soluble human insulin resulted in peak plasma insulin levels at 105 min. Injection of the analogue produced a rapid early peak in insulin levels at 30 min. Peak plasma levels were approximately four-fold greater for the analogue compared with the soluble human insulin administration. The post-prandial rise in plasma glucose levels was significantly lower between 15 and 210 min following the administration of INA AspB9, GluB27 than soluble human insulin (Fig. 4). The cumulative area under the incremental glucose curve for the analogue was 55% that observed for the soluble human insulin. In comparison with the reference soluble human insulin, INA AspB9, GluB27 administration resulted in rapid increase in plasma insulin levels and markedly reduced post-prandial glycaemic excursions.

The higher plasma insulin levels observed following the administration in normals and IDDs of INA AspB9, GluB27, compared with soluble human insulin, result from the three-fold faster absorption and a lower metabolic clearance rate for the analogue [50, 52]. The metabolic clearance rate for the analogue is approximately 30% that of human insulin [52], which precludes direct comparison of plasma insulin levels following the administration of the two insulins. However, "correction" of the analogue levels in plasma, based on the metabolic clearance rate, sugests that the plasma insulin profile following the administration of the analogue approaches the normal physiologic meal-related insulin secretion [52].

Advances in recombinant DNA technology and protein engineering have enabled the development of a series of insulin analogues with a reduced tendency to self-associate compared with the parent human insulin. Comparison of the subcutaneous absorption of soluble human insulin and the insulin analogues demonstrates that the rate of absorption is inversely correlated to the degree of self-association of the insulins. The absorption from the subcutis of monomeric insulins is substantially faster than the reference hexameric insulin, especially during the initial 20 – 30 min following injection. The availability of the monomeric insulins has also contributed significantly to our understanding of the processes involved in subcutaneous insulin absorption. Monomeric insulins follow a monoexponential absorption course from the time of injection. The initial lag-phase in the absorption of soluble insulin, that is, the delay in attaining maximal absorption rate, can now be

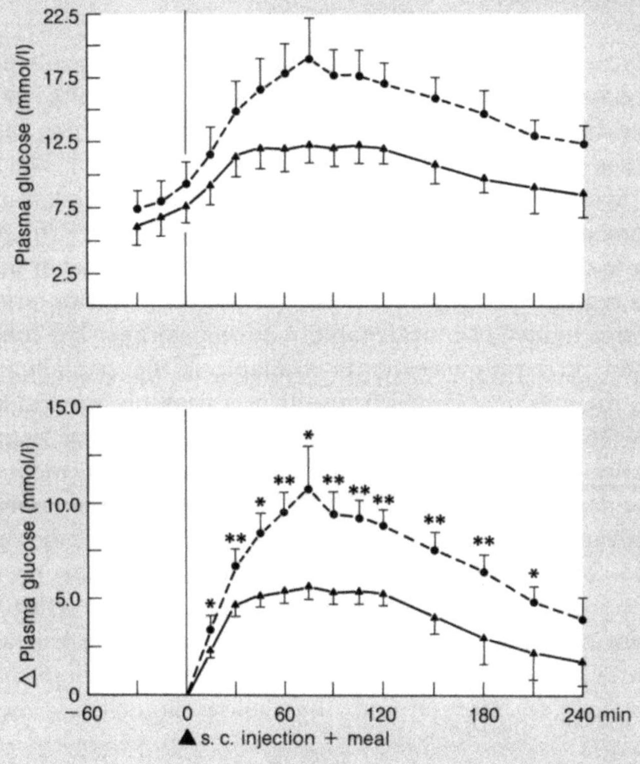

Fig. 4 Mean (± SEM) absolute and incremental plasma glucose levels following the ingestion of a 500 kCal meal and the subcutaneous injection of 10 U soluble human insulin (● — — — ●) or INA AspB9, GluB27 (▲ — — — ▲) at time = 0 min.
* $P < 0.05$ ** $P < 0.01$.

explained as the time required for sufficient dilution and dissociation of the hexameric unit of the injected insulin into monomers or dimers prior to absorption. The faster absorption of the monomeric insulin analogues results in reduced post-prandial glycaemic excursion compared with soluble human insulin, when both preparations are injected immediately prior to meal ingestion. Further improvement in post-prandial glycaemic control may be obtained by the administration of the analogues 10–15 min prior to meal ingestion. The data summarised above suggest that monomeric insulins are potential candidates for rapid insulin delivery by the subcutaneous route and may minimise post-prandial hyperglycaemia and delayed hypoglycaemia in insulin-dependent diabetics.

Prolonged-action insulins

Improved glycaemic control with bolus-basal regimens depends not only on rapid meal-related increments in plasma insulin levels but also on a constant and reproducable absorption of intermediate- and long-acting insulin preparations utilised to fulfill basal insulin requirements [16–20]. The absorption of currently available insulin preparations with protracted action is characterisied by considerable intra- and inter-subject variation [19, 21–23, 34], contributing to the day-to-day variation in glycaemic control in IDDs. These preparations require special precautions, such as resuspension prior to injection, and posses limited chemical stability during storage. The longest acting human insulin preparation currently available is the crystalline ultralente formulation, the injection of which results in a peak plasma insulin levels at between 12–16h [53]. In some patients, the duration of action of this preparation does not provide adequate basal insulin supplementation when injected once daily and, therefore, results in fasting hyperglycaemia [54].

A major advance in subcutaneous insulin therapy would be the development of prolonged-action insulin preparations with a slow rate of absorption requiring once-daily injection with reduced intra- and inter-subject variation in absorption, resulting in a stable and reproducible basal insulin supply. Soluble protracted-action insulin preparations would obviate the need for resuspension prior to injection and, thus, allow the delivery via pen-jector devices.

Soluble prolonged-acting insulins have been developed by the manipulation of the isoelectric pH of the parent human insulin [55–57]. An increase in the isoelectric pH of insulin would result in derivatives with low solubility at the pH of the subcutaneous tissue. The isoelectric pH of insulin of 5.4 is shifted to 6.2, 6.8 and 7.7 by the addition of 1,2, and 3 positive charges, respectively, to the molecule. The development of tryptic transpeptidation of insulin and the expression and export in yeasts of single-chain insulin precursors allows the modification of the C- and N-terminals of the B-chain of insulin [55]. Addition of positive charges relative to human insulin, by substitution with basic amino acids at the terminals of the B-chain and by blocking of the C-terminal carboxyl group of the B-chain (B30) by amidation, results in prolonged-acting insulins without substantial reduction of in-vivo biological potency [55]. The prolonged action of such derivatives is attributed to the readiness to crystallise and low solubility when the pH of an acid solution is adjusted to the isoelectric pH of the derivative, such as on injection into the subcutaneous tissue. The increased crystallization and reduced solubility results from either improved hexameric packing or enhanced α-helical conformation in the C-terminal. The duration of action of the B30 substituted insulins can be further prolonged by introduction of positive changes within the A- or B-chains of the human insulin molecule [56, 57]. Increased positive charge relative to insulin can be achieved by the substitution of acidic amino acid residues with neutral counterparts, by site-specific mutagenesis. In order to retain biological potency, the sites for substitutions in the derivatives were chosen by comparison of human insulin with insulins from other mammalian species [56]. Substitutions have been carried out for the A17, A21, B8, B13, B23, B27 and B30 sites [56, 57].

In absorption studies in pigs, the disappearance of radiolabelled preparations of the derived analogues demonstrate T50% (time to 50% initial radioactivity) of between 5–24 hours [56]. The largest increase in the protraction of absorption with a single amino acid substitution was obtained with the ArgB27 substitution. The slowest rate of disappearance from subcutaneous injection sites was observed with a GlnB13, ArgB27, the ThrB30–NH_2 analogue, with three positive charges relative to human insulin. Retention of the ThrB30 carboxyl group, however, results in analogues with comparatively faster absorption. The degree of protraction of most of the analogues developed can be increased by the addition of zinc ions to the formulation [56]. Initial animal studies demonstrated that the duration of action of the ArgB27, ThrB30–NH2 analogue, formulated with 6 zinc ions per hexamer, results in plasma insulin levels suitable for the provision of basal insulin requirements when injected once daily. However, acid solutions of the insulins are chemically unstable as the A21 residue of asparagine of the human insulin readily deamidates to aspartic acid and participates in the formation of covalent dimers of insulin [57]. The incorporation of an additional substitution of glycine for asparagine at the A21 position produces chemical stability of the prolonged action analogues during storage as slightly acidic solutions [57,

58]. The in-vitro potency of the GlyA21, ArgB27, ThrB30 – NH_2 analogue is similar to human insulin [57]. Unlike other prolonged action analogues, the rate of absorption from the subcutaneous tissue of the GlyA21, or ArgB27, ThrB30 – NH_2 derivative is independent of the concentration of zinc ions in the formulation [57].

Clinical studies in insulin-dependent diabetics have compared the subcutaneous absorption of the GlyA21, ArgB27, ThrB30 – NH_2 analogue with that of the ultralente preparation of human insulin [59]. Following subcutaneous adminstration, the disappearance of radiolabelled preparations of the analogue and the ultralente preparation were examined by external monitoring of the residual radioactivity over the injection site for a period of 100 hrs. The time to 50% initial radioactivity (T50%) was 35 h for the analogue and 26 h for the ultralente preparation. Intra-patient variation for T50% was lower for the analogue, at 18.4%, compared with 44.5% for the reference ultralente preparation. Inter-patient variation for T50 was, however, similar for the two preparations. The reduced intra-subject variation of the GlyA21, ArgB27, ThrB30 – NH_2 analogue probably reflects the lack of effect of the zinc ion concentration in the formulation on the rate of dissolution of the crystals of the derivative, formed on injection within the subcutaneous tissue.

The development of such soluble prolonged-action insulin analogues may, in future, result in an insulin preparation which adequately fulfills basal insulin requirements. The improved absorption characteristics, with reduced intra-patient variation compared with current long-acting preparations, should provide stable and reproducible basal plasma insulin concentrations.

Intranasal administration of insulin

Subcutaneous adminstration of soluble insulin results in peak plasma insulin levels of 90 – 150 min after injection [19, 21 – 23]. Thereafter plasma insulin concentrations remain inappropriately elevated for approximately 120 min prior to declining gradually [19, 21 – 23]. By comparison, meal ingestion in normal subjects produces an early rise in plasma insulin concentrations with peak levels at 30 – 60 min followed by a rapid decline to basal values by 120 – 180 min [9, 10, 13 – 15] (see Section I). This delay in the absorption of subcutaneously administered soluble insulin results in early post-prandial hyperglycaemia and delayed hypoglycaemia. The characteristics of subcutaneous absorption of soluble insulin, with considerable intra- and inter-patient variation, and the social stigma attached with parenteral injection therapy, have resulted in a search for alternative routes of insulin administration.

Intranasal delivery of insulin is an attractive alternative on the basis of the large surface area available for absorption, due to numerous microvilli present on the epithelial surface and highly vasculised subepithelial layer. Absorption of the intranasally administered drugs occurs within the respiratory region of the nasal cavity, which is covered by numerous mobile cilia over which is a thin continuous mucus layer [60]. Intranasal absorption of drugs is highly dependent on the inhaled particle size. Particles smaller than 1 micron in diameter are inhaled into the lungs, whilst those of 15–50 micron are deposited within the nasal mucus layer and are available for absorption. The oscillatory action of the cilia produces an anterior to posterior mucus flow rate of approximately 5 mm/min [60]. Therefore, particles within the mucus layer are cleared form the nasal cavity within approximately 15 min and is a major contributory factor in the loss of drugs from potential absorption surfaces. This rapid clearance, and possible enzymatic degradation of peptides within the mucus layer, results in low bioavailabilities of intranasally administered drugs, particularly for comparatively large molecules such as insulin.

Absorption enhancers have been used to overcome the inefficient intranasal absorption of insulin. Animal and human studies have demonstrated that insulin can be delivered across the nasal mucosa when formulated with hydrophobic bile salts [61–66] and nonionic detergents [62, 67]. Studies in normal subjects, insulin-dependent and non-insulin dependent diabetics have mainly utilised sodium glycocholate or polyoxyethylene-9-lauryl ether as surfactants [63–67]. The precise mechanism of the enhanced nasal absorption of insulin when formulated with these adjuvants is unknown. However, it has been proposed that hydrophobic bile salts increase the membrane permeability to insulin by producing high juxta-membrane concentrations of insulin by solubilisation of insulin monomers and dimers within bile salt micelles [66]. Adjuvants may also reduce the viscosity of the mucus, allowing easier diffusion, and inhibit degrading enzyme systems.

Aerosolized intranasal administration of soluble insulin to normal and diabetic subjects results in peak plasma insulin levels within 10–30 min [61, 64, 67]. Plasma insulin levels, thereafter, decline rapidly to reach basal values by 60–90 min following administration. Similar results have been reported for nasal adminstration of droplets of the insulin-adjuvant formulation [63]. In fasting normal subjects, intranasal insulin results in a nadir in plasma glucose at 45–50 min post-administration, followed by recovery to basal values by 90 min [63, 67]. The maximal hypoglycaemic effect in fasting IDDs, who omitted their breakfast and usual subcutaneous insulin therapy, was observed at 120 min [67]. Intranasal insulin administration to fasted non-insulin dependent diabetics (NIDDs) produced a plasma glucose nadir at 50 min, followed by a recovery phase, compared with a slow continual decline in plasma glucose levels for approximately 5 h following subcutaneous injection of insulin [64]. As expected from these results, intranasal insulin administered at the start of a meal reduced post-prandial glycaemic excursions compared with subcutaneous insulin injection, in both IDDs and NIDDs [64, 67]. Multiple intranasal adminstrations within the first 60 min of commencing a meal produced further improvement in post-prandial hyperglycaemia in NIDDs [64].

The above studies have, however, consistently reported 10–20% bioavailability of intranasal insulin compared with subcutaneous soluble insulin injection [61, 63, 64, 67]. Therefore, preprandial intranasal administration requires large quantities of insulin, ranging between 0.4 to 1.5 U/kg [61, 64, 67]. In order to reduce the volume of the insulin-adjuvant formulation administered, U250 and U500 strength insulin preparations have been utilised [61, 64, 65, 67]. Long term use over 3–4 months of preprandial bolus administration of intranasal insulin as a component of bolus/basal regimens results in identical [67] or a deterioration [65] in glycaemic control compared with subcutaneously injected soluble insulin. In the former study, however, the dosage of basal component of long-acting insulin varied considerably but was maintained constant by the latter group. Both studies, however, reported marked increases in the pre-prandial dosage of insulin when administered intranasally compared with subcutaneous injections of soluble insulin [65, 67]. Local irritation, such as nasal stinging, congestion and rhinorrhoea, were common amongst these subjects. These symptoms were ascribed to the adjuvant utilised in the intranasal insulin formulation.

The data discussed above suggest that the nasal route may be effective for insulin delivery. The pharmokinetics of intranasal delivery of insulin indicate a potential role for this route for preprandial insulin administration. The acceptability of a nasal insulin delivery system requires further refinement, such as the development of an accurate and convenient delivery device and potent absorption enhancers with less irritant properties. Long term clinical studies, relating to the calibre of glycaemic control achieved and the effects of adjuvants on the nasal mucosa, will be required before intranasal delivery can be considered a therapeutic option.

Conclusion

The achievement of normoglycaemia by insulin-dependent diabetics is hindered by the inherent pharmacokinetic properties of the currently available short- and protracted-action insulin preparations. Despite its injection 30–

60 min prior to meal ingestion, the absorption characteristics of soluble insulin allow for the development of early post-prandial hyperglycaemia and delayed hypoglycaemia. The absorption of insulin preparations with protracted action is characterised by marked intra- and inter-patient variation. Preliminary clinical data demonstrates that subcutaneously adminstered monomeric insulins are promising candidates for rapid insulin delivery, thus, limiting excessive post-prandial glucose excursions and delayed hypoglycaemia. The complementary development of new soluble prolonged-action insulin analogues, may fulfill the requirements of a stable and reproducible basal insulin supply. Extensive studies are, however, required to evaluate such preparations, especially their immunogenic properties, prior to the introduction into clinical practice. The development of the insulin analogues represents a major landmark in the evolution of insulin treatment for the insulin-dependent diabetic. These and further advances in subcutaneous insulin therapy should enable the attainment of normoglycaemia in the insulin treated diabetic.

References

[1] Banting F, Best G, Collip CH et al. Pancreatic extracts in the treatment of diabetes mellitus: Preliminary report. Can Med Assoc J 1922; 12: 141–146.

[2] Deckert T, Poulsen JE, Larsen M. Prognosis of diabetics with diabetes onset before the age of thirty-one. Diabetologia 1978; 14: 363–370.

[3] Borch-Johnsen K, Kreiner S, Deckert T. Mortality of type I (insulin dependent) diabetes mellitus in Denmark. Diabetologia 1986; 29: 767–772.

[4] Pirart J. Diabetes mellitus and its degenerative complications: a prospective study of 4,400 patients observed between 1947 and 1973. Diabetes Care 1978; 1: 168–88, 252–63.

[5] Tchobroutsky G. Relation of diabetic control to development of microvascular complications. Diabetologia 1978; 15: 143–52.

[6] Siperstein MD. Diabetic microangiopathy and the control of blood glusose. N Engl J Med 1983; 309: 1577–79.

[7] Hanssen KF, Dahl-Jorgensen K, Lauritzen T et al. Diabetic control and microvascular complications: the near-normoglycaemic experience. Diabetologia 1986; 29: 677–84.

[8] Unger RH. Meticulous control of diabetes: benefits, risks and precautions. Diabetes 1982; 31: 479–83.

[9] Eaton RP, Spencer W, Schade DS et al. Diabetic glucose control: matching plasma insulin concentrations to diet and stress hyperglycaemia. Diabetes Care 1978; 1: 40–44.

[10] Eaton RP, Allen C, Schade DS et al. "Normal" insulin secretion: The goal of artificial insulin delivery systems. Diabetes Care 1980; 3: 270–73.

[11] Schade DS, Eaton RP, Spencer W. Normalisation of plasma insulin profiles in diabetic subjects with programmed insulin delivery. Diabetes Care 1980; 3: 9–14.

[12] Malharbe C, DeGasparo M, De Hertogh R. et al. Circadian variations of blood sugar and plasma insulin levels in man. Diabetologia 1969; 5: 397–404.

[13] Genuth SM. Plasma insulin and glucose profiles in normal obese and diabetic persons. Ann Intern Med, 1973; 79: 812–22.

[14] Hansen A, Johansen K. Diurnal patterns of blood glucose, serum fatty acids, insulin, glucagon, and growth hormone in normal and juvenile diabetes. Diabetologia 1970; 6: 27–33.

[15] Ahmed M, Gannon MC, Nuttall FQ. Post-prandial plasma glucose, insulin, glucagon and triglyceride responses to a standard diet in normal subjects. Diabetologia 1976; 12: 61 – 67.
[16] Mirouze J, Selam JL, Pham TC et al. Evaluation of exogenous insulin haemostasis by the artificial pancreas in insulin-dependent diabetes. Diabetologia 1977; 13: 273 – 278.
[17] Rizza RA, Gerich JE, Haymond MW et al. Control of blood sugar in insulin dependent diabetes: Comparison of an artificial endocrine pancreas, continuous subcutaneous insulin infusion, and intensified conventional insulin therapy. N Eng J Med 1980; 303: 1313 – 18.
[18] Pickup JC, Keen H, Parsons JA et al. Continuous subcutaneous insulin infusion: an approach to achieving normoglycaemia. Br Med J 1978; 1: 204 – 07.
[19] Skyler JS, Miller NE, O'Sullivan MJ et al. Use of insulin in insulin-dependent diabetes mellitus. In: Skyler JS, ed. Insulin Update 1982, Princeton, NJ, Excerpta Medica 1982; 125 – 56.
[20] Turner RC, Phillips M, Jones R et al. Ultralente-based insulin regimens in insulin-dependent diabetes. In: Skyler JS, ed. Insulin Update 1982, Princeton, NJ, Excerpta Medica 1982; 157 – 74.
[21] Galloway JA, Spradlin CT, Nelson RL et al. Factors influencing the absorption, serum insulin concentration, and blood glucose responses after injections of regular insulin and various insulin mixtures. Diabetes Care 1981; 4: 366 – 76.
[22] Owens DR. Human insulin. Clinical pharmacological studies in normal man. Thesis. University of Wales, Cardiff MTP Press, Lancaster U.K., Hingham MA, 1986.
[23] Binder C, Lauritzen T, Faber O et al. Insulin pharmacokinetics. Diabetes Care 1984; 7: 188 – 99.
[24] Pehring G, Tessari P, Gerich JE. Abnormal meal carbohydrate disposal in insulin-dependent diabetes. J Clin Inves 1984; 74: 985 – 991.
[25] Van Haeften TW. Clinical significance of insulin antibodies in insulin-treated diabetic patients. Diabetes Care 1989; 12: 641 – 48.
[26] Kinmonth AL, Baum JD. Timing of pre-breakfast insulin injection and post-prandial metabolic control in diabetic children. Br Med J 1980; 280: 604 – 06.
[27] Dimitriades GD, Gerich JE. Importance of timing of pre-prandial insulin administration in the management of diabetes mellitus. Diabetes Care 1983; 6: 374 – 77.
[28] Taylor R, Home PD, Alberti KGMM. Plasma free insulin profiles after administration of insulin by jet and conventional syringe injection. Diabetes Care 1981; 4: 377 – 79.
[29] Pehling GB, Gerich JE. Comparison of plasma insulin profiles after subcutaneous administration of insulin by jet spray and conventional needle injection in patients with insulin dependent diabetes mellitus. Mayo Clinic Proc 1984; 59: 751 – 54.
[30] Edsberg B, Herly D, Hildebrandt P et al. Insulin bolus given by sprinkler needle: Effect on absorption and glycaemic response to a meal. Br Med J 1987; 294: 1373 – 76.
[31] Linde B. Dissociation of insulin absorption and blood flow during massage of a subcutaneous injection site. Diabetes Care 1986; 9: 570 – 74.
[32] Owens DR, Vora JP, Birtwell J et al. The influence of aprotinin on regional absorption of soluble human insulin. Br J Clin Pharmac 1988; 10: 470 – 72.
[33] Menon RK, Gaylarde PM, Hyden AM et al. Insulin absorption accelerated by adrenergic blockade at injection site. Diabetes Care 1987; 10: 470 – 72.
[34] Binder C. Absorption of injected insulin. Acta Pharmac Tox 1969; 27 (suppl 2): 1 – 87.
[35] Schlichtkrull J. The absorption of insulin. Acta Paediatr Scand 1977; suppl 207: 97 – 102.
[36] Hildebrandt P, Sejrsen P, Nielsen SL et al. Diffusion and polymerization determines the insulin absorption from subcutaneous tissue in diabetic patients. Scand J Clin Lab Invest 1985; 45: 685 – 90.
[37] Blundell T, Dodson G, Hodgkin D et al. Insulin: The structure in the crystal and its reflection in chemistry and biology. Ad Protein Chem 1972; 26: 279 – 402.
[38] Binder C. A Theoretical model for the absorption of soluble insulin. In: Brunetti P, Alberti KGMM, Albisser AM et al, eds. Artificial Systems for Insulin Delivery. New York: Raven Press, 1983, 53 – 57.

[39] Ribel U, Jorgensen K, Brange J et al. The pig as a model for subcutaneous insulin absorption in man. In: Diabetes 1985, Serrano-Rios, Lefebvre PJ, eds. Amsterdam: Elsevier, 1986, 891–96.
[40] Goldman J, Carpenter FH. Zinc binding, circular dichroism, and equilibrium sedimentation studies on insulin (bovine) and several of its derivatives. Biochemistry 1974; 13: 4566–74.
[41] Jones DH, McMillan AJ, Fersht AR. Reversible dissociation of dimeric tyrosyl-tRNA synthetase by mutagenesis at the subunit interface. Biochemistry 1985; 24: 5852–57.
[42] Brange J, Ribel U, Hansen JF et al. Monomeric insulins obtained by protein engineering and their medical implications. Nature 1988; 333: 679–82.
[43] Brange J, Diers I, Hansen J et al. Monomeric insulins by protein engineering. Protein Engn 1987; 1: 250.
[44] Brange J, Diers I, Hansen J et al. Prompt insulin: Monomeric insulins are absorbed three times faster from subcutis than human insulin. Diabetes 1987; 36 (suppl 1): 77A.
[45] Gammeltoft S. Insulin receptors: Binding kinetics and structure-function relationship of insulin. Physiol Rev 1984; 64: 1321–78.
[46] Ribel U, Drejer K, Moller U et al. Insulin analogs and human insulin: Equivalent in vivo biological activity in spite of widely different in vitro potencies. Diabetes Res Clin Pract 1988; 5 (suppl 1): S368.
[47] Volund A, Meador M, Watanabe R et al. Insulin analogs with altered absorption kinetics exhibit metabolic effects similar to native insulin. Diabetes Res Clin Pract 1988; 5 (suppl. 1): S369.
[48] Drejer K, Kruse V, Larsen UD. Insulin analogs: Binding to the human liver cell line, HEP G2. Diabetes Res Clin Pract 1988; 5 (suppl 1): 231.
[49] Brange J, Ribel U, Hansen JF et al. The significance of insulin self-association for the absorption of dissolved insulin. Diabetes Res Clin Pract 1988 b; 5 (suppl 1): S609.
[50] Vora JP, Owens DR, Dolben J et al. Recombinant DNA derived monomeric insulin analogue: Comparison with soluble human insulin in normal subjects. Br Med J 1988; 297: 1236–39.
[51] Kang S, Owens DR, Burch A et al. The association state of insulin determines the rate of absorption of soluble insulin in normal man. Diabetes 1989; 22 (suppl 2): 79A.
[52] Kang S, Owens DR, Vora J et al. Comparison of insulin analogue B9Asp B27Glu and soluble human insulin in insulin-treated diabetes. Lancet 1990; 335: 303–306.
[53] Owens DR, Vora JP, Heding LG et al. Human, porcine and bovine ultralente insulin: subcutaneous administration in normal man. Diabetic Medicine 1986; 3: 326–329.
[54] Francis AJ, Hanning I, Alberti KGMM. Human ultralente insulin: A comparison with porcine lente insulin as a twice daily insulin in insulin dependent diabetics with fasting hyperglycaemia. Diabetes Res 1986; 3: 263–8.
[55] Markussen J, Hougaard P, Ribel U et al. Soluble, prolonged acting insulin derivatives. 1. Degree of protraction and crystallizability of insulins substituted in the termini of the B-chain. Protein Engineering 1987; 1: 205–213.
[56] Markussen J, Diers I, Engesgaard A et al. Soluble, prolonged-acting insulin derivatives. II. Degree of protration and crystallisability of insulin substituted in positions A17, B8, B13, B27 and B30. Protein Engineering 1987; 1: 215–223.
[57] Markussen J, Diers I, Hougaard P et al. Soluble, prolonged acting insulin derivatives. III. Degree of protraction, crystallizability and chemical stability of insulins substituted in positions A21, B13, B23, B27 and B30. Protein Engineering 1988; 2: 157–166.
[58] Langkjaer L, Kornfelt T, Markussen J et al. Stable insulin solutions with prolonged action. Diabetologia 1988; 31: 512A.
[59] Jorgensen S, Vaag A, Langkjaer L et al. Novosol Basal: pharmacokinetics of a novel soluble long acting insulin analogue. Br Med J 1989; 299: 415–9.
[60] Illum L. Drug delivery systems for nasal application. Arch Pharm Chemi 1987; 94: 127–135.
[61] Moses AC, Gordon GS, Carey MC et al. Insulin administered intranasally as an insulin-

bile salt aerosol. Effectiveness and reproducibility in normal and diabetic subjects. Diabetes 1983; 32: 1040–1047.
[62] Hirai S, Ikenaga T, Matsuzawa T. Nasal absorption of insulin in dogs. Diabetes 1978; 27: 296–99.
[63] Pontiroli A, Alberetto M, Secchi A et al. Insulin given intranasally induces hypoglycaemia in normal and diabetic subjects. Br Med J 1982; 284: 303–306.
[64] Frauman AG, Jerums G, Louis WJ. Effects of intranasal insulin in non-obese type II diabetics. Diabetes Research 1987; 3: 197–202.
[65] Frauman AG, Cooper ME, Parsons BJ et al. Long term use of intranasal insulin in insulin-dependent diabetic patients. Diabetes Care 1987; 10: 573–78.
[66] Gordon GS, Moses AC, Silver RD et al. Nasal absorption of insulin: Enhancement of hydrophobic bile salts. Proc Natl Acad Sci 1985; 82: 7419–7423.
[67] Salzman R, Manson JE, Griffing GT et al. Intranasal aerosolized insulin: Mixed meal studies and long-term use in Type I diabetes. N Engl J Med 1985; 312: 1078–84.

Diabetogenic drugs

H. Lithell, C. Berne

Introduction

The propensity of certain drugs to produce diabetes mellitus or impaired glucose tolerance is a significant clinical problem. In the National Diabetes Data Group's criteria for the classification and diagnosis of diabetes mellitus, drugs and chemical agents were officially recognized as important factors in the precipitation of diabetes mellitus or impaired glucose tolerance [1].

The possibility of predicting the risk of developing drug-induced diabetes is, with few exceptions, limited in clinical practice. Certain situations, however, such as drug treatment of women with gestational diabetes, obese patients or those with close relatives with diabetes mellitus provide the practising physician with the opportunity to avoid agents which may precipitate diabetes. In essential hypertension, the increased awareness of the association between hypertension, diabetes mellitus and lipid abnormalities [2] may lead to a more cautious attitude and avoidance of drugs which derange carbohydrate and lipid metabolism when the choice of appropriate antihypertensive treatment is made.

It is sometimes difficult to establish a clear link between a specific drug and the development of diabetes, since many diseases of varying severity are in themselves diabetogenic. Inflammatory diseases [3, 4], acute infections [5], the stress of trauma and sepsis [6] as well as hypertension [2] are all associated with insulin resistance and a risk of developing glucose intolerance or diabetes mellitus.

Diabetes mellitus and impaired glucose tolerance may be produced by different mechanisms. Insulin release may be inhibited either directly by the drug or indirectly as a consequence of enhanced secretion of hormones, which reduce insulin release. Extrapancreatic effects on hepatic glucose production or peripheral glucose disposal may impair glucose tolerance and cause diabetes. Furthermore, a direct toxic action on the pancreatic B-cells may lead to loss of B-cells and cause insulin-dependent diabetes mellitus. Finally, it is likely that the precipitation of diabetes by drugs requires a susceptible individual, with a hereditary predisposition to the disease.

Rather than going into reports of possible associations between diabetes mellitus and a wide variety of drugs, which may be retrieved in standard texts which monitor the drug side effects, we have tried to focus on some clinically relevant situations in which the diabetogenic action of drugs may require serious judgement by the physician. We have also tried to cover the different mechanisms underlying the diabetogenicity of drugs.

Antihypertensive drugs

In a Swedish study [7] the prevalence of diabetes mellitus was found to be six times higher among middle-aged women who had been treated with diuretics for about 12 years than among non-hypertensive women of the same age. However, not all of the original cohort of hypertensive women had been treated with diuretics but instead with propranolol and in that group the prevalence of diabetes was also about six times higher than in the background population. In Uppsala, a group of more than 2,300 50 year-old men have been followed for 10 years. Among those treated for moderate hypertension, the prevalence of diabetes was about six times higher than in a group of normotensive men matched for body-mass index, intravenous glucose tolerance, serum-triglyceride and cholesterol concentrations [8]. Treatment with antihypertensive drugs (beta-blockers and/or diuretics) was still associated with a significant risk for diabetes mellitus after inclusion of other significant risk factors such as anthropometric characteristics, plasma insulin, blood glucose and blood pressure at the start of the trial [9]. These data indicate that treatment with beta-blockers and/or thiazide diuretics may in itself be a factor that contributes to the development of impaired glucose tolerance and diabetes mellitus.

Ever since the thiazide diuretics were introduced for treatment of hypertension in 1957, many clinical observations and results in prospective trials have raised the question whether this type of treatment is associated with an increased risk for development of impaired glucose tolerance and non-insulindependent diabetes mellitus [10].

In the Medical Research Council's study [11] about 18,000 men and women (age 35–64 years) were studied, one-fourth of them during treatment with bendrofluazide (10 mg per day). After about two years of active treatment, impaired glucose tolerance was reported to be four to seven times more frequent in the group treated with bendrofluazide than in the placebo-treated control group. Eighty percent of all cases developed during the first treatment year. Regression of the impaired glucose tolerance was reported in 60% of the patients within the year following cessation of treatment.

In the European Working Party for Treatment of Hypertension in the Elderly Study [12], the patients averaged 72 years of age when invited to take part in a study with hydrochlorothiazide (25 – 50 mg) and triamterene (50 – 100 mg). Fasting blood glucose was increased by 0.5 mmol/l after two years in the actively treated group in comparison with the placebo-treated group. The patients followed for three to four years had an even larger increase in blood glucose levels and the increase seemed to be proportional to the duration of the treatment period.

Studies specifically investigating effects on glucose metabolism and insulin secretion in treatment of hypertension

Thiazide diuretics

Fifty patients with mild to moderate hypertension were enrolled in a controlled, randomized, double-blind, double-dummy crossover trial comparing the effects of hydrochlorothiazide and captopril; each active treatment period of 18 weeks' duration [13]. It could be demonstrated that during thiazide treatment insulin-sensitivity index decreased by 16%. This decrease in insulin sensitivity was also reflected in a significantly increased plasma-insulin concentration in the fasting state and at 90 min. of an intravenous glucose tolerance test (IVGTT). Furthermore, both the fasting plasma-glucose concentration and the glucose concentrations during the IVGTT were significantly higher during thiazide treatment than during placebo treatment and HbA_{1c} increased from 4.6 to 5.3% ($p < 0.001$). No dose-effect relationship could be demonstrated with regard to insulin sensitivity, insulin concentrations or glucose values. Furthermore, it could be demonstrated that the decrease in insulin sensitivity was long-lasting and could be demonstrated also after one month of placebo + five months of captopril treatment.

The mechanism underlying the diabetogenic effect of thiazide diuretics is unclear. Hypokalemia may impair both insulin secretion and sensitivity. However, in our study there was no relationship between changes in insulin sensitivity and changes of serum potassium. It cannot be excluded that low intracellular concentrations of potassium and magnesium may contribute to the diabetogenicity of thiazides.

Diazoxide

Diazoxide is a thiazide derivative which strongly inhibits insulin secretion [14]. The drug lacks diuretic properties. It also tends to produce sodium retention and edema with long-term use [15]. The intravenous preparation of the drug is used as a potent antihypertensive agent, mainly in emergency situations, to treat grossly elevated blood pressure or hypertensive crisis. The hyperglycemic properties of diazoxide have been clinically utilized as an interim solution to elevate blood glucose in patients with insulinomas waiting for operation [15]. In the acute situation, hyperglycemia is seldom a problem since the medication is swiftly changed once the acutely raised blood pressure is under control. The mechanisms of action of diazoxide have recently been clarified. It was found that the inhibitory effects on the glucose-induced insulin release are mediated through selective activation of ATP-sensitive potassium channels, leading to a hyperpolarization of the pancreatic B-cell membrane [16,17].

Beta-blockers

In a recent study [18] we have shown that during metoprolol treatment (200 mg/day] insulin-sensitivity index was reduced by 27%, whereas during treatment with atenolol (50 mg/day] the insulin-sensitivity index was reduced by 23% in comparison with the value during the run-in placebo period. The two drugs did not differ significantly from each other in this respect. During both regimes serum-insulin concentrations and plasma-glucose concentrations in the fasting state and during the IVGTT were significantly increased. Thus, this study demonstrates that treatment with selective beta-blockers is associated with a decreased insulin sensitivity and hyperinsulinemia of similar magnitude to that reported for thiazide-diuretic treatment.

In a recent study (to be published) a comparison was made between the effect of propranolol (160 mg/day) and pindolol (10 mg/day) in 40 hypertensive patients. During propranolol treatment insulin-sensitivity index was reduced by 30% but significantly less so during pindolol treatment (reduction of 17%).

Calcium-channel blockers

In one study [19], 58 patients were randomized for active treatment with either diltiazem (mean dose 329 mg/day) or atenolol (mean dose 67 mg/day) for six months. It could be demonstrated that during diltiazem treatment neither insulin sensitivity nor insulin or glucose values were affected by the treatment. In a recent study (unpublished results) insulin-sensitivity index during nifedipine treatment was significantly reduced. In fact, case-reports on the development of diabetes during treatment with nifedipine may have their explanation in effects on insulin sensitivity as reported here. Thus calcium-channel blockers seem to differ with respect to the effects on carbohydrate metabolism. Variable effects on the calcium-dependent insulin secretion or varying activation of the sympato-adrenal system may explain the effects.

ACE-inhibitor

During treatment with captopril [13] the insulin-sensitivity index was improved by 18% compared with the results obtained during the placebo run-in period. The insulin concentrations were lower in the fasting state and during the late part of the IVGTT. Similar improvements were reported during treatment of NIDDM patients with captopril [20].

Alpha-1 blockers

Prazosin treatment was associated with improvements in insulin-sensitivity index and this improvement was reflected in significantly lower insulin concentrations in the fasting state and during the late part of the IVGTT [21].

Table 1 Summary of metabolic effects of antihypertensive drugs

	Thiazide	Metoprolol and atenolol	Prazosin	Diltiazem	Captopril
Fasting insulin	↑	↑	–	–	–
Fasting glucose	↑	↑	↓	–	–
Insulin sensitivity	↓	↓	↑	–	↑
Triglyceride	↑	↑	–	–	–
Total cholesterol	↑	–	–	–	–
LDL cholesterol	↑	–	–	–	–
HDL cholesterol	–	↓	–	–	–
Potassium	↓	–	–	–	↑
Uric acid	↑	(↑)	–	–	(↓)

↑ = increase; ↓ = decrease; – = no change; ( ) = no consistent change

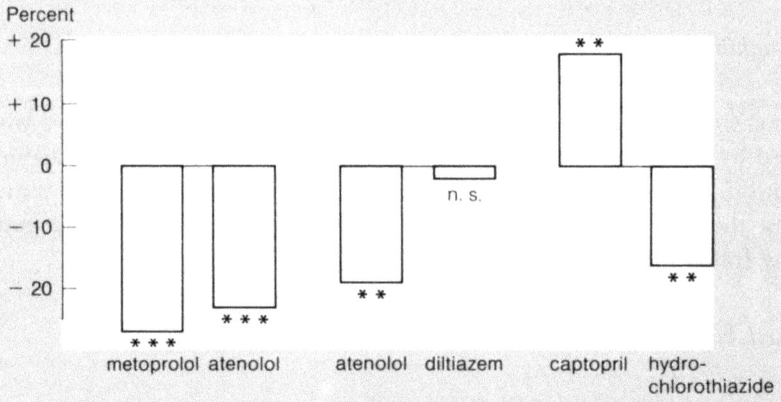

Fig. 1 Mean percentage changes in insulin sensitivity index during different antihypertensive treatments in prospective trials, compared with the run-in placebi-treatment results.

In conclusion

During treatment with both thiazide diuretics, selective and non-selective beta-blockers and non-selective beta-blockers with ISA, the insulin sensitivity decreased (Table 1 and Fig. 1). These findings were associated with increases in insulin and glucose concentrations as well as HbA_{1c} and provide a reasonable explanation for the epidemiological findings. In contrast, during treatment with diltiazem (a calcium-channel blocker), with captopril (an ACE-inhibitor) or with prazosin (an alpha-1 blocker), insulin sensitivity was unchanged or improved. This may indicate a smaller risk for development of diabetes than with thiazides or beta-blockers, although epidemiological studies in support of this are lacking.

Lipid-lowering agents

Since official guidelines for the treatment of hypercholesterolemia and hypertriglyceridemia have been introduced during the latter part of the eighties, it may be foreseen that in the future a considerable part of the population will also be subjected to drug treatment for hyperlipidemia. It is therefore of great importance that such drugs are also well characterized with regard to effects on glucose metabolism in analogy with the case for antihypertensive drugs. There are presently four major categories of drugs on the market, namely bile-acid binding resins (colestipol or cholestyramine), niacin (or derivatives thereof), fibrates and HMGCoA-reductase inhibitors. The first three categories have had representatives on the market for 20 years or more and some of them have been the subject for investigations of effects on carbohydrate metabolism.

Bile-acid binding resins

In the Lipid Research Clinics Study [22] 3,806 men were recruited and followed for up to nine years (average follow-up time seven years). There has been no report of an excess of diabetes mellitus in the actively treated group in comparison with the placebo-treated group. In short-term dose-response studies [23] it has been reported that insulin concentrations in the fasting state were significantly higher during treatment with colestipol than during the run-in period. Unfortunately, no investigations specifically addressed to investigate insulin sensitivity have been carried out with these agents.

Fibrates

A large number of fibrates are used in today's medicine for treatment of hyperlipidemia, especially in cases where hypertriglyceridemia coexists with low HDL-cholesterol concentrations. They seem to differ from each other with regard to effects on glucose metabolism.

Clofibrate

In the WHO multi-centre study [24] of the effects of clofibrate on the risk for myocardial infarction, an increased incidence of glucosuria was reported among those treated with clofibrate. However, this was not a consistent finding for all centres. In a separate study, however, the long-term effects of clofibrate treatment on diabetes in 50 hyperlipidemic patients followed for six to eight years were favourable [25]. In mode-of-action studies it has been demonstrated that during clofibrate treatment there is no overall improvement in intravenous glucose tolerance but a significant and consistent reduction in fasting and late insulin concentrations (at an intravenous glucose tolerance test) [26,27].

In contrast to these findings, treatment with gemfibrozil does not affect fasting-insulin concentrations [28].

During treatment with bezafibrate, similar effects on insulin concentrations as with gemfibrozil were found [29] and in a recent study using the hyperinsulinemic clamp technique it was demonstrated that there were no significant effects on insulin sensitivity or insulin concentration during bezafibrate treatment [30].

Nicotinic acid

It has been demonstrated that fasting-blood glucose increases and that intravenous glucose tolerance decreases significantly during treatment with niceritrol (pentaerytritrol-tetranicotinate) [27]. Higher fasting and late insulin concentrations (at the end of the IVGTT) were also noted.

Treatment with acipimox, a nicotinic-acid derivative, has been carried out in a large multi-centre study comprising 3,009 outpatients with non-insulin dependent diabetes with hyperlipoproteinemia. Treatment was carried out for at least two months. Fasting blood-glucose and glycated hemoglobin levels showed a slight reduction during the study [31]. These effects on glucose metabolism seem to be related to the decrease in plasma FFA obtained by inhibition of lipids during nicotinic acid treatment. This in turn affects and facilitates the glucose oxidation that was significantly increased in several studies [32,33].

Thus, earlier observations of increases in blood-glucose concentrations may be related to the fact that lipolysis is incompletely inhibited after prolonged fasting. However, the recent experiences with acipimox seem to indicate that neither non-insulin-dependent diabetics nor non-diabetic hypertriglyceridemic patients are adversely affected with regard to glucose metabolism during such treatment.

HMgCoA-reductase inhibitors

This new class of drug for treatment of hypercholesterolemia has not been reported to be associated with any effects on glucose metabolism.

Hormones

Glucocorticoids

It has long been established that the administration of glucocorticoids is associated with impairment of glucose tolerance. The term "steroid diabetes" was introduced 50 years ago to describe hyperglycemia in rats receiving corticosteroids [34].

Large dosages of glucocorticoids are invariably associated with abnormalities of insulin secretion [35] and action [36], although it is likely that a genetic predisposition to diabetes is required for overt diabetes to develop. This is substantiated by the observation that obesity and diabetes in the family were found to be risk factors for steroid diabetes in post transplant patients [37]. Although hyperinsulinemia, a common finding in glucocorticoid excess [38], indicates that insulin resistance is a major factor behind the metabolic effects, experimental data show that the function of the pancreatic B-cells does not escape the influence of glucocorticoids. It was shown early that cortisone induces morphological signs of hyperplasia and increased numbers of pancreatic islets in various species, but the increased B-cell mass was found to be associated with glycogen infiltration of the B-cells (for review, see [39]). A changed metabolism of the B-cells may explain why later studies have shown that the function of the islets may eventually be impaired, since several species of glucocorticoids inhibit insulin release in vitro [40].

Despite the fact that in vitro studies have disclosed that glucocorticoids may impair B-cell function, the earliest finding after administration of glucocorticoids is hyperinsulinemia, indicating that resistance to the insulin action has evolved. Some in vitro studies paradoxically indicated that glucocorticoids increased the number of insulin receptors [41]. However, after co-incubation of cells with glucocorticoids and excess insulin, a strong down-regulating effect of insulin finally resulted in a decreased receptor number [42]. In isolated adipocytes a major effect of dexamethasone was ascribed to a decrease in glucose transport and not to receptor function abnormalities [43]. Both hepatic sensitivity to insulin and the effect of insulin on peripheral glucose disposal are impaired by glucocorticoids [44]. The dominating effect seems to be exerted at the post-receptor level.

In clinical practice, glucocorticoids are used with considerable restraint due to their long-term adverse effects. Their use is limited to severe and disabling disease manifestations, e.g. asthma, rheumatic disease, vasculitides, malignancies, anti-rejection treatment after transplantation and so forth. The treatment of diabetes in these clinical situations is not without problems due to the combined action of the disease and the glucocorticoids on insulin sensitivity. Non-ketotic hyperosmolar coma may occasionally develop, and in children steroid diabetes may be precipitated by glucocorticoids [45,46]. The insulin resistance may be severe and respond poorly to diet alone, requiring sulfonylurea therapy or large dosages of insulin. Steroid diabetes is often characterized by afternoon hyperglycemia, whereas fasting blood glucose is often only moderately increased. Screening for steroid diabetes should therefore include blood-glucose measurements late during the day.

In rare instances, a paradoxical improvement of glucose tolerance after glucocorticoid treatment may be observed. A therapeutically induced decrease in insulin resistance caused by the disease itself, can be alleviated by the antiinflammatory action of the drug treatment, e.g. in rheumatoid arthritis [3].

Gonadal steroids

Hyperandrogenism has been associated with insulin resistance in the polycystic ovarian syndrome [47]. It is known that androgens may decrease insulin action both by influencing receptor binding and by post receptor effects [48]. The clinical use of testosterone is mainly confined to replacement therapy in males. The related compounds, anabolic steroids, which have gained widespread illegal use among athletes, share the same ability to increase insulin resistance, and may therefore precipitate diabetes mellitus in susceptible individuals [49,50].

The effect of female sex hormones will be covered in a later chapter of this volume.

Catecholamines and derivatives

The naturally occurring catecholamines, noradrenalin, adrenalin or dopamine are used in clinical practice only for short-term intravenous treatment of indications such as severe hypotension or shock, anaphylactic reactions or severe asthma. In these situations a diabetogenic action is rarely of clinical significance. Adrenalin is an insulin-antagonistic hormone with a variety of points of action, which act in concert to elevate blood glucose. It stimulates glycogenolysis in the liver, thereby increasing hepatic glucose output and inhibits peripheral glucose uptake primarily by beta$_2$-mediated effects [51,52]. The lipolytic action of adrenalin may also lead to increased insulin resistance through the glucose-fatty acid cycle [53]. Insulin release is strongly inhibited by an alpha$_2$-adrenergic mechanism [54,55]. Noradrenalin has less powerful effects but has been reported to increase insulin resistance [56] and reduce insulin secretion in healthy subjects [57].

Derivatives of catecholamines are frequently used in the long-term treatment of patients and sometimes a diabetogenic action is seen. Clonidine, a central and peripheral alpha$_2$-agonist used in hypertension and in migraine has been reported to induce glucose intolerance, secondary to a defective insulin secretion [58]. Beta$_2$-mimetics used in the treatment of asthma may precipitate diabetes mellitus or impair glucose tolerance [59].

Beta$_2$-mimetics are also used as an effective treatment to inhibit pre-term labour. Special caution is warranted if type 1 diabetic women require this treatment. Worsening of metabolic control even to acute ketoacidosis has been reported [60]. Therefore, if no alternative treatment is available, an increase in the frequency of glucose control and ketonuria testing is mandatory. Tocolytic treatment may also precipitate gestational diabetes in susceptible women and therefore should be accompanied by close monitoring of blood glucose.

Thyroid hormones

Hyperthyroidism is associated with diabetes mellitus, which is explained by the known association of type 1 diabetes mellitus to autoimmune thyroid disease, by changes in catecholamine sensitivity and finally to effects of thyroid hormone excess on the pancreatic B-cells and on insulin action [61]. Since thyroxin is used solely as a replacement therapy, its potential diabetogenic action is rarely a clinical problem. One situation in which the insulin antagonistic effect of thyroid hormones must be taken into account is during initiation of replacement therapy in hypothyroid subjects with diabetes mellitus, when an increase in insulin dosage must follow the return towards euthyroidism.

Growth hormone

Growth hormone has various actions on glucose metabolism and may in some situations exert insulin-like effects [62]. In the human being an increase in insulin resistance follows the administration of growth hormone [62]. With the few limited medical indications for growth hormone therapy today, the hormone is mainly used as replacement therapy in hypopituitarism which presents no real problem. If the indications for therapy with growth hormone are expanded, its diabetogenic action, clinically evident in acromegaly [62], may turn out to cause greater problems.

Drugs causing pancreatic B-cell damage

Streptozotocin

Streptozotocin is a model drug for B-cell cytotoxic agents. Streptozotocin is a nitrosomethylurea derivative coupled to a glucose moiety [63]. It was recognized early that injection of streptozotocin in mice was followed by a rapid depletion of NAD (nicotinamide dinucleotide) in the pancreatic B-cells [63]. Later studies have established that streptozotocin acts through the formation of carbonium ions, which cause alkylation of DNA. The following DNA repair is associated with poly (ADP-ribose) activation, a process which consumes large amounts of NAD. The loss of this important component of oxidative metabolism eventually leads to cell death [64].

Streptozotocin is probably the most widely used agent producing diabetes in experimental animals. It was the first effective anti-tumour agent for treatment of malignant insulinoma. The human use of streptozotocin has been less complicated by diabetes mellitus than might be expected from its effects in rodents [15]. The toxicity of the drug affects both the liver and kidney and limits its dosage, which may explain the relative tolerance to the diabetogenic effect of the drug in human beings.

In this context it should be mentioned that a related nitrosamine, the rodenticide with the generic name Vacor® was reported to cause ketosis-prone diabetes mellitus in humans, who had ingested this agent either unintentionally or in order to commit suicide [65].

Cyclosporine A

The use of cyclosporine A as an immunosuppressive drug was found to be associated with a diabetogenic effect. In the study by Gunnarsson et al. cyclosporine A was found to be associated with a plasma concentration-dependent resistance to insulin [66]. In experimental animals, and in studies of pancreatic islets in vitro, a direct B-cell cytotoxicity was also observed [67]. Recent studies have shown that the triplet immunosuppression (prednisolone, azathioprine and cyclosporine) which is today used in renal allograft transplantation was associated with a 19% incidence of diabetes in the post transplantation period, which is nearly three times higher than when prednisolone was used in combination with only one of the other two drugs [68]. Several studies have confirmed that renal transplant recipients, who receive cyclosporine A require a careful monitoring of blood-glucose for the early detection of diabetes in the post transplant period [69].

Pentamidine

Pentamidine, a rarely used anti-protozoal drug, has received increased attention lately as an agent used for the treatment of Pneumocystosis carinii-pneumonitis in immuno-compromised hosts, e.g. after bone marrow transplantation and in the acquired immune deficiency syndrome (AIDS). Its use has been limited by the appearance of overt diabetes mellitus [70] which is likely to be a result of pancreatic B-cell damage. The glucose changes after administration of the drug are a phase of hypoglycemia followed by hyperglycemia, which resembles the action of streptozotocin [70,71]. The hypoglycemia is probably caused by insulin from destroyed B-cells followed by diabetes mellitus caused by B-cell loss.

L-asparaginase

L-asparaginase is an anti-tumour agent, mainly used in the treatment of acute lymphatic leukemia in children. It was observed that administration of the drug was occasionally associated with the development of transient or permanent diabetes [72,73]. The primary mode of action of L-asparaginase is thought to be an inhibition of protein biosynthesis in the pancreatic B-cells, or more selectively an interference with the biosynthesis of the insulin molecule, which contains L-asparagine [73]. This hypothesis of a primary action on the insulin-producing cells is substantiated by the observation, in humans, of a deterioration in insulin secretion after an oral glucose load [74]. Diabetic ketoacidosis has been reported in several cases [73], which strongly supports the theory that a hypoinulinemic state is induced by L-asparaginase.

Other diabetogenic drugs

Anti-inflammatory drugs

Prostaglandins are involved in the insulin release process. Inhibitors of prostaglandin biosynthesis from the group of non-steroid anti-inflammatory drugs (NSAID) have been reported both to augment [75] and inhibit (indomethacin) the glucose-induced early insulin response [76]. In contrast, acetyl salicylic acid is well known as exerting a hypoglycemic action.

Studies in vitro have shown that chloroquine may directly affect insulin secretion and biosynthesis [77], which could lead to diabetogenic effects. Studies in man, however, show that a putative inhibition of the lysosomal degradation of insulin may ameliorate hyperglycemia in non-insulin-dependent diabetes mellitus [78].

Diphenylhydantoin

The widely used anti-epileptic drug, diphenylhydantoin has been reported as being associated with overt diabetes and even non-ketotic hyperosmolar coma [79]. This is caused by a direct inhibition of insulin release by interference with the transmembrane transport of calcium and sodium [80, 81]. Attempts have been made to use this effect of diphenylhydantoin to control insulin secretion in patients with insulinoma [15]. Hyperglycemia is a rare adverse effect of diphenylhydantoin, probably due to the fact that the dosage is under close supervision with repeated measurements of serum drug levels. Even though studies in patients on long-term diphenylhydantoin therapy have not disclosed an increased incidence in diabetes mellitus, it is recommended that attention be paid to the diabetogenic effect of diphenylhydantoin in patients with risk factors of developing diabetes mellitus [81].

Conclusions

From a population-based perspective, even minor diabetogenic effects produced by pharmacological agents used in asymptomatic patients with prevention of disease as the primary objective may be important for the health of a population. An increase in the prevalence of diabetes mellitus in large groups of patients may increase the morbidity or mortality in atherosclerotic disease, e.g. stroke or myocardial infarction.

Diabetes-related symptoms or the subsequent development of microvascular and macrovascular complications may also decrease the quality of life in patients already stricken with illness. In serious disease states, diabetes mellitus as an adverse effect may even be an acceptable complication to treatment. In contrast, the development of diabetes mellitus or glucose intolerance during the course of treatment for mild hypertension or during oral contraception is much less acceptable.

A separate but important clinical problem is the use of diabetogenic drugs in diabetes mellitus. In insulin-dependent diabetes without endogenous insulin secretion, the induction of insulin resistance by drugs may be counteracted by elevation of the insulin dose. In the long run, however, the resultant increase in plasma free insulin may be a disadvantage. Insulin has been suggested as being a risk factor for macrovascular disease not only in populations [2], but also in subjects treated with exogenous insulin.

From a therapeutic standpoint, non-insulin-dependent diabetes mellitus may be a greater problem, since diabetogenic drugs may lead to the escalation of therapy from diet to sulfonylureas or insulin.

The long-term adverse effects of drug-induced diabetes are essentially the same as those of all other major forms of diabetes irrespective of cause, i.e. nephropathy, retinopathy, neuropathy and macrovascular disease. Since drug-induced diabetes is usually of the non-insulin-dependent variety with associated lipid abnormalities, macrovascular complications must be considered as an important factor following drug-induced diabetes mellitus.

Diabetes mellitus precipitated by drugs is not a minor clinical problem, rather it must be dealt with by many categories of practising physicians. Today, older and more vulnerable patient groups are exposed to potent drug treatment with potential diabetogenic actions. This requires alertness by the physicians handling these drugs, to use them with care and try to avoid exposure of susceptible patients.

References

[1] National Diabetes Data Group. Classification and diagnosis of diabetes mellitus and other categories of glucose intolerance. Diabetes 1979; 28: 1039–1057.

[2] Reaven GM. Role of insulin resistance in human disease. Diabetes 1988; 37: 1595–1607.

[3] Hällgren R, Berne C. Glucose intolerance in patients with chronic inflammatory disease is normalized by glucocorticoids. Acta Med Scand 1983; 213: 351–355.

[4] Svenson KLG, Pollare T, Lithell H et al. Impaired glucose handling in active rheumatoid arthritis. III Relationship to peripheral resistance. Metabolism 1988; 337: 125–130.

[5] Rayfield EJ, Curnow RT, George DT et al. Impaired carbohydrate metabolism during a mild viral illness. New Engl J Med 1973; 618–621.

[6] Frayn KN. Hormonal control of metabolism in trauma and sepsis. Clin Endocrinol 1986; 24: 577–599.

[7] Bengtsson C, Blohmé G, Lapidus L et al. Do antihypertensive drugs precipitate diabetes? Br Med J 1984; 289: 1495–1497.

[8] Skarfors E, Lithell H, Selinus I et al. Do antihypertensive drugs precipitate diabetes in predisposed men? Br Med J 1989; 298: 1147–1152.

[9] Skarfors E. Risk factors for development of diabetes mellitus, hypertension and coronary heart disease with special reference to serum insulin levels. A ten-year follow-up of an Uppsala health survey in middle-aged men. Thesis. Acta Universitatis Upsaliensis 1989; 212.

[10] Furman BL. Impairment of glucose tolerance produced by diuretics and other drugs. Pharmac Ther 1981; 12: 613–649.

[11] Greenburg G. Adverse reactions to bendrofluazide and propranolol for the treatment of mild hypertension. Lancet 1981; II: 539–543.

[12] Amery A, Berthaux P, Bulpitt C et al. Glucose intolerance during diuretic therapy. Results of trial by the European Working Party on hypertension in the elderly. Lancet 1978; I: 681–683.

[13] Pollare T, Lithell H, Berne C. A comparison of the effects of hydrochlorothiazide and captopril on glucose and lipid metabolism in patients with hypertension. New Engl J Med 1989; 321: 868–873.

[14] Milner RDG, Hales CN. The interaction of various inhibitors and stimuli of insulin release studied in rabbit pancreas in vitro. Biochem J 1969; 113: 473–479.

[15] Vinik AI, Moattari AR. Treatment of endocrine tumors of the pancreas. Endocr Metab Clin NA 1989; 18: 483–518.
[16] Trube G, Rorsman P, Ohno Shosaku T. Opposite effects of tolbutamide and diazoxide on the ATP dependent K^+ channel in mouse pancreatic B-cells. Pflügers Arch 1986; 407: 493–499.
[17] Henquin JC. ATP-sensitive K^+ channels may control glucose-induced electrical activity in the pancreatic B-cells. Biochem Biophys Res Comm 1988; 156: 769–775.
[18] Pollare T, Lithell H, Selinus I et al. Sensitivity to insulin during treatment with atenolol and metoprolol: a randomized, double blind study of effects on carbohydrate and lipoprotein metabolism in hypertensive patients. Br Med J 1989; 298: 1152–1157.
[19] Pollare T, Lithell H, Mörlin C et al. Metabolic effects of diltiazem and atenolol: results from a randomized, double-blind study with parallel groups. J Hypertension 1989; 7: 551–559.
[20] Rett K, Lotz N, Wicklmayr M et al. Verbesserte Insulinwirkung durch ACE-Hemmung beim Typ-II-Diabetiker. Deutsch Med Wschr 1988; 113: 243–249.
[21] Pollare T, Lithell H, Selinus I et al. Application of prazosin is associated with an increase of insulin sensitivity in obese patients with hypertension. Diabetologia 1988; 31: 415–420.
[22] Lipid Research Clinics Program. The lipid research clinics coronary primary prevention trial results. I. Reduction in incidence of coronary heart disease. JAMA 1984; 251: 351–364.
[23] Lithell H, Vessby B, Boberg J et al. The effects of colestipol when combined with clofibrate in the treatment of severe hyperlipidemia. Atherosclerosis 1980; 37: 175–186.
[24] Oliver MF, Heady JA, Morris JN et al. A co-operative trial in the primary prevention of ischaemic heart disease using clofibrate. Report from the Committee of Principal Investigators. Brit Heart J 1978; 40: 1069–1118.
[25] Berkowitz D. Long-term treatment of hyperlipidemic patients with clofibrate. JAMA 1971; 218: 1002–1005.
[26] Lithell H, Boberg J, Hedstrand H et al. Effects of clofibrate on glucose tolerance, serum insulin, serum lipoproteins and plasma fibrinogen. Eur J Clin Pharmacol 1977; 12: 51–57.
[27] Lithell H, Vessby B, Hellsing K. Changes in glucose tolerance and plasma insulin during lipid-lowering treatment with diet, clofibrate and niceritrol. Atherosclerosis 1982; 43: 177–184.
[28] Vessby B, Boberg M, Lithell H. Influence of gemfibrozil on lipoprotein composition: triglyceride removal capacity and fatty acid composition of the plasma lipid esters. In: Wood C, ed. Further Progress with Gemfibrozil. Royal Society of Medicine Services International Congress and Symposium Series No. 87, Royal Society of Medicine Services, Ltd. 1986; 1–10.
[29] Vessby B, Lithell H, Hellsing K et al. Effects of bezafibrate on the serum lipoprotein lipid and apolipoprotein composition, lipoprotein triglyceride removal capacity and the fatty acid composition of the plasma lipid esters. Atherosclerosis 1980; 37: 257–269.
[30] Riccardi G, Genovese S, Saldalamacchia G et al. Effects of bezafibrate on insulin secretion and peripheral insulin sensitivity in hyperlipidemic patients with and without diabetes. Atherosclerosis 1989; 75: 175–181.
[31] Lavezzari M, Milanesi G, Oggioni E et al. Results of a phase IV study carried out with acipomox in type Ii diabetic patients with concomitant hyperlipoproteinaemia. J Int Med Res 1989; 17: 373–380.
[32] Fulcher GR, Walker M, Catalano C et al. Overnight suppression of lipolysis with acipomox increases carbohydrate oxidation and lowers fasting blood glucose in type 2 (non-insulin-dependent) diabetes. Abstract. Diabetologia 1989; 32: 489A.
[33] Taskinen M-R, Saloranta C, Hilden H et al. Effects of acipomox on glucose and FFA metabolism in hypertriglyceridemic patients. Abstract. X international symposium on drugs affecting lipid metabolism.

[34] Ingle DJ, The production of glucosuria in the normal rat by means of 17-hydroxy-11-deoxycorticosterone. Endocrinology 1941; 29: 649–657.
[35] Gunnarsson R, Lundgren G, Magnusson G et al. Steroid diabetes: a sign of overtreatment with steroids in renal graft recipients. Scand J Uron Nephrol 1980; 14: 135–139.
[36] Conn JW, Fajans SS. Influence of adrenal cortical steroids on carbohydrate metabolism in man. Metab Clin Exp 1956; 5: 114–121.
[37] Pagano G, Bruno A, Cavallo-Perin P et al. Glucose intolerance after short-term administration of corticosteroids in healthy subjects. Arch Int Med 1989; 149: 1093–1101.
[38] Perley M, Kipnis DM. Effect of glucocorticoids on plasma insulin. New Engl J Med 1966; 274: 1237–1241.
[39] Hellerström C. Growth pattern of pancreatic islets in animals. In: Volk BW, Wellman KF, eds. The diabetic pancreas. New York: Plenum publishing corp, 1977; 61–97.
[40] Pierluissi J, Navas FO, Ashcroft SJH. Effects of adrenal steroids on insulin release from cultured rat islets of Langerhans. Diabetologia 1986; 29: 119–121.
[41] Beck-Nielsen H, DePisso R, Pedersen O. Prednisone increases the number of insulin receptors on monocytes from normal subjects. J Clin Endocr Metab 1980; 50: 1–4.
[42] Fantus IG, Saviolakis GA, Hedo JA et al. Mechanism of glucocorticoid-induced increase in insulin receptors of cultured human lymphocytes. J Biol Chem 1982; 257: 8227.
[43] Olefsky JM. Effect of dexamethasone on insulin binding, glucose transport and glucose oxidation of isolated rat adipocytes. J Clin Invest 1975; 56: 1499–1508.
[44] Rizza RA, Mandarino LJ, Gerich JE. Cortisol-induced insulin resistance in man: impaired suppression of glucose production and stimulation of glucose utilization due to a postreceptor defect of insulin action. J Clin Endocr Metab 1982; 54: 181–138.
[45] Fujukawa LS, Meisler DM, Nozik RA. Hyperosmolar hyperglycemic non-ketotic coma. A complication of short-term corticosteroid use. Ophthalmology 1983; 90: 1239–1242.
[46] Perlman K, Ehrlich RM. Steroid diabetes in the childhood. Am J Dis Child 1982; 136: 64–68.
[47] Burghen GA, Givens JR, Kitabchi. Correlation of hyperandrogenism with hyperinsulinemia in polycystic ovarian disease. J Clin Endocrinol Metab 1980; 50: 113–116.
[48] Peiris AN, Mueller RA, Struve MF et al. Relationship of androgenic activity to splanchnic insulin metabolism and peripheral glucose utilization in premenopausal women. J Clin Endocr Metab 1987; 64: 162–169.
[49] Cohen JC, Hickman R. Insulin resistance and diminished glucose tolerance in powerlifters ingesting anabolic steroids. J Clin Endocr Metab 1987; 64: 960–963.
[50] Woodard TL, Burghen GA, Kitabchi et al. Glucose intolerance and insulin resistance in aplastic anemia treated with oxymetholone. J Clin Endocr Metab. 1981; 53: 905–908.
[51] Cryer PE, Gerich JE. Glucose counterregulation, hypoglycemia, and intensive insulin therapy in diabetes mellitus. New Engl J Med 1985; 313: 232–241.
[52] Lager I, Attwall S, Eriksson BM et al. Studies of the insulin-antagonistic effect of catecholamines in normal man. Diabetologia 1986; 29: 409–416.
[53] Ferrannini E, Barrett Ej, Bevilacqua S et al. Effect of fatty acids on glucose production and utilization in man. J Clin Invest 1983; 72: 1737–1747.
[54] Cerasi E, Luft R, Efendic S. Antagonism between glucose and epinephrine regarding insulin secretion. Acta Med Scand 1971; 190: 411–417.
[55] Nakadate T, Nakaki T, Muraki T et al. Adrenergic regulation of blood glucose levels: Possible involvement of post-synaptic alpha$_2$-type adrenergic receptors regulating insulin release. J Pharmacol Exp Ther 1980; 215: 225–230.
[56] Marangou AG, Alford FP, Ward G et al. Hormonal effects of norepinephrine on acute glucose disposal in humans: a minimal model analysis. Metabolism 1988; 37: 885–892.
[57] Schade RS, Eaton RP. The metabolic response to norepinephrine in normal versus diabetic man. Diabetologia 1978; 15: 433–439.
[58] Metz SA, Halter JB, Robertson RP. Induction of defective insulin secretin and impaired glucose tolerance by clonidine. Diabetes 1978; 27: 554–562.

[59] Main EK, Main EM, Gabge SG. Chronic oral terbutaline tocolytic therapy is associated with maternal glucose intolerance. Am J Obstet Gynecol 1987; 157: 664–647.
[60] Mordes D, Kreutner K, Metzger W et al. Dangers of intravenous ritodrine in diabetic patients. JAMA 1982; 248: 973–975.
[61] Lenzen S, Bailey CJ. Thyroid hormones, gonadal and adrenocortical steroids and the function of the islets of Langerhans. Endocr Rev 1984; 5: 411–434.
[62] Davidson MB. Effect of growth hormone on carbohydrate and lipid metabolism. Endocr Rev 1987; 8: 115–131.
[63] Gunnarsson R, Berne C, Hellerström C. Cytotoxic effects of streptozotocin and N-nitrosomethylurea on the pancreatic B cells with special regard to the role of nicotinamide-adenine dinucleotide. Biochem J 1974; 140: 487–494.
[64] Eizirik DL, Sandler S. Function and metabolism of pancreatic B-cells maintained in culture following induced damage. Pharmacol Toxicol 1989; 65: 163–168.
[65] Prossner PR,Karam JH. Diabetes mellitus following rodenticide ingestion in man. JAMA 1978; 239: 1148–1151.
[66] Gunnarsson R, Klintmalm G, Lundgren G et al. Deterioration in glucose metabolism in pancreatic transplant recipients after conversion from azathioprine to cyclosporine. Transpl Proc 1984; 16: 709–712.
[67] Andersson A, Borg H, Hallberg A et al. Long-term effects of cyclosporin A on cultured mouse pancreatic islets. Diabetologia 1984; 27: 66–69.
[68] Bodreaux JP, McHugh L, Canafax DM et al. The impact of cyclosporine and combination immunosuppression on the incidence of posttransplant diabetes in renal allograft recipients. Transplantation 1987; 44: 376–381.
[69] Roth D, Milgrom M, Esquenazi V et al. Posttransplant hyperglycemia. Increased incidence in cyclosporine-treated renal allograft recipients. Transplantation 1989; 47: 278–281.
[70] Bouchard PH, Sai P, Reach G et al. Diabetes mellitus following pentamidine-induced hypoglycemia in humans. Diabetes 1982; 31: 40–45.
[71] Schen M, Orwoll ES, Conte JE et al. Pentamidine-induced pancreatic beta-cell dysfunction. Am J Med 1989; 86: 726–728.
[72] Land VJ, Sutow WW, Fernbach DJ et al. Toxicity of L-asparaginase in children with advanced leukemia. Cancer 1972; 30: 339–347.
[73] Whitecar JP, Bodey GP, Hill CS et al. Effect of L-asparaginase on carbohydrate metabolism. Metabolism 1970; 19: 581–586.
[74] Lavine RL, Brodsky I, Garofano CD et al. The effect of E. Coli L-asparaginase on oral glucose tolerance and insulin release in man. Diabetologia 1978; 15: 113–116.
[75] Robertson RP, Chen M. A role for prostaglandin E in defective insulin secretion and carbohydrate intolerance in diabetes mellitus. J Clin Invest 1977; 60: 747–753.
[76] Widström A. Influence of indomethacin on glucose-induced insulin response in normal man-role of prostaglandins in the rapid insulin release? Horm Metab Res 1977; 9: 172–175.
[77] Hallberg A, Berne C, Andersson A. Effects of chloroquine on lipid metabolism of mouse pancreatic islets. Biochem Pharmacol 1984; 33: 1465–1470.
[78] Smith GD, Amos TAS, Mahler R et al. Effect of chloroquine on insulin and glucose homeostasis in normal subjects and patients with non-insulin dependent diabetes mellitus. Br Med J 1987; 294: 465–467.
[79] Farriss BL,Lutcher CL. Diphenylhydantoin-induced hyperglycemia and impaired insulin release. Diabetes 1971; 20: 177–181.
[80] Malherbe C, Burill KC, Levin SR et al. Effect of diphenylhydantoin on insulin secretion in man. New Engl J Med 1972; 286: 339–342.
[81] Cummings NP, Rosenbloom AL, Kohlere W et al. Plasma glucose and insulin responses to oral glucose with chronic diphenylhydantoin therapy. Pediatrics 1973; 51: 1091–1093.

Treatment of NIDDM patients with peroral antidiabetic drugs

– sulfonylureas, biguanides and new pharmacological approaches –

H. Beck-Nielsen

Introduction

Non-insulin dependent diabetes mellitus (NIDDM) is a very frequent metabolic disorder in Europe. About 5–10% of subjects between 60 and 70 years of age suffer from this disease [1]. The overall mortality rate in NIDDM is approximately twice as high as that of non-diabetics. Thus, those who acquire NIDDM before the age of 50 may expect the loss of 5–10 years of life. The average loss of longevity is greater in women than in men. It decreases markedly with age and is about 3 years in those who develop diabetes after the age of 70 and is negligible at age 75. The main causes of death in NIDDM are cardiovascular and cerebrovascular diseases. The prevention of nephropathy and microangiopathy are closely related to duration in control of the metabolic disorder as in IDDM, although varying in severity. The prognosis of the disease is not only dependent on the quality of control of glucose metabolism, but also on the correction of frequently associated disorders such as hypertension, obesity, lipid abnormalities and adverse lifestyle, especially smoking.

Diabetes specific symptoms may be relieved and diabetes specific complications may be prevented by correction of the metabolic disorder. Therefore, near normal control of metabolism is desirable. However, it is important not to induce hypoglycemia especially in elderly people where prevention of long term complication plays a minor role. It is important to treat not only metabolic disorders but also hypertension and lipid abnormalities. However, that is not the topic of this review.

Pathophysiology of NIDDM

Most patients with NIDDM are characterized by impaired insulin sensitivity in both liver and peripheral tissues as well as an abnormal pancreatic B-cell response to glucose [2]. Insulin secretion may be elevated in mild diabetes but reduced in patients with high blood glucose values. However, frank diabetes mellitus does not develop in subjects where the B-cell capacity is able to compensate for the insulin resistant state. Opposite to the heterogeneity in insulin secretion, all non-insulin dependent diabetics exhibit insulin resistance. Recent studies have indicated that a certain degree of insulin resistance is inherited [3]. Insulin resistance can also be induced e. g. by obesity, overconsumption of fat and reduced exercise. This environmental insulin resistance, added to the genetic resistance, may precipitate diabetes mellitus. Since insulin resistance and inappropriate insulin secretion both play a physiological role, an ideal anti-diabetic drug should of course tend to ameliorate both of these abnormalities. In fact, there is currently substantial evidence that sulfonylureas, in patients with NIDDM, increases insulin secretion and decreases insulin resistance (in both hepatic and extrahepatic tissues). On the other hand, biguanides only seem to affect insulin resistance.

Treatment of the metabolic disorder NIDDM

An algorithm for the therapeutic management of non-insulin dependent diabetes mellitus obtained from the European Consensus Report is outlined in Fig. 1 [4]. As can be seen from this figure, it is important to define individual aims of therapy. The aims may differ between young and old diabetics and between complicated and uncomplicated forms. Furthermore, the degree of obesity must be taken into consideration. Targets for metabolic control are outlined in Table 1, again referring to the European Consensus Report.

Diet treatment plays an important role in especially obese subjects in order to avoid overweight, but all patients with non-insulin dependent diabetes mellitus need dietary education. However, that is not the topic of this review. In case diet treatment is not sufficient to normalize the metabolism, peroral antidiabetics are recommended as the first drug of choice and later on insulin treatment may be considered. In lean diabetics sulfonylureas are the first drug of choice where biguanides may be the first drug of choice for severely obese subjects. Combination of biguanides and sulfonylureas may be considered in many obese patients with NIDDM.

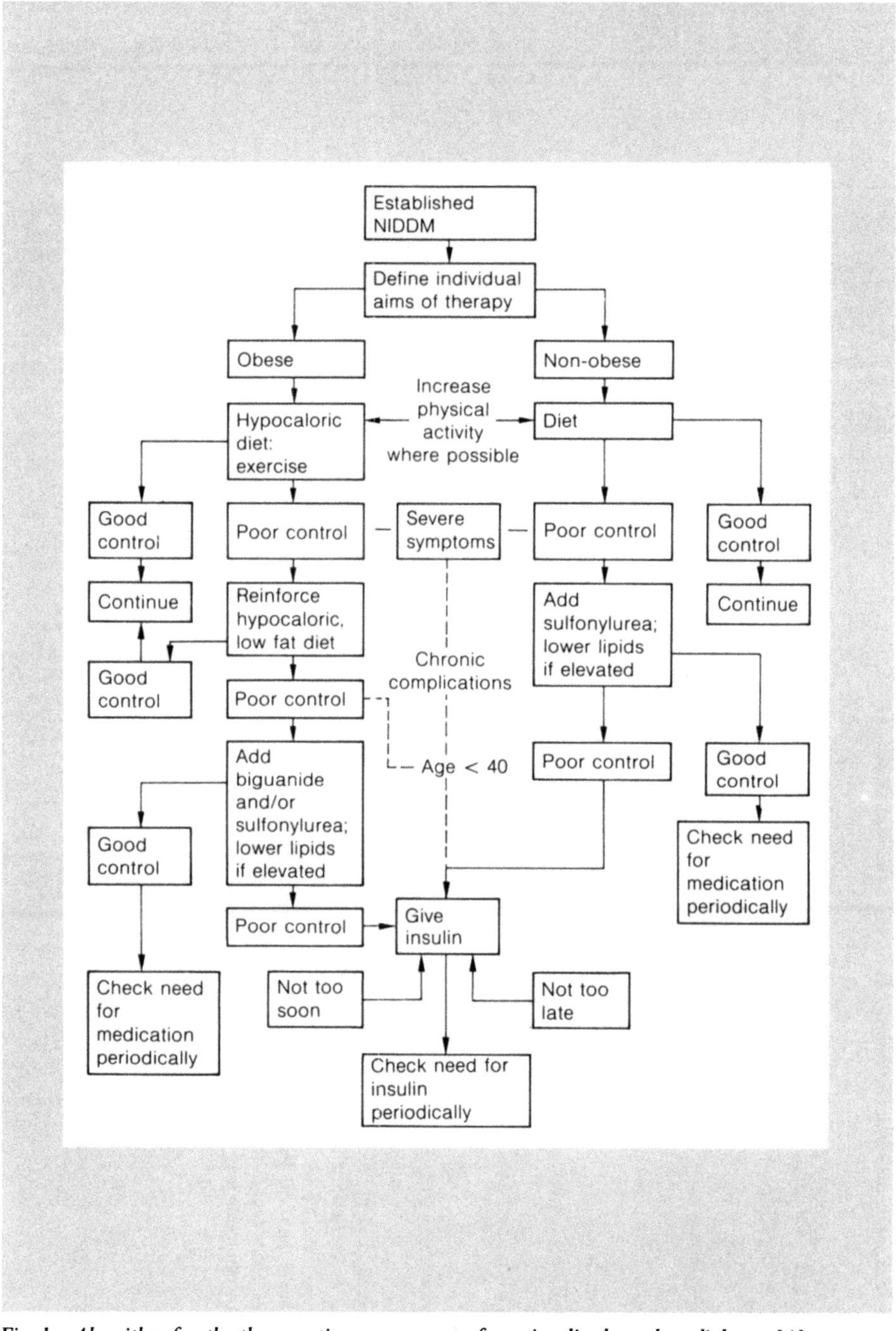

Fig. 1 Algorithm for the therapeutic management of non-insulin dependent diabetes [4]

Table 1 Targets for metabolic control; European Concensus Group [4]

		Good[a]	Acceptable	Poor
Blood glucose				
Fasting	mg/dl	80–120	<140	>140
	mmol/l	4.4–6.7	<7.8	>7.8
Post-prandial	mg/dl	80–160	<180	>180
	mmol/l	4.4–8.8	<10	>10
HbA_1[b]		<Mean + 2 S.D.	<Mean + 4 S.D.	>Mean + 4 S.D.
Urine glucose %		0	<0.5	>0.5
Total cholesterol[c]	*mg/dl*	*<200*	*<250*	*>250*
	mmol/l	*<5.2*	*<6.5*	*>6.5*
HDL-cholesterol	*mg/dl*	*>40*	*>35*	*<35*
	mmol/l	*>1.1*	*>0.9*	*<0.9*
Fasting triglycerides	*mg/dl*	*<150*	*<200*	*>200*
	mmol/l	*<1.7*	*<2.2*	*>2.2*
Body mass index ♂	*kg/m^2*	<25	<27	>27
Body mass index ♀		<24	<26	>26

a) This is the ideal and may be difficult, impossible or unnecessary to achieve in certain patients (see objectives)
b) Reference ranges for HbA_1 vary greatly so targets expressed as mean + standard deviation of mean
c) Lower targets may be desirable in younger patients

In the following, the pharmacology of sulfonylureas and biguanides will be discussed in more detail. Furthermore, new drugs under investigation will be mentioned.

Sulfonylurea treatment

Sulfonylureas consist of a phenyl-SO4-NH-C-NH-core with substitutions on either end which convey certain pharmacokinetic and pharmacological differences. They were introduced for treatment of diabetes in the mid nineteen-sixties. The first four compounds were tolbutamide, acetohexamide, tolazamide, chlorpropamide – first generation drugs. Later on, a new generation of sulfonylureas known as second generation drugs were introduced. The major difference between the first and second generation drugs is that second generation drugs are more potent. The most used second generation drugs are glibenclamide, glipizide, gliclazide, and gliquidone (see Table 2).

Currently, around forty per cent of all diabetics in Europe treated with peroral antidiabetics. Glibenclamide is the most used drug.

Mechanism of action

Pancreatic effects: Sulfonylureas stimulate insulin release not only in vivo but also in vitro [5]. The main effect in vivo is to increase B-cell sensitivity to release stored insulin in response to glucose. There are no indications of a direct effect on insulin synthesis [5]. When islet B-cells are studied histologically, sulfonylureas treatment results in a depletion of the secretion granules and sulfonylurea appeared to stimulate the release of already synthesized insulin. The mechanism of action for different sulfonylureas seems to be essentially identical, confirming a new theory that all sulfonylureas seem to inhibit K+ efflux from pancreatic B-cells in vitro. High-affinity sulfonylurea receptors have been demonstrated on cell lines derived from pancreatic B-cells: the order of potency of sulfonylurea binding to B-cells approximates their potency in stimulating insulin release and inhibiting K+ efflux [6] (Fig. 2). The sulfonylurea receptor has been shown to be closely linked to, or part of the ATP sensitive K+ channel, and inhibition of K+ efflux by sulfonylureas leads to depolarization of the B-cell membrane [7]. The consequence of this is that Ca++ channels on B-cells are opened permitting Ca++ entry. It is likely that the increased intercellular calcium concentration conveys an increased binding of calcium to the carrier protein calmodulin which results in mocrofilament contraction, and exocytosis of granules in which insulin is stored. However, it must be emphasized that sulfonylurea receptors have not been shown in human B-cells until now.

Table 2 Some pharmacological properties of the most used sulphonylurea drugs

Drug	Average daily dose (range) (mg)	Plasma half-life*	Duration of action*	Route of elimination	Active metabolite*	Severe hypoglacaemia
Acetohexamide	1000 (250–1500)	Medium	Medium	Hepatic	+	
Chlorpropamide	375 (100–500)	Very long	Very long	Hepatic and renal	+	1.0
Tolazamide	500 (100–1000)	Short	Medium	Hepatic	+	
Tolbutamide	1500 (500–2000)	Short	Short/medium	Hepatic		0.2
Glibenclamide	10 (2.5–20) 7 (3.5–14)***	Very short	Long	Hepatic	?	1.1
Gliclazide	160 (40–240)	Medium	Medium	Hepatic		
Glipizide	10 (2.5–20)	Very short	Short/medium	Hepatic		0.5
Gliquidone	60 (15–180)	Long	Long	Hepatic	+	

* Very short = 0–3 h, short = 3–6 h, medium = 6–12 h, long = 12–24 h and very long = over 24 h.
** Active metabolites are renally excreted, and so accumulate in patients with poor renal function.
*** New formulation.

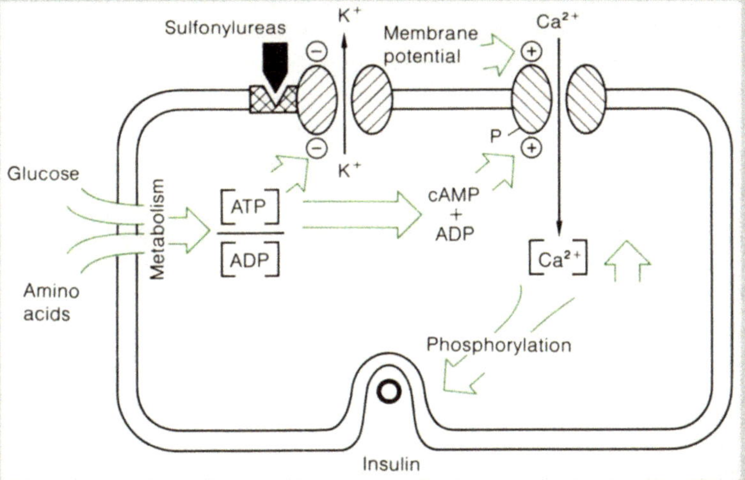

Fig. 2 The sulfonylurea receptor

During chronic treatment with sulfonylureas the insulin response to oral glucose often returns to pretreatment levels [8]. This finding led to the idea that sulfonylureas only have an effect on insulin secretion in the acute phase of treatment. This conclusion however, is false since the insulin responses will of course decline in parallel with the decline in plasma glucose values during treatment.

Added to the direct effect on B-cells, sulfonylureas may reduce extraction of insulin in the liver and may also inhibit glucagon secretion [9]. However, these two effects may play only a minor clinical role.

Extrapancreatic effects: Sulfonylurea receptors have not been identified in peripheral tissues. However, there is no doubt that sulfonylureas also have a pronounced extrapancreatic effect. The clinical experience with sulfonylurea treatment shows that primarily fasting plasma glucose values are reduced, whereas the glucose increments after a meal are only slightly effected [10]. These data are in accordance with the conclusion that sulfonylureas exert the major effects on the liver by improving insulin mediated glycogen formation and inhibiting glycogenolysis and gluconeogenesis [11].

In vivio studies show that glucose disposal in muscles may be facilitated by sulfonylurea treatment, but it has never been normalized by these drugs and in some diabetic patients glucose disposal is uneffected [10]. Accordingly, plasma glucose increments after meals are only slightly improved by sulfonylureas.

The effect of sulfonylureas on glucose metabolism in fat cells has no major impact on the overall plasma glucose concentration. However, reduction in lipolysis may improve glucose oxidation and reduce gluconeogenesis through a reduction of plasma FFA levels [12]. Sulfonylureas seem to affect insulin binding, glucose transport and glucose metabolism in fat cells [13]. Stimulation of lipogenesis may explain the weight-gain which is observed in many subjects treated with sulfonylureas [12, 13].

As discussed, sulfonylureas appear to improve both insulin secretion and action. The events take place at the same time and may influence each other. Improvement in insulin action results in reduced plasma glucose values, which again improves the glucose sensitivity of the B-cells and consequently increases insulin secretion. On the other hand, improved insulin secretion may result in a reduction in plasma glucose concentration. The decrease in plasma glucose will be followed by a reduction in insulin resistance. Conceivably, the two events are closely related. It has often been discussed which of the two variables is of greater importance for the hypoglycemic effects of sulfonylureas and which one initiates the events. The answer seems to be that the variables play a different pathogenic role in different diabetic patients and thus improved insulin secretion may be the primary event in some subjects, whereas improved insulin action may initiate the events in others. Since the variables run in parallel, it is impossible to determine which one is of greatest importance, but the general opinion is that the effect of sulfonylureas on B-cells is crucial [11].

Clinical pharmacology

The clinical pharmacology of sulfonylureas has been outlined schematically in Table 2 [14]. Sulfonylureas differ in potency (first and second generation drugs), duration of action, metabolism, side effects and other pharmacological properties. All are well absorbed even when taken with food and there is no reason to take the drug 30 minutes before meals as previously outlined [15]. Peak serum concentration is usually observed 2–4 hours after intake. Sulfonylureas are extensively bound to plasma proteins and can be displaced by other compounds which play a role in side effects and drug interactions. Sulfonylureas are metabolized mainly in the liver and metabolites may be excreted in the urine.

Tolbutamide: The least potent and shortest acting sulfonylurea is tolbutamide (Table 2). Half of the dose is eliminated in about four hours and the effective duration of action is from 6 to 10 hours. Therefore, it may be given 2 to 3 times daily. Though it was one of the first sulfonylureas introduced into the market it is still very popular due to the low frequency of serious side effects [14, 16, 17].

Chlorpropamide: This drug is the longest acting sulfonylurea. It may require up to 3 days until it is metabolized in the liver, but 20% is excreted unchanged in the urine which means that impaired renal function must be taken into consideration when the drug is used, as severe hypoglycemical attacks may be provoked [17]. Chlorpropamide has the greatest frequency of serious side effects of which prolonged hypoglycemia is the most important. But severe hyponatremia and antibuse-like reaction may also be mentioned [14, 16, 17]. Today the drug is not often used and the general opinion from The European Consensus Report is that chlorpropamide treatment should be avoided [4].

Glibenclamide: This is the most used sulfonylurea in Europe. Some of the metabolites are potentially excreted in the urine. Therefore, care must be taken in patients with renal diseases [18]. The half-life of glibenclamides is calculated differently in different papers, because there seem to be two phases. The effective duration of action is up to 24 hours [19]. The drug is mainly divided into two dosages.

Glipizide: Like glibenclamide, glipizide is around 100 times more potent than tolbutamide on a molar basis. It is very rapidly eliminated. The effective duration of action is up to 10 hours [20]. The drug is metabolized mainly in the liver and only a small part is excreted unchanged with the urine. The drug is usually divided into 2 dosages daily.

Gliclazide: One of the newest second generation sulfonylureas with both a medium plasma half-life and a medium duration of action [20]. This means that the pharmacokinetics lie somewhere between glibenclamide and glipizide. It is metabolized mainly in the liver and is often divided into 2 dosages, but like glibenclamide, one dose may be enough in long term treatment.

Adverse effects

Hypoglycemia is the most common adverse effect of sulfonylureas [17, 21–23]. Although serious hypoglycemia is uncommon, it is more likely in patients who are taking chlorpropamide or glibenclamide than tolbutamide [23]. Furthermore, there is special risk in elderly patients with renal insufficiency or acute intercurrent illness where food intake is reduced. Therefore, we recommended in the European Consensus Report that long-acting sulfonylureas should not be used in elderly patients [4]. The risk of severe hypoglycemic attacks is approx. 0.2 per 1000 patients per year [21]. It is important to emphasize that hypoglycemic attacks in elderly people treated with sulfonylureas may differ from the well known symptoms in insulin treated insulin dependent diabetics. More often, psychiatric and neurologic symptoms such as paresis and mental disturbances e. g. confusion are reported.

In some sulfonylureas, especially chlorpropamide, hyponatremia has been described due to increased sensitivity to the antidiuretic hormone [24].

After publication of the University Group Diabetes Programme study it has been a matter of speculation if tolbutamide may impair cardiac function due to induction of cardial infarction, but this conclusion has not been emphasized by recent studies [25]. In fact, a new study from Sweden claims that tolbutamide may have a cardioprotective effect in patients with glucose intolerance [26]. The truth is still uncertain and hopefully the problem will be cleared up by the UK prospective study. More uncommon side effects may be mentioned i. e. gastrointestinal discomfort, dermatologic hypersensitivity and affection of the bone marrow. These unusual phenomena are described during the first weeks of treatment.

In respect to treatment with chlorpropamide, the antibuse-like reaction must be mentioned, however it is rather uncommon.

Drug interactions

From a safety point of view, one must be particularly aware of drugs which enhance the hypoglycemic action of sulfonylureas, for example pharmacokinetic interactions, which display them from plasma protein binding sites.

Some of these will reduce the metabolism of sulfonylureas or decrease their urinary elimination.

The most important drugs affecting sulfonylureas are listed in Table 3.

Table 3 Pharmacodynamic interactions which augment the hypoglycemic action of sulfonylurea

- Drugs that displace sulfonylureas from plasma preoteins:
  phenylbutazone, salicylates, sulfonamides and clofibrate.
- Drugs that reduce hepatic metabolism:
  monamine oxidase inhibitors, and phenylbutazone.
- Drugs that decrease urinary excretion:
  allopurinol, probenecid, phenylbutazone, salicylates, and sulfonamides.
- Drugs with intrinsic hypoglycemic activity:
  insulin, alcohol, beta adrenergic blockers; salicylates, monamine oxidase inhibitors.

Which drug to use and when

In accordance with the European Consensus Report, sulfonylureas are indicated as the first drug of choice in lean diabetics where diet treatment alone is not sufficient. In obese diabetics, sulfonylurea may be selected as the first drug of choice, but it seems to be more logical to begin with biguanides and add sulfonylureas if the effect of biguanides is not sufficient.

It is important when using sulfonylureas to begin with small dosages in order not to induce hypoglycemia. Furthermore, the patients must be followed intensively in the first weeks of treatment. The dose may be increased with time in order to avoid side effects. After treatment for 6 months or one year, reduction of the dose or completely withholding of the treatment must be considered.

In elderly people, tolbutamide is recommended because it is safe and since it often is potent enough to bring glucose values down to acceptable levels in these elderly people. In younger people especially, second generation drugs are recommended. There does not seem to be a major difference between glibenclamide, glipizide and gliclazide in respect to effects and side effects. However, the tendency today is to recommend drugs with a short duration due to the risk of inducing hypoglycemia. It is, however, important to emphasize that we still need comparable studies to help in the selection of drugs. My personal view is that the doctor must be familiar with the drug he employs, and this concept may be more important than differences between drugs.

Sulfonylureas should not be used in patients with severe liver disease and should not be given to alcoholics.

If these guidelines are used the risk of inducing hypoglycemic attacks is rather low. If the first generation drug is not effective a second generation drug may be considered. However, there is no guarantee of a better effect with second generation drugs, although it has been claimed [27]. If not, insulin may be the drug of choice.

Very few patients are "primary failures" to sulfonylureas and represent approx. 10%. However, during treatment secondary failures develop in about 20 per cent of patients treated (see chapter X). The apparent loss of sulfonylurea effectiveness may be due to weight gain, concomitant illness or stress. However, in most patients it results from a deterioration of B-cell function due to progression of the disease.

Biguanides

Around 25 per cent of the non-insulin dependent diabetes mellitus patients treated with peroral antidiabetics get biguanides [28]. They were introduced to the market in the mid nineteen-fifties. However, due to induction of lactic acidoses in some cases, they were withdrawn from the market in the U.S.A. and are still not used there. They are now under investigation for a possible come-back. In Europe there seems to have been an increase in the use of biguanides during the last few years.

Biguanides are derivates of guanidine in which two molecules are linked together with the elimination of an aminogroup [29]. Three compounds have been on the market: phenformin, buformin, metformin. Today, only metformin is used in most countries.

Mechanism of action

Metformin differs from sulfonylureas in several important aspects. It does not affect insulin secretion in B-cells but works mainly by affecting insulin action. This means that the drugs are not hypoglycemic agents since they do not affect non-diabetics [30].

The mechanism of action is poorly understood, and the effects are probably multifactorial. The following mechanism has been suggested:

1. Increase of glucose uptake in skeletal muscle
2. Decrease of gluconeogenesis
3. Decrease of intestinal glucose absorption [28, 31, 32].

The effect of metformin on glucose absorption in the abdomen is not major but may explain why metformin can provoke diarrhea in some patients. Concerning the effects of hepatic glucose production in the liver, only in vitro studies with animal tissue have shown that large pharmacological concentrations of metformin may suppress hepatic gluconeogenesis [33]. It is, however, not established whether a similar effect is generated by therapeutic dosages in man. Only in 1 of 3 published studies in man was the hepatic glucose production reduced by metformin and in that study the results must be questioned due to technical problems [34]. Therefore, the major effect seems to be on peripheral insulin action i. e. in skeletal muscle. Several studies have shown that metformin improves the insulin mediated glucose uptake in skeletal muscle [33]. Therefore, metformin seems to improve one of the major problems in non insulin dependent diabetes mellitus, the reduced glycogenesis. However, more studies are needed for further evaluation of the mechanism of action, especially concerning the cellular effects where the results until now indicate that metformin works on the postreceptor post transporter step. An increase in non oxidative glucose metabolism has been demonstrated recently (unpublished data from our lab).

Clinical pharmacology

Biguanides are almost completely absorbed from the abdomen. Metformin is not metabolized in the liver and is not bound to serum proteins and has a mean plasma half life in humans of 1.5–2.8 hours [31, 35]. This means that the drug must be given 2–3 times a day.

Adverse effects

Lactic acidosis, a potentially lethal condition, has been reported in patients taking biguanides [31, 32]. Biguanides stimulate production of lactate in muscle and/or in the abdomen. Therefore, many patients taking biguanides have slightly elevated lactate levels. However, lactate acidosis seems to develop only in patients with reduced elimination of biguanides and lactate, or in patients with increased production i. e. reduced renal function, liver diseases, alcoholism and cardiorespiratory insufficiency.

Especially phenformin is associated with lactate acidosis. In Sweden, lactic acidosis was calculated at 0.05 cases per 1000 patient year for metformin [36]. This means that the risk for lactic acidosis is very small, especially if the contraindications are taken into consideration when the drug is used. In

Canada where the drug is commonly used, no cases of lactic acidosis have been reported until now.

It is important to emphasize that metformin should not be given to patients with elevated serum creatinine levels.

Further adverse effects have gastrointestinal symptoms including nausea, discomfort and diarrhea [31]. These side effects are present in approx. 10 per cent of the patients at the beginning of treatment, and some must discontinue treatment due to gastrointestinal discomfort.

Very few other averse effects have been reported but they are not of clinical relevance.

Clinical use of metformin

Metformin is indicated for the treatment of NIDDM patients in whom satisfactory control of blood glucose cannot be obtained by diet alone and where no specific contraindication is present. Since metformin also reduces the appetite it is mainly used for obese NIDDM patients. In severe obesity it is the first drug of choice.

Metformin has been shown to reduce the diurnal plasma glucose values, but the general opinion is that it is not potent enough to normalize blood glucose values in most diabetics. In combination with diets however, it may reduce the fasting blood glucose values aroune 3–5 mmoles per liter. A survey by Herman [30] reported that 80 per cent of metformin treated patients had either good or very good response to the drug.

It is also claimed that metformin has an anorexic effect which may help the patient to stick to the diet. Therefore weigt reductions seem to be higher in the group treated with metformin than in a control group.

Metformin also has a beneficial effect on lipid metabolism resulting in reduction of low density lipo-proteins (LDL) [37].

Metformin should be given 2–3 times a day together with a meal. It is important to start with a small dose and to increase with time. If patients do not tolerate the drug they will react immediately with nausea and diarrhea, in which case their dose must be reduced or the drug must be withdrawn. Around 10 per cent of the NIDDM patients will not tolerate the drug. However, in many patients the gastrointestinal side effects are transient. It is important to remember to stop treatment or reduce the dosage if the patients develop kidney, liver, or severe cardiopulmonary diseases during treatment.

In conclusion it is important to emphasize that the risk of developing severe lactic acidosis when using metformin is not higher than the risk of inducing severe hypoglycemia in subjects treated with sulfonylureas.

Combination therapy of sulfonylureas and biguanides

Since sulfonylureas mainly stimulate insulin secretion and metformin mainly improves insulin action, it may be a good idea to combine the two drugs. The combination will not increase the risk of side effects and there is no negative interaction between the two drugs. Several clinical studies have shown a beneficial effect of this combination in respect to reducing blood glucose values in NIDDM patients [38].

New pharmacological approaches in the treatment of non-insulin dependent diabetes mellitus

As stated above, neither sulfonylureas nor biguanides are ideal peroral antidiabetic drugs since glucose and lipid metabolism is only normalized in few patients, and since both groups of drugs may induce severe side effects. Therefore, we need new approaches to the treatment of NIDDM patients, especially in respect to more potent and safer drugs. Until now, no new drug types have been introduced into the market, but several pharmacological compounds are under consideration. Among the new drugs being developed to treat NIDDM patients are agents that can:
1. Directly stimulate or augment insulin secretion.
2. Mimic some of the effects of insulin on target tissues.
3. Inhibit gluconeogenesis.
4. Reduce postprandial elevation of the blood glucose values.

Insulin secretaogues

Some of the newly discovered agents that increase insulin release act through mechanisms that are still poorly understood. These include pyridine derivates. In isolated rat islets pyridine derivatives seem to facilitate the metabolism of glucose, which may be the stimulus for insulin secretion [39]. These drugs therefore seem to improve the basic defects in B-cells, namely the ability to respond to a higher ambient glucose concentration by increasing the amount of insulin release. However, the major effect of pyridine derivatives seems to be on glucose processing in peripheral tissue.

Drugs that promote target tissue effects similar to insulin

Pyridine derivatives have been shown to stimulate the oxidative metabolism of glucose in peripheral tissue. Since that pathway seems to be resistant to insulin in NIDDM patients, pyridine derivates also seem to improve one of the major defects in insulin action [3, 39]. Despite these beneficial effects of pyridine derivatives, they do not seem to be useful clinically due to side effects such as liver function abnormalities and seizures.

Another attractive new compound is dechloroacetate. Dechloroacetate has been shown to stimulate pyruvate dehydrogenase in peripheral tissues, leading to increased oxidation of pyruvate [39]. This compound also seems to have side effects such as neurologic lesions, testicular degeneration and development of cataracts in animal studies.

Inhibitors of gluconeogenesis

To inhibit fat oxidation in non-insulin dependent diabetics, new drugs have been developed which inhibit the enzyme carnitine acyltransferase which is of importance for transport of FFA into mitochondria. These drugs have been shown to be potent in respect to reducing plasma glucose values, but unfortunately they have also been shown to be toxic. Chroic administration of one of the enzyme inhibitors, methyl-2-tetradecylglycidate, in mice has been found to induce myocardial hyperthrophy [39]. A new nicotinic acid derivate, acipimox, has been found to severely inhibit lipolysis in both healthy subjects and NIDDM patients. Consequently, not only glucose oxidation but also non-oxidative glucose metabolism is improved [40]. However, it is not possible to keep lipolysis down, and after treatment for about 8 hours there will be a breakthrough of lipolysis resulting in an increase in fat oxidation and inhibition of glucose oxidation. Therefore these drugs, despite the potent effect on glucose metabolism in acute studies, may not to be useful in chronic treatment. If drugs with a retarded effect can keep lipolysis down, a potent tool in the treatment of NIDDM patients has been developed.

Conclusion on new peroral antidiabetic drugs

Despite the potent effect of many of these new drugs and in spite of their ability to reverse the metabolic defect in non-insulin dependent diabetics, they still seem to have too many side effects to be used in clinical practice. However, other tolcrable derivatives may be developed. Therefore, it is important to encourage not only drug companies, but also clinical researchers to continue these promising investigations.

References

[1] Damsgaard EM, Faber OK, Frøland A et al. Prevalence of fasting hyperglycaemia and known non-insul dependent diabetes mellitus classified by plasma C-peptide: Fredericia survey of subjects 60–74 yr old. Diabetes Care 1987; 10: 26–32.

[2] Beck-Nielsen H, Hother-Nielsen O. Insulin resistance: The Diabetes Annual 1988; 4: 565–591. Elsevier Science Publishers, B.V.

[3] Beck-Nielsen H. Insulin resistance in skeletal muscles of patients with diabetes mellitus. Diabetes/Metabolism Reviews 1989; 5 (No. 6): 487–493.

[4] Alberti KGMM, Gries FA. Management of non-insulin-dependent diabetes mellitus in Europe: A concensus view. Diabetic Medicine 1988; 5: 275–281.

[5] Grodsky G, Epstein G, Fonska R et al. Pancreatic action of sulfonylureas. Fed Proc 1977; 36: 2714–2719.

[6] Schmid-Antomarchi H, DeWeele J, Fosset M et al. The receptor for the antidiabetic sulfonylureas controls the activity of the ATP-modulated K+ channel. J Biol Chem 1987; 262: 14840–14844.

[7] Gaines K, Hamilton S, Boyd A. Characterization of the sulfonylurea receptor on beta-cell membranes. J Biol Chem 1988; 263: 2589–2592.

[8] Duckworth WC, Solomon S, Kitabchi AE. Effect of chronic sulphonylurea therapy on plasma insulin and pro-insulin levels. J Clin Endocrinol Metab 1972; 35: 585–591.

[9] Scheen AJ, Lefebvre PH, Luyckx AS. Glipizide increases plasma insulin but not C-peptide level after a standardized breakfast in type 2 diabetic patients. Eur J Clin Pharmacol 1984; 26: 471–474.

[10] Hother-Nielsen O, Schmitz O, Andersen PH et al. In vivo action of glibenclamide in obese subjects with mild type 2 (non-insulin-dependent) diabetes. Diabetes Res 1988; 8: 63–70.

[11] Beck-Nielsen H, Hother-Nielsen O, Pedersen O. Mechanism of action of sulphonylureas with special reference to the extrapancreatic effect: An overview. Diabetic Medicine 1988; 5: 613–620.

[12] Bolinder J, Ostman J, Arner P. Reversal of insulin resistance in adipose tissue of non-insulin-dependent diabetics by treatment with diet and sulphonylurea. Acta Endocrinol 1985; 108: 85–90.

[13] Maloff BL, Lackwood DH. In vitro effects of a sulphonylurea on insulin action in adipocytes. J Clin Invest 1981; 68: 85–90.

[14] Ferner R, Chaplin S. The relationship between the pharmacokinetics and the pharmacodynamic effects of oral hypoglycemic drugs. Clin Pharmacokinetics 1987; 12: 379–401.

[15] Faber OK, Beck-Nielsen H, Binder C et al. Sulfonylurea drugs, which and why? Diabetes Care 1990; (In Press.)

[16] Balant L. Clinical pharmacokinetics of sulphonylurea hypoglycaemic drugs. Clin Pharmacokinetics 1981; 6: 215–241.

[17] Jackson J, Bessler R. Clinical pharmacology of sulfonylurea hypoglycemic agents. Drugs 1981; 22: 211–245, 295–320.

[18] Fabre J, Balant J, Lautan L et al. Hypoglycemic activity of th main metabolite of glibenclamide: influence of renal insufficiency. Kidney international 1978; 13: 435.

[19] Pearson J, Antal E, Raehl C et al. Pharmacokinetic disposition of 14C-glyburide in patients with varying renal function. Clin Pharmacol Ther 1986; 39: 318–324.

[20] Melander A. Clinical pharmacology of sulfonylureas. Metabolism 1987; 36 (Suppl. 1): 12–16.

[21] Berger W. Incidence of severe side effects during therapy with sulfonylureas and biguanides. Horm Metab Res 1985; 17: (Suppl. 15): 111–115.

[22] Jennings A, Wilson R, Ward J. Symptomatic hypoglycemia in NIDDM patients treated with oral hypoglycemic agents. Diabetes Care 1989; 12: 203–208.

[23] Ferner R, Niel H. Sulfonylureas and hypoglycemia. Brit Med J; 296: 949–950.

[24] Kadowaki T, Jagura R, Kajnuma KH et al. Chlorpropamide-induced hyponatremia: incidence and risk factors. Diabetes Care 1983; 6: 468–472.

[25] Seltzer H. A summary of criticisms of the findings and conclusions of the University Groups Diabetes Program (UGDP). Diabetes 1972; 21: 976–979.

[26] Sartor G, Scherstein B, Calstrom S et al. Ten-year follow-up of subjects with impaired

glucose tolerance: prevention of diabetes by tolbutamide and diet regulation. Diabetes 1980; 29: 41–49.
[27] Cohen KL, Harris S. Efficacy of glyburide in diabetics poorly controlled on first-generation oral hypoglycemics. Diabetes Care 1987; 10: 555–557.
[28] Bailey C, Nattras M. Treatment-metformin. Baillere's Clinical Endocrinol and Metab 1988; 2: 455–476.
[29] Davidoff F. Guanidine-derivatives in medicine. N Engl J Med 1973; 278: 141–46.
[30] Herman L. Metformin: a review of its pharmacologic properties and therapeutic use. Diabete et Metabolisme 1975; 5: 233–245.
[31] Vigneri R, Goldfine I. Role of metformin in treatment of diabetes mellitus. Diabetes Care 1987; 10: 118–122.
[32] Schafer G. Biguanides. A review of history, pharmacodynamics and therapy. Diabete et Metabolisme 1983; 9: 148–163.
[33] Hother-Nielsen O, Schmitz O, Andersen PH et al. Metformin improves peripheral but not hepatic insulin action in obese patients with type II diabetes. Acta Endocrinologica (Copenh) 1989; 120: 257–265.
[34] Jackson R, Hawa M, Jaspan J et al. Mechanism of metformin action in noninsulin-dependent diabetes. Diabetes 1987; 36: 632–640.
[35] Tucker G, Casey C, Phillips P et al. Metformin kinetics in healthy subjects and in patients with diabetes mellitus. Br J Clin Pharmacol 1981; 12: 235–246.
[36] Bergman U, Boman G, Wiholm BE. Epidemiology of adverse drug reactions to phenformin and metformin. Br Med J 1978; 2: 464–66.
[37] Rains SGH, Wilson GA, Richmond W et al. The reduction of low density lipoprotein cholesterol by metformin is maintained with long-term therapy. Journal of the Royal Society of Medicine 1989; 82: 93–94.
[38] Rains S, Wilson G, Richmond W et al. The effect of glibenclamide and metformin on serum lipoproteins in type 2 diabetes. Diabetic Medicine 1988; 5: 653–658.
[39] Rifkin H et al. Diabetes Mellitus. Theory and practice. Fourth Edition. Chapter 54. 887–895.
[40] Beck-Nielsen H. The effect of a new antilipolytic drug Acipimox on glucose metabolism in skeletal muscle. Diabetes (In press.)

Modulation of intestinal glucose absorption: postponement of glucose absorption by α-glucosidase inhibitors

M. Toeller

Introduction

The goals of the therapy of diabetes mellitus are to achieve physiological blood glucose and haemoglobin $A1_c$ levels, to maintain desirable body weight and serum lipids, to avoid hyperinsulinaemia and specific diabetic complications and to retard the development of atherosclerosis [1]. The ultimate aim of intervention in diabetic patients is a healthy individual with a good quality of life and normal longevity.

Present nutrition and drug therapy practices in diabetes have only resulted in a rather incomplete achievement of these goals. Therefore, new therapeutic concepts in diabetes must be tested. One new treatment concept is the postponement of intestinal glucose absorption by α-glucosidase inhibitors [2–7].

Theoretically, slowing down the rate of absorption should lead to lower blood glucose and insulin responses in support of improved control of carbohydrate and lipid metabolism in diabetes. The first available α-glucosidase inhibitor, acarbose, has now been approved by the regulatory authorities of 9 countries. The following chapters summarize the therapeutic potential of acarbose in diabetic patients and whether or not α-glucosidase inhibitors are able to take a step forward in the treatment of the disease.

Slowing down the rate of glucose absorption by dietary modifications

Prior to the description of the pharmacological approach, the concept of how to reduce the rate of glucose absorption by dietary modification will be briefly reviewed (Table 1). The principle of delaying carbohydrate absorption by dietary modification has been followed for many years [8–17]. Postponement of glucose absorption by dietary modification is helpful in avoiding a rapid and high increase in blood glucose following food intake in insulin-dependent

Table 1 Dietary modification to avoid rapid carbohydrate absorption with subsequent blood glucose peaks in diabetic patients

Prefer:	< Frequent small servings
	< Complex carbohydrates
	< CHO-containing foods rich in soluble fibre (e. g. legumes, oats, barley)
	< CHO-containing foods with low glycaemic index (e. g. beans, apples, oranges, skim milk, pasta)
	< CHO together with fat and protein
Avoid:	> Simple sugars (mono- and disaccharides, e. g. in beer, fruit juice)
	> Added sucrose (e. g. in soft drinks, sweets, desserts)
	> Large servings

diabetic patients where the physiological availability of exogenous insulin is impaired, as well as in non-insulin dependent diabetic patients where insulin secretion is delayed and insulin action is insufficient [18, 19]. Even if an oral hypoglycaemic agent like a sulphonylurea is given before a meal, the glucose from the diet is usually absorbed by the small intestine much faster than it takes the oral agent to become effective. Therefore it was hypothesised that one major problem, postprandial hyperglycaemia, in diabetic patients could be solved by means of slowing down the rate of glucose absorption from the small intestine [20, 21].

Frequent small meals

Considerable attention has been paid to the concept of spreading the nutrient load throughout the day. The advantage of nibbling versus gorging on glucose tolerance and serum lipid levels was described by Gwinup et al. in the early sixties [8]. These results have also been confirmed by Jenkins et al. [21]. The phenomenon had already been observed by Staub-Traugott, who found that one carbohydrate meal improves the response to the next meal; the shorter the interval between the meals, the better the subsequent tolerance. Consequently, nutritional recommendations for individuals with non-insulin-dependent diabetes and for diabetic patients treated with conventional insulin therapy include the advice that food intake should be distributed as evenly as possible throughout the day and large meals should be avoided [1, 18, 19].

Preference of complex carbohydrates

Since it is well known that simple carbohydrates from commonly used foods tend to raise blood glucose more than complex carbohydrates from starchy foods, diabetic patients are advised to eat foods which are rich in complex carbohydrates and to avoid foods which contain mainly simple sugars.

Although glucose, maltose and sucrose produce large increases in blood glucose, fructose does not. Fructose, which is metabolized without requiring insulin, produces only minimal increases in blood glucose [11, 13]. Therefore, fructose plays an important role as a sweetener for individuals with diabetes.

Sucrose use has traditionally been restricted in the diabetic diet. Though it has been shown recently that small amounts of additional sucrose in mixed meals do not worsen blood glucose control in generally well-controlled diabetic patients, most diabetologists do continue to recommend the avoidance of sugar as a table-sweetener, specifically in obese patients who are not well-controlled [18, 19, 22]. The Diabetes and Nutrition Study Group of the European Association for the Study of Diabetes has suggested in their Statement that the total intake of additional sucrose should be limited to 30 g/day until more information is available on its long-term metabolic effect [19].

Increase of soluble fibre

Fibre has been suggested as a means of slowing down carbohydrate absorption. Increasing the fibre intake in the diet has been shown to reduce fasting blood glucose, glycosylated haemoglobin and serum lipid levels [16, 19, 21]. However, there is some evidence that this effect is only present in high carbohydrate, high fibre diets. Only the soluble, gel-forming fibres in fibre-rich foods or the fibre supplements, such as guar or pectin, reduce postprandial glycaemia, whereas insoluble cereal fibres have little or no effect. Problems with compliance and with long-term effectiveness set a limit on the therapeutic potential of soluble fibre foods and soluble fibre supplements.

Low glycaemic index foods

It has been shown that complex carbohydrates in different forms evoke different glycaemic responses [17, 22]. Bread and potatoes raise blood glucose more than beans for example. In the past many researchers have compared the glycaemic responses to different foods rich in complex carbohydrates [9, 11, 15, 17]. Foods were ranked according to what degree equal amounts of carbohydrate raise the blood glucose. Jenkins et al. introduced the term 'glycaemic index'. The index may be considered an indicator of the glucose absorption rate. The glycaemic index appears to be useful in identifying foods likely to be beneficial in terms of glycaemic control. However, concern has arisen from the absence of an effect when foods with differing glycaemic impact were compared in mixed meals [17, 21]. Most dietary sugars and virtually all of the starches are eaten in natural form or as processed foods together with other foods in a mixed meal. The acute glycaemic response which is seen when various carbohydrate containing foods are tested individually has little relevance as a predictor of glycaemic response following mixed meals.

Carbohydrates in mixed meals

The nature and the source of dietary carbohydrate as well as their physical and chemical properties have an influence on the blood glucose response. Toasting and cooking, for example, modify the rise of blood glucose following a meal.

Many years ago it was also pointed out that bread with butter produces a smaller rise in blood glucose concentration than bread alone. It has been suggested that fats and protein reduce the glycaemic response to carbohydrates mainly by increasing insulin secretion followed by improved glucose assimilation in response to hyperglycaemia [12, 13]. This moderating effect of fat and protein does not occur in untreated IDDM patients and is reduced in NIDDM patients with impaired insulin secretion and insulin resistance. Delaying gastric emptying may also play a role when carbohydrates are ingested together with fat and protein.

Pharmacological approach to reducing the rate of glucose absorption: α-glucosidase inhibitors

Though all principles of dietary modification for the postponement of glucose absorption have been shown to be beneficial for improved glycaemic control, they are far from having solved the problems which result from frequent postprandial hyperglycaemia in diabetic patients.

A new pharmacological approach to achieving the metabolic benefits of a reduced rate of carbohydrate absorption has been introduced by Puls et al. [2]. The idea was to prevent or to reduce postprandial hyperglycaemia by slowing down the digestion of nutrient carbohydrates and consequently the absorption of monosaccharides, essentially glucose. Therefore, it was attempted to modify the activities of intestinal α-glucosidases with specific inhibitors. Acarbose and its homologs were isolated from fermentation of various actinoplanes strains [7, 24]. Acarbose, a pseudo-tetrasaccharide of microbial origin, is a competitive and reversible inhibitor of intestinal α-glucosidase activity [4, 6, 7]. No other microbial α-glucosidase inhibitor to date has been so thoroughly researched and developed with respect to fermentation conditions, isolation procedures, chemical and biochemical characterization and modification, pharmacology, safety profile and clinical efficacy. Only a few other α-glucosidase inhibitors have reached the stage of clinical development as antidiabetic drugs. One of them is miglitol, a monosaccharidic 1-deoxyno-jirimycin derivative.

Effect of α-glucosidase inhibitors on intestinal carbohydrate digestion and absorption

α-Glucosidases are located in the luminal brushborder formed by enterocytes. Since only monosaccharides are readily taken up from the intestine, all other carbohydrates (disaccharides and polysaccharides) have to be broken down by glucosidases before they can be absorbed [25]. In this process α-glucosidase inhibitors are able to delay carbohydrate digestion, thus leading to delayed glucose absorption. Absorption of glucose itself is not influenced by acarbose [4]. Carbohydrates which are not digestible (like cellulose), not cleaved by an α-glucosidase (like lactose), or directly absorbed (like glucose, fructose and Sorbitol) are not affected by the drug. Thus, the efficacy of α-glucosidase inhibitors as modulators of the postprandial blood glucose levels depends strongly on the carbohydrate composition of the meals.

Nutritional intake in affluent countries often contains large amounts of refined sugars which are quickly absorbed in the uppermost part of the small intestine, whereas the digestion of traditional foods with slowly digested and absorbed carbohydrates also involves lower segments of the small intestine [24–27]. Considerable enzymatic activity is usually present in this part of the digestive tract also. α-Glucosidase inhibitors lead to retardation of digestion and to partial displacement of absorption into the lower intestine [5].

The inhibitory potency of acarbose is highest for glucoamylase, followed by sucrase, maltase and isomaltase whereas lactase is not inhibited [4, 25]. Jenkins et al. have confirmed these in vitro results with studies in man where a dosage of 200 mg acarbose resulted in a markedly reduced response to starch and sucrose loads, a slight reduction after maltose, but no effect following the administration of lactose and glucose [28, 29]. In a study in healthy volunteers, the extent of sucrose absorption was 90% within 200 minutes under control conditions and 60% within 400 minutes following administration of 100 mg acarbose [29, 30].

Certain studies have shown that the modulation of carbohydrate assimilation by α-glucosidase inhibitors is dose-dependent [5, 20, 25]. Radziuk et al. observed in C^{14} isotope studies that acarbose dose-dependently reduces glucose absorption rates and postprandial blood glucose increases [30].

It has been suggested that the dose dependent effects of α-glucosidase inhibitors are also influenced by the individual pattern of intestinal α-glucosidase activities which have reportedly shown rather large variations [5, 7, 31, 32].

Acarbose itself is absorbed in the active form only in very small amounts (a maximum of 1 – 2%). Acarbose can be broken down by the bacteria of the large intestine. Most of the inactive breakdown products are excreted in the faeces and only small amounts are eliminated in the urine. Unlike acarbose, miglitol is extensively absorbed from the gastrointestinal tract [24].

The elimination half-life of acarbose is about 2.8 hours. However, there is some evidence for a more slowly declining terminal phase with half-life of about 9 hours.

Carbohydrate malabsorption

In a number of studies, hydrogen breath analysis has verified that carbohydrate absorption is decreased in the presence of α-glucosidase inhibitors and that the amount of fermentable carbohydrate reaching the colon is increased [33, 35]. This suggests that malabsorption of carbohydrates could be a problem, especially with large dosages of acarbose [33]. However, there is evidence that the carbon and energy content of sucrose and other carbohydrates which are metabolized by the microflora of the colon may not be lost [30, 36 – 38]. Malabsorption may also occur with foods rich in undigestible fibre, fructose and Sorbitol.

Effect of α-glucosidase inhibitors on postprandial blood glucose, gastrointestinal hormones and triglyceride concentrations

Animal studies and studies in man have clearly demonstrated that acarbose is able to reduce the postprandial increase of blood glucose, insulin and triglycerides [5 – 7, 24]. Acarbose does not exhibit the hypoglycaemic effects of either insulin or ß-cytotropic sulphonylurea. It influences the secretion of insulin indirectly, since less insulin is released with the smaller increase in blood glucose after carbohydrate administration. The reduction in serum triglycerides seems to result from the reduction of carbohydrate-driven, insulin-mediated synthesis of very low density lipoproteins.

Studies in healthy volunteers evaluating the hormonal response to test meals have shown that acarbose administration significantly reduces insulin, c-peptide, gastrin and pancreozymin, while somatostatin levels were significantly increased [20, 39, 40]. A number of investigators have studied gastric inhibitory polypeptide responses to test meals under acarbose administration. They reported that GIP was significantly decreased in parallel with insulin in healthy volunteers receiving acarbose [39, 40].

Clinical trials with α-glucosidase inhibitors

The efficacy of α-glucosidase inhibitors has been studied in NIDDM and IDDM patients as well as in patients with dumping syndrome, reactive hypoglycaemia and hyperlipoproteinaemia [41]. The number of studies in dumping syndrome, reactive hypoglycaemia and type IIb and IV hyperlipoproteinaemias is limited with rather small numbers of patients.

Just a single dose of acarbose was able to improve the clinical symptoms of dumping syndrome [42]. In one study, the magnitude of hypoglycaemic and insulin response to an oral sucrose load was significantly reduced with 100 mg acarbose compared to placebo [29]. A few studies have already shown that α-glucosidase inhibitors have the potency to significantly reduce serum triglycerides in hypertriglyceridaemic patients [29, 41, 43]. However, no marked effect was seen in hypercholesterinaemia.

Most of the studies with α-glucosidase inhibitors have been carried out to evaluate the therapeutic potential in diabetic patients.

Studies in NIDDM patients

The studies with acarbose and miglitol in NIDDM patients were recently reviewed by Clissold and Edwards (1988), Willms (1988), Sachse (1988), Tuomilehto (1988) and Rosak (1988) [29, 44–47]. Therefore, only a summary of the main findings will be given here. In addition, a few new and as yet unpublished data will be presented.

With α-glucosidase inhibitors generally improved metabolic control was achieved regardless of whether acarbose or miglitol were administered in addition to oral antidiabetic agents or to diet alone [41, 43–50]. The most significant finding was the reduction of postprandial blood glucose concentrations. Some studies also showed a reduction in glycosylated haemoglobin and a few studies demonstrated a decrease in fasting blood glucose and serum triglycerides. There was also evidence that serum insulin could be reduced [51–53].

Acarbose therapy was found to be comparably effective in the treatment with guar, with biguanide and, in one study, with glisoxepide and glibenclamide [29, 49].

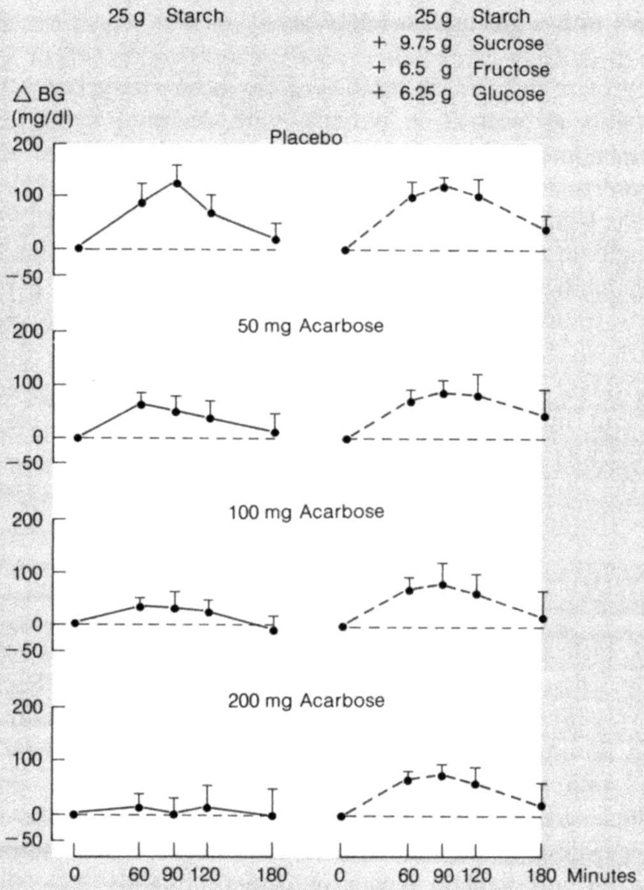

Fig. 1 Blood glucose response after 25 g starch (mashed potatoes) and after 25 g starch plus 9.75 g sucrose, 6.5 g fructose and 6.25 g glucose (orange juice) with acarbose (50 mg/100 mg/200 mg) compared to placebo in 3 NIDDM patients.

Coniff and Innerfield have presented promising first data from a double-blind, placebo controlled multi-centre study of the long-term efficacy and safety of acarbose in NIDDM patients inadequately controlled by sulphonylurea or diet alone [52, 53]. In this study, 167 NIDDM patients on sulphonylurea and 217 patients on diet alone were randomly assigned to either acarbose or placebo for 6 months. Treatment started after a 6-week lead-in period and the study was followed by a 6-week wash-out period. All metabolic parameters were improved with acarbose, which had been titrated step-wise from 50 mg to a maximum of 300 mg/day. Specifically, the authors were able to show a significant reduction of glycosylated haemoglobin and of postprandial insulin concentrations.

Puls et al. have pointed out that the principle of glucosidase inhibition is effective in all humans. However, it has also been reported that in some patients, little or no postprandial blood glucose lowering effects were seen. This could have been due to insufficient intake of carbohydrates, specifically starch which is the main substrate, the digestion of which is influenced by α-glucosidase inhibitors. Another reason could have been that the meals contained predominantly monosaccharides and lactose where digestion and absorption is not influenced by α-glucosidase inhibitors.

We investigated the blood glucose response of NIDDM patients to meals with 25 g starch and to meals with 25 g starch, 6.25 g glucose, 6.5 g fructose and 9.75 g sucrose under different dosages of acarbose compared to placebo (Fig. 1). Postprandial blood glucose concentrations following the starch meals were dose-dependently decreased by acarbose. However, when monosaccharides and disaccharides were added to the starch meals, blood glucose concentrations in the same patients were still reduced as compared to placebo, but the obvious dose-dependency seen with starch was lost. Higher dosages of acarbose were not able to blunt the powerful blood glucose elevating effect of the added monosaccharides and disaccharides which were about 50% of the given carbohydrates [27].

Thus, it is extremely important in acarbose treatment that diabetic patients follow the dietary guidelines which advise the intake of complex carbohydrates instead of simple sugars [19, 26].

Willms et al. reported interesting findings on the blood glucose response to isocaloric meals. A standard breakfast and a muesli breakfast were randomly ingested with and without miglitol by 24 NIDDM patients. With placebo the blood glucose increase was significantly lower after the muesli than after the standard breakfast. With miglitol, a similar decrease of blood glucose concentrations was achieved with both breakfast meals. Thus the blood glucose lowering effect of miglitol was more obvious with the standard breakfast [44]. This was probably due to less starch and more lactose in the muesli breakfast as compared to the standard breakfast. However, the study could clearly show that α-glucosidase inhibitors do have an additive potential in reducing postprandial blood glucose concentrations to the dietary modifications following the concept of delaying carbohydrate absorption.

We were able to show that not only blood glucose but also insulin concentrations following a standard meal were markedly reduced in NIDDM patients by acarbose (100 mg) compared to placebo (Fig. 2). The test meals with 56% carbohydrate and 63% of CHO as starch were randomly ingested with the drug or placebo, respectively (Table 2). The study confirmed that α-glucosidase inhibitors are able to decrease undesirable postprandial hyperinsulinaemia in NIDDM patients.

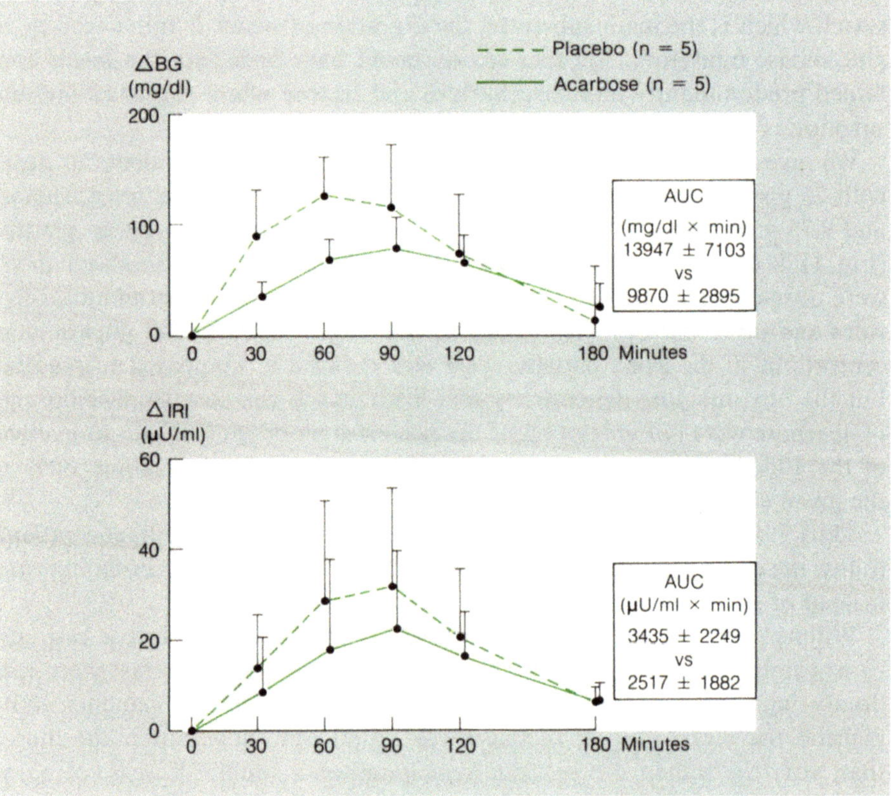

Fig. 2 Blood glucose and insulin responses after a standard meal with acarbose (100 mg) compared to placebo in 5 NIDDM patients.

Table 2 Standard meal

Energy	418 Kcal	*in:*
Protein	14.4 g (14%)	90 g Rye bread
Fat	13.5 g (30%)	20 g Low-fat margarine
CHO	57.5 g (56%)	20 g Cheese "Edam" (30% Fat)
Fibre	4.5 g	12 g Cherry jam
Starch	36.3 g (63% of CHO)	100 g Unsweetened orange juice
Sucrose	11.4 g	2 g Evaporated milk (4% Fat)
Lactose	2.9 g	300 ml Decaffeinated coffee
Fructose	3.0 g	
Glucose	2.6 g	
Saturated fatty acids	4.8 g	
Linolic acid	3.6 g	
Cholesterol	15 mg	

Table 3 Dietary intake and body mass index of 15 NIDDM patients who were assigned to 3 months treatment with the α-glucosidase inhibitor, miglitol, in a randomised, double-blind, placebo-controlled, cross-over trial with a 4-week lead-in and a wash-out period.

$\bar{x} \pm SD$	Preperiod	After the 3 months treatment period with	
		Miglitol	Placebo
Energy (Kcal)	1729 ± 597	1636 ± 403	1708 ± 444
Protein (g)	83 ± 27 (20%)	73 ± 17 (19%)	75 ± 20 (19%)
Fat (g)	71 ± 34 (39%)	68 ± 34 (40%)	74 ± 31 (41%)
CHO (g)	169 ± 63 (41%)	162 ± 34 (41%)	163 ± 40 (40%)
Alcohol (g)	0.6 ± 2	1.0 ± 4	0.3 ± 1
Glucose (g)	10 ± 6	10 ± 4	10 ± 5
Fructose (g)	20 ± 13	20 ± 13	21 ± 13
Lactose (g)	12 ± 8	12 ± 9	11 ± 8
Sucrose (g)	11 ± 9	11 ± 4	12 ± 7
Maltose (g)	4 ± 4	4 ± 6	3 ± 1
Starch (g)	84 ± 34	82 ± 23	79 ± 22
Fibre (g)	21 ± 8	21 ± 6	24 ± 8
PUFA (g)	13 ± 7	11 ± 9	14 ± 11
SAFA (g)	29 ± 16	28 ± 20	33 ± 13
Cholesterol (mg)	333 ± 205	306 ± 252	236 ± 138
Body Mass Index (kg/m^2)	26 ± 2	26 ± 2	26 ± 2

It has sometimes been argued that treatment with α-glucosidase inhibitors may be accompanied by an alteration of the dietary intake towards a more atherogenic diet with reduced carbohydrate and increased fat intake, especially in case of concomitant gastrointestinal side effects. We have demonstrated that no significant changes occurred in the proportion of nutrients in 15 NIDDM patients in the 3 month treatment period with miglitol compared to placebo and to the lead-in period [27, 54] (Table 3). This was also true in the 4 of 15 patients who complained of permanent gastrointestinal symptoms under miglitol treatment. Fig. 3 shows the average postprandial decrease in blood glucose concentration over the 12-week study period.
In 5 of 15 NIDDM patients in this study, no or only very little effect on postprandial blood glucose was observed under treatment with miglitol.

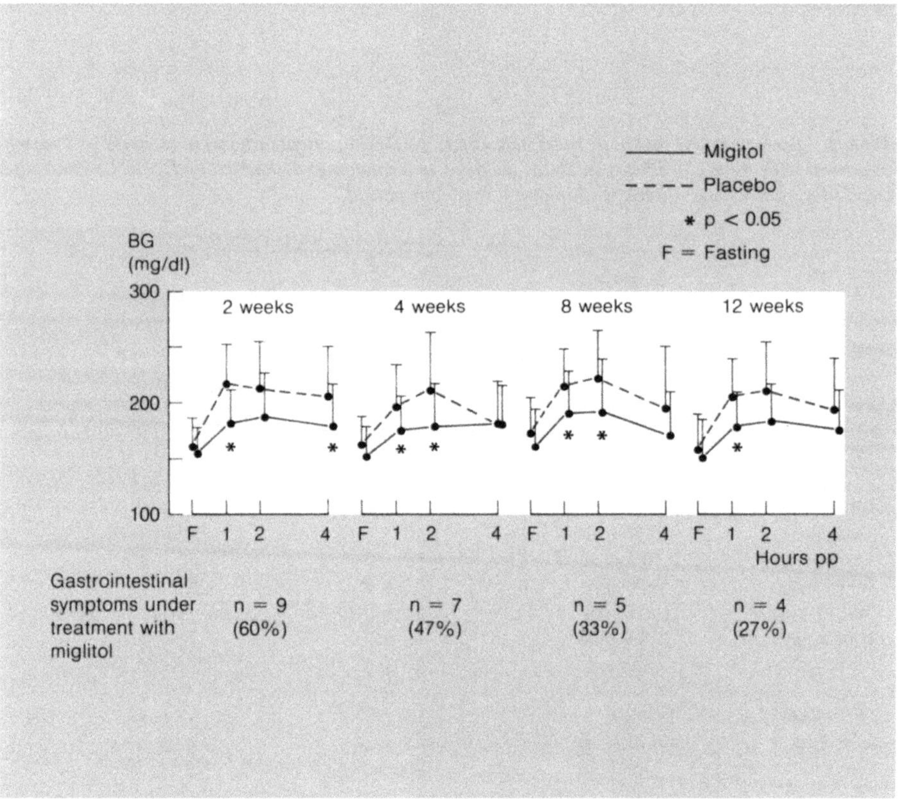

Fig. 3 Blood blucose values ($\bar{x}$) and gastrointestinal symptoms (flatulence) under treatment with the α-glucosidase inhibitor, miglitol, compared to placebo in 15 NIDDM patients.

When we analyzed the dietary intake of these patients compared to those who showed a significant decrease in postprandial blood glucose values under miglitol, it became obvious that in one case the reason for non-efficacy probably was the very high intake of lactose (milk), and in the 4 others the very low intake of starch, together with the rather high intake of maltose (beer) and fructose.

Side effects

Four of the patients not responding to miglitol had continuous gastrointestinal symptoms (flatulence) under miglitol treatment which could be explained by the very low amounts of starch together with high amounts of monosaccharides and disaccharides. Knowing this, it is very important to advise patients that gastrointestinal symptoms may occur from inadequate nutritional intake. Some authors have also reported a high incidence of uncomfortable abdominal symptoms after the ingestion of large amounts of sucrose together with acarbose [20, 28, 41].

Adverse effects like flatulence, abdominal distension or diarrhoea may occur if malabsorbed carbohydrates reach the colon and are fermented by colonic bacteria to short chain fatty acids, CO_2 and H_2. However, since the assimilation within the large bowel is very effective there is no faecal loss of calories [25]. Indeed the studies in healthy subjects as well as in diabetic patients did not reveal significant weight loss during treatment with α-glucosidase inhibitors [41, 54].

Most studies have demonstrated that gastrointestinal symptoms have an obvious tendency to decrease with treatment time [41]. It is not known whether this is due to reduced gas production with time or other adaptation mechanisms.

Efficacy and gastrointestinal side effects of α-glucosidase inhibitors depend on certain factors, some of which can be controlled by the physician and the patient, like the dosage of α-glucosidase inhibitors and the dietary intake, and others which are beyond their influence, such as the individual pattern of intestinal α-glucosidase activities and the quality of the colonic flora [7, 27, 55].

The amount and composition of nutrient carbohydrates are of special importance for minimizing side effects. Thus the patient's diet should include sufficient complex carbohydrates, namely starch, the main substrate for inhibitor action.

It is also important that all carbohydrates which can be cleaved by α-glucosidases are fully digested and absorbed while still in the small intestinal tract. This means that the individual dose for optimal efficacy without causing side effects must be determined in the co-operation of the physician and the diabetic patient. This also means that treatment with α-glucosidase inhibitors has to start with a low dose and with educating the patient on proper dietary intake according to the recommendations given by diabetes associations.

Due to their antihyperglycaemic mechanism of action, α-glucosidase inhibitors do not provoke hypoglycaemia. However, the hypoglycaemic episodes sometimes seen in insulin-treated and sulphonylurea-treated patients may also occur when acarbose is administered as an adjunct to these hypoglycaemic agents.

Results from large clinical studies have demonstrated that acarbose does not produce any clinically significant adverse effects on biochemical and haemotological parameters even after treatment for up to 5 years [41]. Only isolated increases in liver enzymes have been documented.

In two studies where the effects of acarbose on the absorption and metabolism of other nutrients and minerals were investigated, only a significant reduction of serum iron concentration was observed [29]. No adverse drug-drug-interactions have been reported so far. This was specifically investigated with digoxin, propranolol and glibenclamide. Toxicology and long-term carcinogenicity studies with acarbose did not give any indication that acarbose is toxic or carcinogenic [50].

Studies in IDDM patients

The studies with acarbose and miglitol in IDDM patients were summarized in 1988 by Raptis and by Clissold and Edwards [29, 56]. Most studies have shown that postprandial blood glucose concentrations were reduced with α-glucosidase inhibitors. Smoother diurnal blood glucose profiles and, in some cases, a reduction in daily insulin requirements were observed [56, 57]. In one study where acarbose was administered at night, the rate of nocturnal hypoglycaemias was reduced.

However, it should be pointed out that most of the studies in IDDM patients have included only small numbers of patients and a few studies did not show significant beneficial effects of α-glucosidase inhibitors on glycaemic control.

Current treatment modalities

Acarbose has now been approved by regulatory authorities in 9 countries as a drug for the treatment of adult diabetic patients in combination with diet and with other oral antidiabetic drugs or insulin. Registration was first obtained in Switzerland (1986) followed by Czechoslovakia (1987), Uruguay (1988), Luxembourg (1988), Columbia (1989), The Netherlands (1990) and Germany (1990).

The drug is available in 50 mg and 100 mg tablets. Tablets should be administered together with meals [43, 58]. Treatment should begin with a low dose regimen at breakfast and possibly at dinner and lunch. The dose should be increased under blood glucose control until optimal efficacy is achieved without causing gastrointestinal symptoms. The maximum suggested dose is 3 x 200 mg/day. So far, there is insufficient data to give recommendations for children or pregnant women.

Acarbose may be the first line drug in NIDDM patients when diet alone fails to achieve good metabolic control, specifically because the drug, unlike sulphonylurea, does not stimulate endogenous insulin production and secretion which is undesirable in hyperinsulinaemic NIDDM patients [1, 27, 51]. The degree of metabolic abnormality determines whether, and for what length of time, acarbose will be able to normalize elevated postprandial blood glucose concentrations in these patients. In several trials, acarbose was able to reduce postprandial blood glucose values by about 40 mg/dl and glycosylated haemoglobin by up to 1% [29, 41, 52, 53]. A few studies demonstrated decreased postprandial hyperinsulinaemia by about 20–30% [27, 51, 55].

Acarbose may also be used in addition to sulphonylurea and/or biguanide therapy in case good control is not achieved with either one or both of these drugs. Acarbose may also be tried as a measure to flatten blood glucose profiles in insulin-treated NIDDM and IDDM patients, though many of them may achieve good control with intensified insulin therapy without requiring additional drugs.

Monotherapy with α-glucosidase inhibitors does not cause hypoglycaemia. However, it is important to advise the patient to use glucose and not sucrose for the treatment of possible hypoglycaemic episodes when acarbose is administered in combination with sulphonylurea or insulin treatment.

Dietary education is absolutely essential in the treatment with acarbose to achieve good drug efficacy and to minimize gastrointestinal symptoms. When treatment with acarbose fails to show therapeutic effects or causes consistent gastrointestinal side effects, the dietary intake of the patient should be analyzed in order to exclude the possibility that this was caused by insufficient complex carbohydrate and too much simple sugars in the diet.

Therapeutic perspectives of α-glucosidase inhibitors

As pointed out, carbohydrate absorption from the small intestine may be delayed in various ways which all may result in reduced postprandial blood glucose concentrations and concomitantly improved diabetic control. Dietary modification to frequent small meals, the preference for complex carbohydrate, increased intake of soluble fibre and of foods with a low glycaemic index have been shown to contribute to better metabolic control specifically in NIDDM but also in IDDM patients. However, in the course of the disease, glycaemia cannot be sufficiently controlled in most patients by dietary modification alone. Therefore, pharmacological postponement of glucose absorption by α-glucosidase inhibitors is a promising step forward in the therapy of diabetic patients where postprandial hyperglycaemia is insufficiently controlled.

As has been shown, α-glucosidase inhibitors are able to contribute to reaching the goals of diabetic therapy by reducing not only postprandial hyperglycaemia and by lowering glycosylated haemoglobin, but also by a decrease in postprandial hyperinsulinaemia and hypertriglyceridaemia. However, fasting blood glucose is generally insignificantly decreased and obesity is not reduced by the treatment with α-glucosidase inhibitors. It is far too early to speculate as to whether α-glucosidase inhibitors will really contribute to the prevention of diabetic complications and to the retardation of the development of atherosclerosis. So far, a few animal studies have shown rather interesting results [60].

First data from a randomised, placebo-controlled long-term study show that the quality of life can be improved in NIDDM patients with better metabolic control under acarbose treatment. The data strongly suggest that effective treatment with α-glucosidase inhibitors depends on the following conditions:

- Postprandial hyperglycaemia is a problem of control.
- Postprandial hyperglycaemia is not sufficiently controlled by dietary modification.
- Postprandial hyperglycaemia is in the range of the therapeutic potential of α-glucosidase inhibitors.
- The diabetic patient has been given sufficient dietary advice.
- The diabetic patient eats sufficient complex carbohydrate (starch $\geq$ 100 g, simple sugars $\leq$ 40% of total carbohydrate).
- The dose of α-glucosidase inhibitors has been adapted to individual needs.
- The diabetic patient has been trained in self control.

References

[1] Alberti KGMM, Gries FA and the European NIDDM Policy Group. Management of non-insulin-dependent diabetes mellitus in Europe: A consensus view. Diabetic Med 1988; 5: 275–281.
[2] Puls W, Keup U. Influence of an α-amylase inhibitor (BAY d 7791) on blood glucose, serum insulin and NEFA in starch loading tests in rats, dogs and man. Diabetologia 1973; 9: 97–101.
[3] Puls W, Keup U, Krause HP et al. Glucosidase inhibition: a new approach to the treatment of diabetes, obesity and hyperlipoproteinaemia. Naturwissenschaften 1977; 64: 536–537.
[4] Puls W, Keup U, Krause HP et al. Pharmacology of a glucosidase inhibitor. Front Hormone Res 1980; 7: 235–247.
[5] Puls W, Bischoff H. The pharmacological rationale of diabetes mellitus therapy with acarbose. In: Creutzfeldt W, ed. Acarbose for the treatment of diabetes mellitus. 2nd International Symposium on Acarbose. Berlin, Heidelberg, New York: Springer-Verlag, 1988; 29–38.
[6] Truscheit E, Hillebrand I, Junge B et al. Microbial α-glucosidase inhibitors: Chemistry, biochemistry, and therapeutic potential. In: Progress in clinical biochemistry and medicine. Vol 7, Berlin-Heidelberg: Springer-Verlag, 1988; 17–99.
[7] Müller L. Chemistry, biochemistry and therapeutic potential of microbial α-glucosidase inhibitors. In: Demain AL, Somkuti GA, Hunter-Cevera IC et al., eds. Novel Microbial Products for Medicine and Agriculture. Society for Industrial Microbiology, 1989; 109–116.
[8] Gwinup G, Byron R, Roush W et al. Effect of nibbling versus gorging on glucose tolerance. Lancet 1963; II: 165–167.
[9] Otto H, Bleyer G, Pennartz M et al. Kohlenhydrataustausch nach biologischen Äquivalenten. In: Otto H, Spaethe K, eds. Diätetik bei Diabetes mellitus. Bern: Verlag-Huber, 1973; 41–50.
[10] Crapo PA, Insel J, Sperling M et al. Comparison of serum glucose, insulin and glucagon responses to different types of complex carbohydrate in non-insulin-dependent diabetic patients. Am J Clin Nutr 1981; 34: 184–190.
[11] Jenkins DJA, Ghafari H, Wolever TMS et al. Relationship between rate of digestion of foods and post-prandial glycaemia. Diabetologia 1982; 22: 450–455.
[12] Collier G, Mc Lean A, O'Dea K. Effect of co-ingestion of fat on the metabolic responses to slowly and rapidly absorbed carbohydrates. Diabetologia 1984; 26: 50–54.
[13] Nuttall FQ, Gannon MC, Wald JL et al. Plasma glucose and insulin profiles in normal subjects ingesting diets of varying carbohydrate, fat and protein content. J Am Coll Nutr 1985; 4: 437–450.
[14] Elsenhaus B, Caspary WF. Absorption of carbohydrates. In: Caspary WF, ed. Structure and function of the small intestine. Amsterdam, Excerpta Medica 1987; 139–163.
[15] Jenkins DJA, Wolever TMS, Collier GR et al. The metabolic effects of a low glycemic index diet. Am J Clin Nutr 1987; 46: 968- 975.
[16] Willms B, Arends J. Vergleich von isolierten (Guar) und natürlichen (Müsli) Ballaststoffen in der Therapie des Typ II-Diabetes. Med Klin 1987; 82: 429–431.
[17] Hollenbeck CB, Coulston AM, Reaven GM. Comparison of plasma glucose and insulin responses to mixed meals of high-, intermediate-, and low-glycemic potential. Diabetes Care 1988; 11: 323–329.
[18] American Diabetes Association. Nutritional recommendations and principles for individuals with diabetes mellitus 1986. Diabetes Care 1987; 10: 126–132.
[19] Diabetes and Nutrition Study Group of the European Association for the Study of Diabetes. Statement. Nutritional recommendations for individuals with diabetes mellitus. Diab Nutr Metab 1988; 1: 145–149.

[20] Lembcke B. Control of absorption: delaying absorption as a therapeutic principle. In: Caspary WF, ed. Structure and function of the small intestine. Amsterdam: Excerpta Medica, 1987; 263–280.
[21] Jenkins DJA, Jenkins AL, Wolever TMS et al. Aims of diet in diabetes management. In: Creutzfeldt W, Lefèbvre P, eds. Diabetes mellitus: Pathophysiology and Therapy. Berlin, Heidelberg, New York: Springer-Verlag, 1989; 299–308.
[22] Toeller M, Lion S. Survey of the management of diet in 26 diabetes centres in Europe. Diabetic Med 1987; 4: 129–134.
[23] Behall KM, Scholfield DJ, Canary JJ. Effect of starch structure on glucose and insulin responses in adults. Am J Clin Nutr 1988; 47: 428–432.
[24] Müller L, Puls W. Pharmacology of α-glucosidase inhibitors. In: Caspary WF, ed. Structure and function of the small intestine. Amsterdam: Excerpta Medica, 1987; 281–300.
[25] Caspary WF. Inhibitors influencing carbohydrate absorption. In: Creutzfeldt W, Lefèbvre P, eds. Diabetes mellitus: Pathophysiology and Therapy. Berlin, Heidelberg, New York: Springer-Verlag, 1989; 172–191.
[26] Toeller M. Kohlenhydrate in der Diabeteskost. Ernährungs- Umschau 1989; 36: 363–368.
[27] Toeller M. Dietary treatment and α-glucosidase inhibitors in NIDDM. Diab Nutr Metab 1990 (suppl. 1) (in press).
[28] Taylor RH, Jenkins DJA, Barker HM et al. Effect of acarbose on the 24-hour blood glucose profile and pattern of carbohydrate absorption. Diabetes Care 1982; 5: 92–96.
[29] Clissold SP, Edwards C. Acarbose. A preliminary review of its pharmacodynamic and pharmacokinetic properties, and therapeutic potential. Drugs 1988; 35: 214–243.
[30] Radziuk J, Kemmer F, Morishima T et al. The effects of an alpha-glucoside hydrolase inhibitor on glycemia and the absorption of sucrose in man determined using a tracer method. Diabetes 1984; 3: 207–213.
[31] Rosenzweig NS, Herman RH. Dose response of jejunal sucrase and maltase activities to isocaloric high and low carbohydrate diets in man. Am J Clin Nutr 1970; 23: 1373- 1377.
[32] Levin RJ. Dietary carbohydrate and the kinetics of intestinal functions in relation to hexose absorption. In: Dobbing J, ed. Dietary Starches and Sugars in Man: A Comparison. Berlin, Heidelberg, New York: Springer-Verlag, 1989; 91–117.
[33] Caspary WF. Sucrose-malabsorption in man after ingestion of α-glucosidase hydrolase inhibitor. Lancet 1978; I: 1231- 1233.
[34] Bond JH, Levitt MD. Use of pulmonary hydrogen (H_2) measurements to quantify carbohydrate absorption. J Clin Invest 1972; 51: 1219–1225.
[35] Wolever TMS, Cohen Z, Thompson LU et al. Ileal loss of available carbohydrate in man: Comparison of a breath hydrogen method with direct measurement using a human ileostomy model. Am J Gastroenterol 1986; 81: 115–122.
[36] Cummings JH. Short chain fatty acids in the human colon. Gut 1981; 22: 763–779.
[37] Scheppach W, Fabian C, Ahrens F et al. Effect of starch malabsorption on colonic function and metabolism in humans. Gastroenterology 1988; 95: 1549–1555.
[38] Wilson PC, Greene HL. The gastrointestinal tract: portal to nutrient utilization. In: Shils ME, Young VR, eds. Modern Nutrition in Health and Disease. 7th ed. Philadelphia: Lea and Febinger, 1988; 481–499.
[39] Fölsch UR, Ebert R, Creutzfeldt W. Response of serum levels of gastric inhibitory polypeptide and insulin to sucrose ingestion during long-term application of acarbose. Scand J Gastroenterol 1981; 16: 629–632.
[40] Uttenthal LO, Ukpoumwam OO, Ghiglione M et al. Acute and short term effects of intestinal alpha-glucosidase inhibition on gut hormone responses in man. Digestive Diseases and Sciences 1987; 32: 139–144.
[41] Hillebrand I, Boehme K. Clinical studies on acarbose during 5 years. In: Creutzfeldt W, ed. Proceedings of the First International Symposium on Acarbose. Amsterdam: Excerpta Medica, 1982; 445–450.

[42] Lyons TJ, Mc Loughlin JC, Shaw C et al. Effect of acarbose on biochemical responses and clinical symptoms in dumping syndrome. Digestion 1985; 31: 89–96.
[43] Fölsch UR, Lembcke B. The clinical use of α-glucosidase inhibitors. In: Caspary WF, ed. Structure and function of the small intestine. Amsterdam: Excerpta Medica, 1987; 301–318.
[44] Willms B. Acarbose in non-insulin-dependent diabetes mellitus: Short-term studies in combination with oral agents. In: Creutzfeldt W, ed. Acarbose for the treatment of diabetes mellitus. 2nd International Symposium on Acarbose. Berlin, Heidelberg, New York: Springer-Verlag, 1988; 79–91.
[45] Sachse G. Acarbose in non-insulin-dependent diabetes – Long- term studies in combination with oral agents. In: Creutzfeldt W, ed. Acarbose for the treatment of diabetes mellitus. 2nd International Symposium on Acarbose. Berlin, Heidelberg, New York: Springer-Verlag, 1988; 92–101.
[46] Tuomilehto J. Acarbose monotherapy in the treatment of non- insulin-dependent diabetes mellitus – a review. In: Creutzfeldt W, ed. Acarbose for the treatment of diabetes mellitus. 2nd International Symposium on Acarbose. Berlin, Heidelberg, New York: Springer-Verlag, 1988; 104–116.
[47] Rosak C. Acarbose treatment and sulfonylurea secondary failure. In: Creutzfeldt W, ed. Acarbose for the treatment of diabetes mellitus. 2nd International Symposium on Acarbose. Berlin, Heidelberg, New York: Springer-Verlag, 1988; 156–161.
[48] Samad AHB, Willing TST, Alberti KGMM et al. Effects of BAY m 1099, a new alpha-glucosidase inhibitor, on acute metabolic responses and metabolic control in NIDDM over 1 Mo. Diabetes Care 1988; 11: 337–344.
[49] Mies R, Spengler M. Efficacy of the glucosidase inhibitor acarbose compared to the sulphonylurea glisoxepid on metabolic control of type 2 (non-insulin-dependent) diabetes. (abstract) Diabetologia 1987; 30: 557A.
[50] Schwedes U, Petzoldt R, Hillebrand I et al. Comparison of acarbose and metformin treatment in non- insulin-dependent diabetic out-patients. In: Creutzfeldt W, ed. Proceedings of First International Symposium on Acarbose. Amsterdam: Excerpta Medica, 1981; 275–281.
[51] Hanefeld M, Fischer S, Schulze J et al. Therapeutical potentials of acarbose as first line drug in non-insulin-dependent diabetics insufficiently treated with diet alone. Diabetes Care 1990 (submitted for publication).
[52] Coniff RF, Innerfield RJ. A multi-center, double-blind, placebo-controlled study of long-term efficacy and safety of acarbose (BAY g 5421) and SFU in the Rx of NIDDM inadequately controlled by maximal SFU. (abstract) Diabetes 1990; 39 (Suppl. 1): 109A.
[53] Innerfield RJ, Coniff RF. A multi-center, double-blind, placebo-controlled study of long-term efficacy and safety of acarbose (BAYg 5421) in the Rx of obese patients with NIDDM Rxed by diet alone. (abstract) Diabetes 1990; 39 (Suppl. 1): 211A.
[54] Toeller M, Klischan A, Schleppinghoff B et al. Delayed absorption by the α-glucosidase inhibitor, miglitol, does not lead to alterations of the dietary intake. A 6 month randomised double-blind cross-over trial in type 2 (NIDDM) patients. (abstract) Diabetes Research and Clinical Practice 1988; 5 (Suppl.): 612.
[55] Seiberling M, Toeller M, Baunack AR et al. Does the amount of carbohydrate of a meal influence the effects of acarbose on the insulin- and blood glucose response? (abstract) Archives of Pharmacology 1989; 339 (Suppl.): 76.
[56] Raptis S, Dimitriadis G, Hadjidakis D. Acarbose treatment in insulin dependent (type 1) diabetes mellitus. In: Creutzfeldt W, ed. Acarbose for the treatment of diabetes mellitus. 2nd International Symposium on Acarbose. Berlin, Heidelberg, New York: Springer-Verlag, 1988; 141–152.
[57] Gérard J, Luyckx AS, Lefèbvre PJ. Improvement of metabolic control in insulin dependent diabetes treated with the alpha- glucosidase inhibitor acarbose for two months. Diabetologia 1981; 21: 446–457.

[58] O'Dea K, Turtle J. Optimum effectiveness of intestinal alpha- glucosidase inhibitors: importance of uniform distribution through a meal. Am J Clin Nutr. 1985; 41: 511–516.
[59] Schlüter G. Toxicology of acarbose, with special reference to long-term carcinogenicity studies. In: Creutzfeldt W, ed. Acarbose for the treatment of diabetes mellitus. 2ndInternational Symposium on Acarbose. Berlin, Heidelberg, New York: Springer-Verlag, 1988; 5–14.
[60] Axen KV, Sclafani A. Acarbose decreases insulin resistance in a rat model of NIDDM. (abstract) Diabetes 1990; 39 (Suppl. 1): 49A.

Combining insulin with oral antidiabetic agents (including problems of secondary failure)

N. Lotz, W. Bachmann, H. Mehnert, E. Standl

Introduction

In recent years, a dualistic concept has been adopted for the pathogenesis of non-insulin dependent or type 2 diabetes mellitus: although the specific biochemical abnormalities are still unknown, a large body of evidence has been accumulated indicating that impaired insulin action on the one hand, and decreased insulin secretion on the other, account for the disturbances in carbohydrate and lipid metabolism seen in NIDDM [1–6]. Whereas insulin resistance remains as a prominent feature throughout the duration of diabetes, insulin secretion gradually decreases over the years leading to secondary failure of oral therapy. There are, however, still considerable amounts of endogenous insulin left circulating in blood at this latter point of time [7–11]. Based on this pathophysiological understanding, combining insulin with sulphonylurea treatment has become increasingly accepted as an alternative therapeutical approach for patients with true secondary failure. Such patients otherwise frequently require insulin doses far in excess of all estimates for daily insulin production in non-diabetic individuals [11–14]. Thus, combination therapy has come a long way since an early phase of interest following the introduction of sulphonylureas into clinical medicine in the 1950s [15, 16]. The present chapter attempts a critical review of the pros and cons with respect to combining insulin with sulphonylurea therapy and provides guidelines for its practical use.

Pathogenetic background

Non-insulin dependent diabetes mellitus (NIDDM) is presently considered as a probably heterogeneous disease entity emerging in predisposed individuals over years [1, 2, 5, 6]. Insulin resistance seems to be a prominent feature long before the clinical onset of NIDDM, while a relatively decreased insulin secretion occurs gradually later on [1, 3, 7, 9–11, 17, 18]. The mutual contribution of insulin resistance and decreased insulin secretion to the development of hyperglycemia appears to vary considerably among patients [18]. Current therapeutic approaches to the management of NIDDM patients, therefore, are directed at increasing insulin action, endogenous insulin secretion (even exogenous substitution, if necessary), or both and treatment modalities have to be tailored to the individual patient.

Insulin resistance

Insulin resistance is characterized by inadequately high amounts of insulin necessary for a normal insulin response of insulin target tissues. Although several abnormalities of the insulin signal transmission chain have been described at the insulin receptor kinase and glucose transporter level in patients with NIDDM, it is still undecided whether these are primary or secondary pathogenetic events [3, 4]. Figures 1 and 2 outline some of these

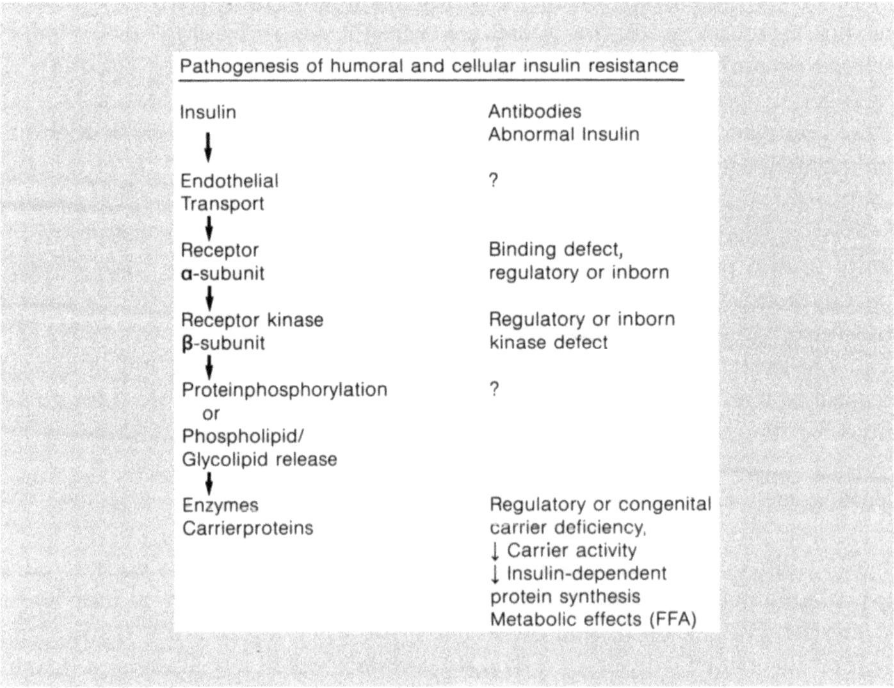

Fig. 1 Schematic diagram of the signal transmitting chain of insulin action and of some defects in this chain leading to insulin resistance. Adapted from ref. [3 and 4].

defects of mechanisms leading to insulin resistance. Moreover, glucose toxicity induced by chronic hyperglycemia seems to also have a negative impact on cellular insulin sensitivity, perhaps by impairing glycogen synthesis [19]. Consecutively to insulin resistance, hyperinsulinemia may be present in many subjects with NIDDM, especially in the preclinical phase and at onset of NIDDM, possibly augmented by metabolic effects of hypertension [1, 2, 5, 6, 9, 20, 21]. In a recent survey of a true random sample of NIDDM in a caucasian population in southern Germany, we have found evidence for marked hyperinsulinemia in every other patient at the clinical onset of NIDDM. This was in close association with hypertension which was observed in 80% of all patients at this point of time [21] (Table 1). Insulin resistance remains a significant problem throughout the duration of NIDDM, also when patients eventually indeed require insulin treatment for metabolic compensation [7, 8, 11, 13]. Many of those patients inject unusually high insulin

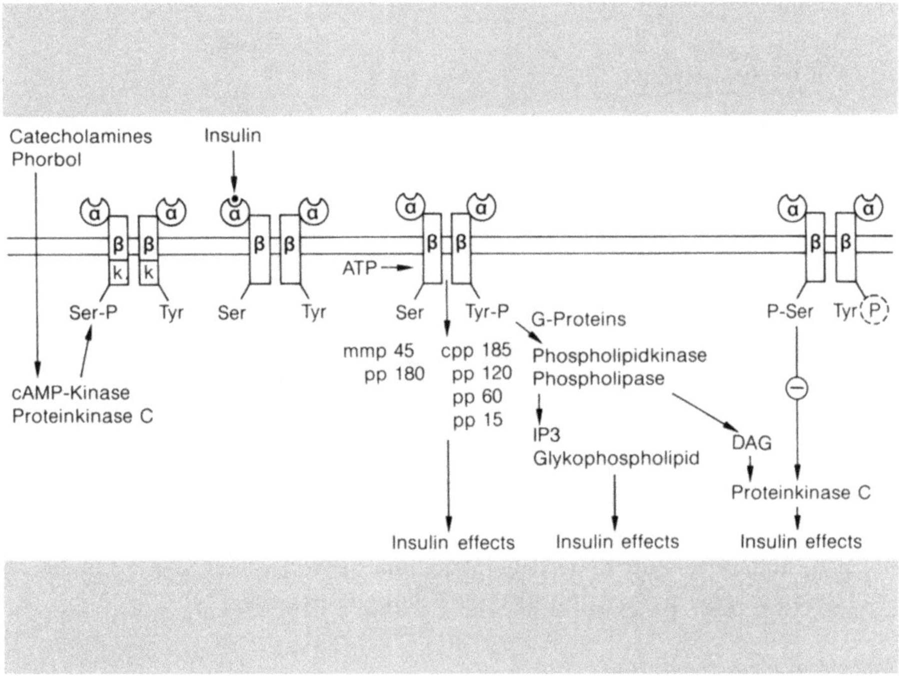

Fig. 2 Model for induction of insulin resistance by inhibition of receptorkinase due to serinphosphorylation. The normal insulin signal transmission through activation of receptorkinase by tyrosinephosphorylation to postkinase levels is inhibited by a reversible serinphosphorylation of receptorkinase induced by cAMPkinase or proteinkinase C. Adapted from ref. [4].

Table 1 The GP-Program in the Greater Munich Area

A. Risk profile in 2 random samples of 41 recently diagnosed and 290 NIDDM patients of all durations of diabetes

	"recent"	"all"
$HbA_{1c} \geq 8\%$	18***	49
Hypertension	78(*)	65
Micro- and Macroalbuminuria	41	42
Hypertriglyceridemia (>200 mg/dl)	78(*)	64
Hypercholesterinemia (>250 mg/dl)	37	39
Fasting C-peptide (>1.4 pmol/ml)	50***	18
BMI (male >24; females >25)	83	77
Factor VIII R: Ag (>130%)	70	73

*** $p < 0.001$; (*) $p < 0.1$ vs. total group

B. Significant correlations of hypertension with other "risk" parameters in a random sample of NIDDM with recent onset of diabetes

	Significance p-value
Fasting C-peptide	<0.001
β_2-microglobulin in serum	<0.001
BMI	<0.01
– HDL-cholesterol i. s.	<0.01
Cholesterol i. s.	<0.05
Microalbuminuria	<0.05
F VIII R: Ag	<0.05
Triglycerides i. s.	<0.05

doses per day, far in excess of all normal "physiological" needs, and in marked contrast to the fact that they still exhibit almost normal endogenous serum insulin or C-peptide levels, although proinsulin instead of insulin secretion may account somewhat for this latter observation [22, 23]. Obesity, physical inactivity, and hypertriglyceridemia obviously aggravate insulin resistance in a large proportion of type 2 diabetic patients [24].

Impaired insulin secretion

On the other hand, major disturbances of insulin secretion have also been described in patients with NIDDM. In particular, a loss of the first phase insulin peak after intravenous, but also oral glucose administration has been found, despite retention of acute phase responses to other insulin stimuli such as intravenous arginine, isoproterenol, and tolbutamide [1, 5, 6, 9, 25, 26]. The acute insulin responses to glucose can be partially restored by improved glycemic control, so that whether this defect is secondary to hyperglycemia or part of the primary lesion of NIDDM [6, 19] must still be substantiated. Recent interest has focused on alterations in the phosphoinositide metabolism of the pancreatic β-cell as a mechanism of glucose toxic abnormalities in insulin secretion [19]. Furthermore, the normal meal-related periodicity or pulsatility of insulin secretion has been found blunted in NIDDM, a phenomenon which might be due to sustained hyperglycemia [27–29]. But even in the fasting state defective patterns of insulin secretion and loss of feedback control can be detected [17, 30]. This may have particular implications for hepatic glucose output during fasting, which is primarily regulated by insulin, yet excessively high in NIDDM and specifically so in patients in so-called secondary failure of oral therapy [1, 2, 17].

Investigations into the disordered insulin secretion in NIDDM have been complicated by the fact that a gradual loss of pancreatic β-cell mass evolves over the years in many patients [31, 32]. The mechanisms behind this process are still obscure, but the capacity to secrete insulin inevitably deteriorates in many patients year after year. Recent interest has concentrated on the possibility that amyloid-like material which often, yet not exclusively, is found in islets of patients with NIDDM may be of significance in the degenerative or destructive sequence occurring in the islets of Langerhans [33]. But little is known about the pathobiochemistry of pancreatic β-cell exhaustion.

Secondary failure

Agreement seems to exist, however, that the insulin secretion capacity reaches a critical level in many patients after years of NIDDM. Beyond this point of time exogenous substitution will be required for glucose control within the individually set target range [13, 14, 17]. Even maximal sulphonylurea therapy on top of appropriate dietary management will not be sufficiently effective [34]. This phenomenon is called secondary failure of oral therapy and 5 to 10% of all NIDDM patients will undergo this phase every year, with a maximum around 12–15 years after known duration of diabetes [34]. Due to a lack of anabolic insulin effects and poor metabolic control with gross glycosuria, body weight has declined to normal in most patients with secondary failure, indicating that secondary failure is commonly diagnosed too late. The same holds true for the initiation of insulin therapy.

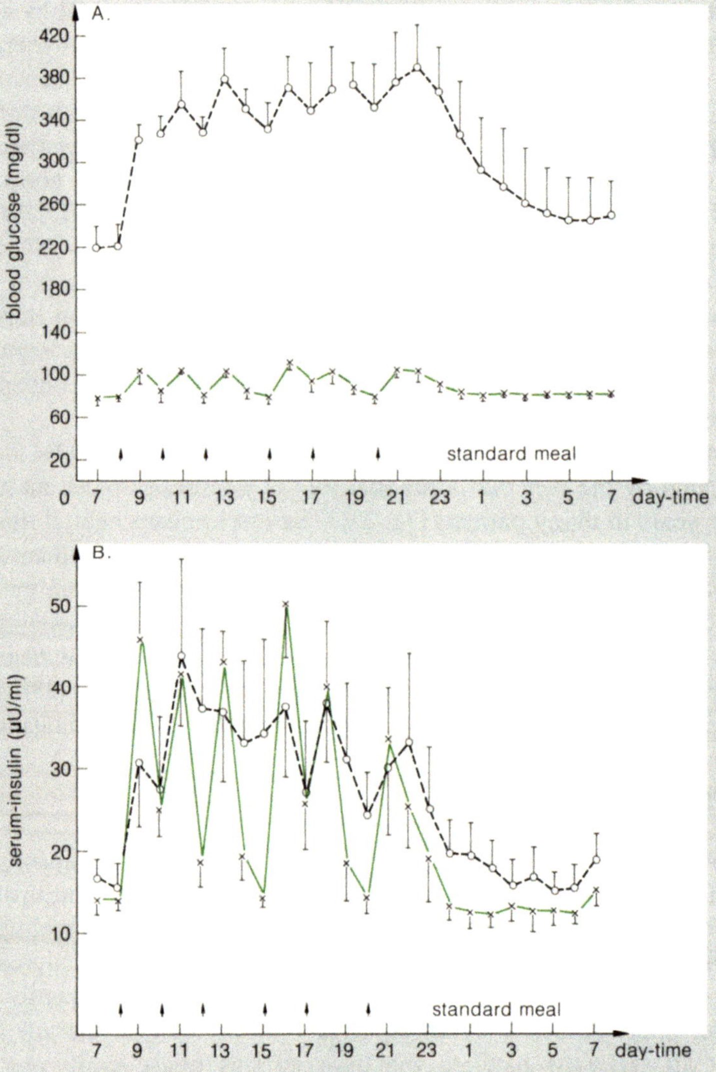

Fig. 3 A 24-h-blood glucose profile in type 2 diabetics with secondary failure to sulfonylureas (o– – –o; n = 5) and in age matched controls (×———×; n = 5).
B 24-h-serum insulin profile in type 2 diabetics with secondary failure to sulfonylureas (o– – –o; n = 5) and in age matched controls (×———×; n = 5).

On the other hand, even in true secondary failure, type 2 diabetics appear to be markedly insulin resistant. In fact, we were able to demonstrate, that compared to non-diabetics with the same or somewhat higher body mass, type 2 diabetics in secondary failure show normal fasting levels and postprandial peaks of serum insulin, underscoring the major contribution of insulin resistance to the sustained hyperglycemia. Figure 3 displays this recent experience of our group. Similar results – yet less detailed – have also been obtained by others [9, 11].

Aside from the insulin resistance of peripheral insulin target tissues, especially skeletal muscle, increased hepatic glucose output seems to be the most important determinant of fasting hyperglycemia in secondary failure [1, 2, 35]. Physiologically, hepatic glucose output is controlled by hepatic insulinisation, particularly via the portal route. Through its position in the blood circulation system, the liver is the central organ exposed to the insulin released from the pancreas and, in fact, takes up and eliminates 50% of all insulin secreted. In secondary failure, lack of insulin, but also effects induced by increased growth hormone and free fatty acid concentrations seem to gear the liver metabolism towards markedly increased glucose production [17, 35].

Treatment approaches

It is in this complex pathogenetic setting of NIDDM that all therapeutical measures have to reveal their effectiveness. A rational treatment approach must aim at a reduction of insulin resistance on one side and insulin substitution – if necessary – on the other, while hyperinsulinemia has to be avoided, since this may turn on insulin resistance or potentially accelerate atherogenesis [36]. A decrease of insulin resistance can be achieved by means of a low caloric diet, physical exercise, biguanides, and carbohydrate absorption inhibitors like acarbose, where was available insulin to the body can be increased by sulphonylureas and insulin administration. Although several studies have suggested that, in chronic use, sulphonylureas lower blood glucose also through mechanisms other than stimulation of endogenous insulin secretion [34, 37–39], in terms of combination therapy the insulin secretagogic action of sulphonylureas seems to be by far the most important effect (see below). Extrapancreatic effects of sulphonylureas have been attributed to a potentiation of the insulin action on the liver, enhanced peripheral sensitivity to insulin, suppression of glucagon secretion and perhaps also a reduction of the hepatic clearance of insulin [37–40].

All therapeutic measures may encounter typical difficulties when applied to patients with NIDDM. Dietary compliance is often a problem, physical

Table 2 Main results of six studies investigating the effects of the addition of sulfonylurea to insulin therapy on the metabolic control and on both insulin secretion and insulin action in type 2 diabetic patients with secondary failure to sulfonylureas. Adapted from [69]

Reference	Evaluation of efficacy			Analysis of the mechanism(s): effects on		Conclusion: efficacy results from improvement in insulin
	Insulin dose	Glucose profile	HbA_{1c}	Insulin secretion Plasma C-peptide response	Insulin action Peripheral glucose disposal	
Lardinois et al. [47]	=	↓	↓	↑ (meal)	↑ (clamp)	action > secretion
Allen et al. [48]	↓ (3/6)	↓ (4/6)	?	no ↑ (OGTT)	↑ (i. v. ITT)	action
Groop et al. [49]	=	↓	↓	↑ (meal)	no ↑ (i. v. ITT)	secretion
Gutniak et al. [50]	↓	=	=	{ ↑ (meal) no ↑ (glucagon)	no ↑ (clamp)	secretion
Simonson et al. [51]	↓	↓	↓	↑ (glucagon)	no ↑ (clamp)	secretion
Castillo et al. [52]						
– Responders	↓	↓	↓	↑ (glucagon)	↗ (clamp)	
– Non-responders	↓	↑	↑	↗ (glucagon)	no ↑ (clamp)	secretion

OGTT: oral glucose tolerance test; i. v. ITT: intravenous insulin tolerance test.

activity faces serious limitations in patients with already existing cardiovascular complications or severe hypertension. Biguanide therapy is hampered by a whole series of contraindications, sulphonylureas are often abused as a substitution of dietary compliance, and α-glucosidase inhibition, e. g. by acarbose, although promising, is a very recent approach which still needs to find its final place. Insulin therapy in NIDDM builds up frequently to excessive daily doses, due to the apparent insulin resistance and superimposed by the peripheral hyperinsulinemia resulting from subcutaneous insulin delivery [14].

Syndrome X

High serum insulin concentrations, however, have been implicated to be atherogenic [7, 8, 36, 41]. The hyperinsulinemia/insulin resistance syndrome as part of the so-called syndrome X seems to be closely related with accelerated atherogenesis in subjects without and especially with NIDDM, as has been shown by several prospective studies in caucasoid populations including the Schwabing Study of our group on macrovascular disease in diabetes mellitus [8, 42–46]. Whether high insulin concentrations indeed carry direct atherogenic risk or rather are "only" an established predictive risk marker of macrovascular disease remains an issue still to be resolved, but for the time being it seems prudent that good diabetes control is targeted also to reduce the amount of circulating insulin where feasible. At the same time, this approach will effectively counteract the problems associated with weight gain and overinsulinisation.

It is in this pathophysiological context of true secondary failure, strive for appropriate metabolic compensation, and avoidance of hyperinsulinemia where a combination therapy with sulphonylureas and insulin might offer some benefits.

Survey of clinical trials

In recent years, a number of clinical trials have been set up to investigate the mechanism of action by which sulphonylurea and insulin treatment may exert its potentially beneficial effects [12–14, 77]. Originally designed to take advantage of the extrapancreatic effects of sulphonylureas in the early 1980s [37, 38], it now appears to be established that the increasing insulin release into the natural route towards the liver is probably the decisive factor for the effectiveness of combination therapy. Table 2 lists several studies in which

Table 3 Controlled studies with double blind crossover (C) or double blind parallel (P) design comparing combination therapy sulfonylurea/insulin vs. insulinmonotherapy in type 2 diabetic patients

Design Features					Results			
Reference	C/P	n	Sulfonylurea	Month of combination	Insulin dose	HbA_{1c}	C-peptide	Hypoglycemic episodes
Mauerhoff [53]	P	22	Glibenclamide	4	↓	?	↑	↑
Quatraro [54]	P	30	Gliclazide	12	↓	↓	↑	?
Reich [55]	P	20	Glibenclamide	4	↓	↓	=	=
Schade [56]	C	16	Glibenclamide	4	↓	↓	↑	↑
Stenman [57]	C	15	Glibenclamide	4	↓	↓	↑	↑
Gutniak [50]	P	20	Glibenclamide	11	↓	=	↑	
Lundershausen [58]	P	79	Glibenclamide	6	↓		↑	
Bachmann [59]	P	68	Glibenclamide	6	↓	=	=	=
Lotz [60]	P	16	Glibenclamide	24	↓	=	↑	
Mezitis [14]	P	12	Glibenclamide	5	↓	=		

↑ increase; ↓ decrease; = no change

systematically and simultaneously the effect both on insulin secretion and insulin action has been assessed [47–52]. The results obtained were strongly in favor of a gain in insulin secretion, although different methodological approaches have been used.

Some caution may be warranted, however, when these principally accepted observations are considered. Hyperglycemia leads to an impairment of insulin secretion and lowering glycemia might by itself increase insulin secretion [19]. In addition, most patients had already been on insulin therapy prior to the study for a variable length of time, and many of them were grossly obese and needed excessively large insulin doses per day. In a sense, they may not represent the typical normal weight type 2 patient in secondary failure. Finally, four of these studies were open label, only two were double-blind and one more had a randomized crossover design.

On the other hand, it should be pointed out that detectable effects and efficacy of combination therapy have been found almost exclusively confined to type 2 diabetics, also in trials in which type 1 and type 2 diabetics have been directly compared [13, 51]. A lack of efficacy in IDDM, however, seems to be in line with the notion that combination therapy is mainly operating through pancreatic, not extrapancreatic sulphonylurea effects.

Long-term efficacy of combination therapy in NIDDM has been evaluated in a series of controlled studies. In Table 3 trials are listed in which the effects of insulin alone versus insulin + sulphonylureas have been compared over a period of 4 months up to 2 years [14, 50, 53–60]. Both double-blind crossover and double-blind parallel design have been used, as indicated in Table 3. It seems noteworthy, however, that only sulphonylurea administration has been blinded, not insulin which usually was adapted to "clinical needs", but without a precise protocol. Of course, there are many more studies [12, 61–65, 77], mainly shorter term, often open-label, and even case reports as early as 1956 and 1957 [66, 67]. Not all of them can be acknowledged in this chapter.

As it is so frequently with clinical studies, they may be extraordinarily heterogenous and difficult to compare with each other. Basically, there are two types: one where patients already were on insulin treatment, commonly on high doses, yet often in poor control, and others where patients were randomly assigned in secondary failure of oral sulphonylurea therapy. Accordingly, individual targets of the various studies have been quite variable, not to mention that often they seemed not to be clearly defined. In patients on high insulin doses, insulin sparing appeared to be an obvious goal, whereas among patients in secondary failure better control was often the primary objective. The outcome of a study, however, may depend largely on the definition of the aim.

With these limitations in mind, the finding of a significantly decreased or lower daily insulin dose was a surprisingly uniform result (Table 3). Apparently, the insulin dose during combination therapy was even frequently not low enough, since an increase in hypoglycemic episodes and a relatively greater weight gain was noted in several studies [53, 56, 57], raising again the issue of appropriate clinical management in such studies. In our experience with the longest published follow up on a prospective parallel design trial, equivalent levels of diabetes control after two years of treatment were achieved with 43 U insulin per day vs. 19 U in the combination group [60]. A 50% lower insulin dose seems to be an attainable aim in most well-designed studies.

Better glycemic control – e. g. as estimated by HbA_{1c} – has turned out to be a more variable result, although often achieved (Table 3). In many instances not expressively defined, "improvement" due to combination could lead to either a reduction in daily insulin doses or a decrease in glycosylated hemoglobin levels (and other measures of glucose control) or both. In contrast to some earlier studies, however, in which an attenuation of the favorable effects of combination therapy on metabolic control has been suggested with time [49, 62], several more recent studies have indicated beneficial long term results up to 2 years [50, 54, 58, 60]. A strong case for longterm metabolic efficacy of combination therapy has also been made by means of prospective withdrawal tests after 6 months of treatment [68]. When either glibenclamide (Fig. 4) or insulin treatment was suspended for 2 weeks, severe metabolic decompensation occurred in all patients. Resumption of combination therapy prompted a rather rapid reinstitution of metabolic control.

Higher C-peptide concentrations – in line with the tentative mode of action – have been regularly found under combination therapy [50, 53, 54, 56–58, 60], whereas plasma-free insulin levels have rarely been measured. Our group has produced some evidence that in particular fasting concentrations may indeed by lower during combination therapy [60, 68].

Changes in serum lipid parameters – if any – appear in most cases to be only minimal in response to combined sulphonylurea/insulin treatment. This applies to serum triglycerides, cholesterol, and HDL-cholesterol [12–14, 69].

With regard to the dosage of the sulphonylurea compound during combination therapy, it has been shown that a maximum dose of glibenclamide (7 mg in the morning, 3.5 mg in the evening) was superior to a treatment scheme with a 3.5 mg dose b. i. d. [70]. In addition, there has also been variation in the insulin treatment approach during combination therapy [12–14]. Patients who had been on excessive amounts of insulin prior to combination usually remained on a split dose regimen in the morning and the evening, whereas true combination patients started in secondary failure,

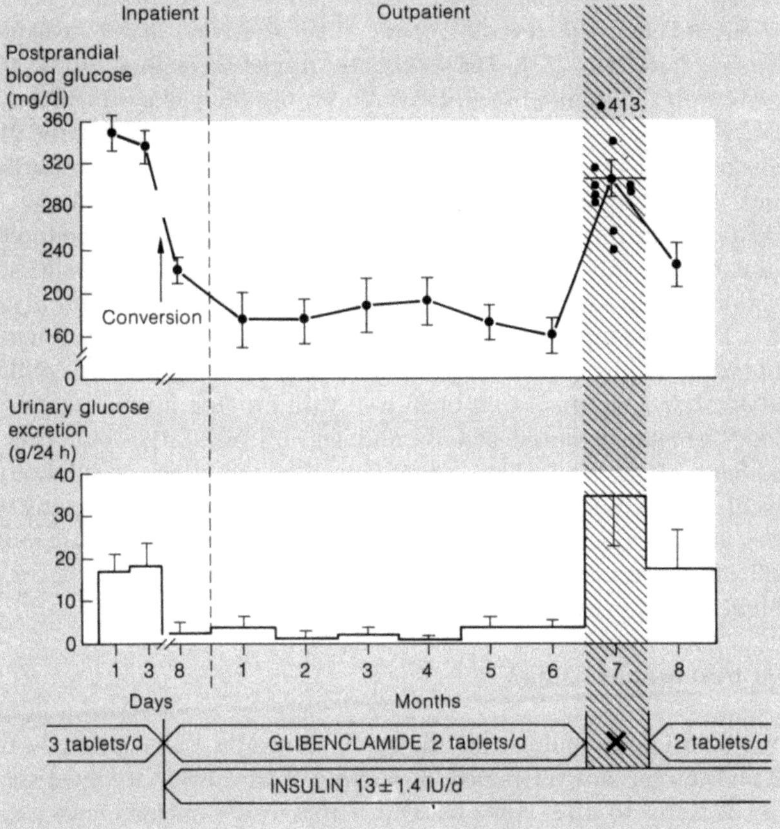

Fig. 4 Changes in postprandial blood glucose and 24-h urinary glucose excretion in type-II diabetics with 'secondary failure of sulphonylurea therapy' during combined insulin/glibenclamide therapy and during the glibenclamide withdrawal test (mean ± SEM). Adapted from ref. [68].

required only one injection (of a small dose) per day in general and significantly less frequently needed a second injection compared to patients with insulin monotherapy (placebo group). In terms of insulin preparations, mainly intermediate-acting NPH has been used, but some experience has also been obtained with regular insulin in patients with very high postbreakfast peaks of blood glucose and with long-acting insulins. Since increased hepatic glucose output appears to be a therapeutical target of primary importance, proinsulin with a tentatively more specific hepatic effect has been under investigation for combined therapy [13]. The metabolic results were favourable, but no randomly assigned comparison proinsulin vs. insulin was performed.

Along the same line of thinking to more effectively control hepatic glucose output, the strategy of evening insulin application has been introduced into combination therapy and evaluated in recent trials [12, 17, 65]. In fact, in the just mentioned proinsulin study, proinsulin had been applied at bedtime. The rationale behind this strategy is the notion that increased hepatic glucose production is mainly an overnight problem which determines fasting glycemia, whereas the postprandial plasma glucose is determined predominantly by insulin-mediated glucose disposal. Hepatic glucose output was significantly decreased after 3 months of an open trial with evening insulin treatment, as was overnight mean blood glucose and plasma free fatty acids [71]. In a double-blind crossover fashion, examining thus the effect of sulphonylurea treatment, glycemic effectiveness of combination therapy with evening insulin has been demonstrated by several studies [65]. No data, however, are available thus far on a direct comparison of morning insulin versus evening insulin in a random order crossover design.

Present treatment modalities

Although until now combination therapy with insulin and sulphonylureas for type 2 diabetes has not yet gained the status of a worldwide accepted standard therapy, it seems to offer some benefits. Obviously, clinicians must decide in their own patients whether the combination approach will be effective and worthwhile. It must be stressed, however, that not any conceivable combination of insulin and sulphonylurea administration does indeed qualify for a rationally based combination therapy. In the light of the discussion of this chapter, there have to be clear cut concepts and strategies [72].

It is also self-evident that combination therapy is no replacement for dietary compliance. On the contrary, if applied properly, it can be of help to reach target control in insulin requiring type 2 diabetics with the lowest possible insulinisation or insulinemia [12]. To succeed in determining the minimal necessary insulin dose, however, may be difficult. The most important rule, above all in combination therapy, is therefore, to start insulin very low and to increase it slowly, if at all. And there is ample time to find the appropriate insulin dose, since the concomitant sulphonylurea treatment will prevent further metabolic decompensation.

Two groups of NIDDM patients seem to benefit the most from combination therapy: 1) patients in true secondary failure of oral sulphonylurea treatment (the by far most appropriate group) and 2) (individual) patients with insufficient glycemic control despite high doses of insulin in a twice-daily injection regimen [12–14]. The concept in the first group of patients is continuation of the oral sulphonylurea therapy, while the small existing insulin deficit is compensated for by small doses of exogenous insulin. The strategy for the second group aims at better insulinisation of the liver, decrease of hepatic glucose production, and unblocking of endogenous insulin secretion suppressed by the large doses of exogenous insulin [12–14, 72].

In patients with imminent secondary failure, combination therapy can be instituted under ambulatory conditions which facilitates the acceptance of insulin therapy and saves costs. The gradual introduction of insulin treatment is very convenient and leaves both doctor and patient enough time for teaching and learning all the necessary items from the injection technique to the selfmonitoring. This approach seems particularly adequate for the often elderly patients and should lead to less mistakes in handling the new therapy, less hypoglycemias, and less weight gain. One final, very important aspect of this type of combination therapy for the patient is that usually it can be accomplished by only one insulin injection a day.

In practical terms before starting combination therapy, proof of true secondary failure should be established which commonly is heralded by recent weight loss and more or less "easy" normalisation of body weight. Of course, significant ketonuria must be absent and warrants rapid insulinisation. Strict hypocaloric diet between 500 and 1000 kcal should then be reinforced to minimize insulin resistance and lower blood glucose. Cooperation of the patient can be sought by explaining that this time limited "dieting approach" is considered as a last attempt to avoid insulin treatment. If after 5 days and despite maximal sulphonylurea dosage, metabolic control remains outside the target range, a lack of endogenous insulin can be assumed [72]. As a consequence, additional treatment with low dose insulin is required.

In imminent secondary failure, hyperglycemia frequently occurs predominantly after breakfast or "postprandially". Hence, insulin therapy is started before breakfast with a dose of 4 to 6 U of an intermediate-acting insulin (NPH or mixture of regular and NPH insulin). Maximal sulphonylurea therapy is continued and the diet may be adjusted to 1000 to 1200 kcal. If necessary, the insulin dose should be increased not earlier than after three days and in steps of no more than two units. Alternatively to the morning insulin concept, insulin therapy can be initiated as a dose of 4 to 6 U NPH insulin between supper and bedtime or at bedtime in case that hyperglycemia is most pronounced in the fasting state in the morning, already before breakfast. Again, cautious adaptations of the insulin dose need to be emphasized.

Obviously, there are certain limits for the simple combination therapy approach in secondary failure: if a patient indeed requires more than 20 U a day or two daily injections, the therapeutic concept must be reconsidered or the patient switched to insulin monotherapy [12].

In contrast to patients with secondary failure, changing patients with insufficient glycemic control despite high insulin doses twice daily to combination therapy must not be attempted under ambulatory conditions. Severe hypoglycemic attacks may occur. Those patients are to be admitted to hospital. After a period of dietary reinforcement, cutting both insulin doses by half an implementation of sulphonylurea treatment may be explored. Controlled by close blood glucose monitoring, insulin is adjusted to the lowest required dose [12].

A major negative aspect of combination therapy consists in the lack of predictability of responders to this therapy. As a group, responders seem to be characterized by higher fasting C-peptides, shorter duration of NIDDM, and somewhat higher body weight, but in the individual patient these parameters do not allow prediction of response [12–14, 69]. If, however, combination therapy is installed early in secondary failure, high positive response rates between 60–80% of all patients can be expected [12, 60, 68]. Long-term effectiveness likewise appears to be high. "Tertiary" failure of initially successful combination therapy seems to occur in about only 5% per year [12, 60, 68].

The issue of combining the risk of side effects of two hypoglycemic drugs as an argument against combination therapy, does not seem to be a serious one. Provided that the indication of true secondary failure is correct, then there should be no higher, but rather a lower risk of hypoglycemia. In terms of drug specific side effects, they appear to be almost neglectable, if human insulin and second generation sulphonylureas are used.

As far as costs are concerned, they are in the meantime lower for combination therapy in most European countries, since the costs for sulphonylureas are more than outweighed by the sparing of costs in decreasing the insulin dose.

Finally, treatment of insulin resistance in NIDDM is not really addressed by combination therapy, aside from the clinically rather minor extrapancreatic effects of sulphonylureas and the impact of better metabolic control on insulin resistance. Combination of biguanides with sulphonylureas or even with insulin treatment principally appears to be an alternative, although biguanide therapy is often unsuitable because of significant contraindications [73, 74].

Future perspectives

The era of unchallenged insulin monotherapy in insulin requiring NIDDM may have come to an end [12–14]. Favorable results can be obtained not only in terms of convenience for patients and doctors, but also with respect to insulin sparing and better control, when sulphonylureas and insulin treatment are combined. Still more studies, however, are needed to substantiate the long-term efficacy and the "tertiary" failure rate of combination therapy more clearly. Triple combinations with the addition of the new oral compound acarbose [75, 76] or biguanides to the sulphonylurea/insulin scheme are being investigated which should reduce hyper insulinemia and insulin resistance further. In addition, blockers of hepatic glucose output are under development. All these combination approaches might be greatly boosted if the hyperinsulinemia/insulin resistance syndrome can indeed be singled out by appropriate prospective intervention studies to directly accelerate macrovascular disease in NIDDM.

References

[1] Bogardus C, Lillioja S, Howard BV et al. Relationship between insulin secretion, insulin action, and fasting plasma glucose concentrations in nondiabetic and non insulin dependent diabetic subjects. J Clin Invest 1984; 74: 1238–46.

[2] De Fronzo RA, Ferrannini E, Koivisto V. New concepts in the pathogenesis and treatment of non insulin-dependent diabetes mellitus. Am J Med 1983; 74: 52–81.

[3] Häring H, Obermaier B, Ermel B et al. Insulin receptor kinase defects as a possible cause of cellular insulin resistance. Diab & Metab 1987; 13: 284–293.

[4] Häring HU, Obermair-Kusser B, Mühlbacher C. Zum Mechanismus der zellulären Insulinwirkung – Rezeptorkinasedefekt beim Typ II-Diabetes. Med Klin 1989; 84: 144–152.

[5] Rasmussen H, Zawalich KC, Ganesan S et al. Physiology and pathophysiology of insulin secretion. Diabetes Care 1990; 13: 655–666.

[6] De Fronzo RA. The Triumvirate: β-cell, muscle, liver: a collusion responsible for NIDDM. Diabetes 1988; 37: 667–687.

[7] Standl E, Janka HU. High serum insulin concentrations in relation to other cardiovascular risk factors in macrovascular disease of type 2 diabetes. Horm Metab Res 1985; Suppl 15: 46–51.

[8] Janka HU, Ziegler AG, Standl E et al. Daily insulin dose as a predictor of macrovascular disease in insulin treated non-insulin-dependent diabetics. Diab & Metab 1987; 13: 359–364.

[9] Zabel-Langhenning R, Lundershausen R, Panzram G. 10-year follow up study in type 2 diabetes: metabolic and vascular findings: 21th EDESG Meeting 1986.
[10] Pontiroli AE, Calderara A, Maffi P et al. Secondary failure to oral hypoglycemic agents in non obese patients with non-insulin-dependent diabetes is related to reduced insulin release. Diab & Metab 1989; 15: 79–84.
[11] Pontiroli AE, Calderara A, Pacchioni M et al. Insulin requirement in elderly patients with non-insulin dependent diabetes mellitus (NIDDM). Aging 1989; 1: 147–152.
[12] Bachmann W, Lotz N, Mehnert H. Insulin/sulphonylurea combination therapy in type II diabetes. Basel: Karger, 1988; 1–159.
[13] Lebovitz HE, Pasmantier RM. Combination insulin-sulfonylurea therapy. Diabetes Care 1990; 13: 667–675.
[14] Bailey TS, Mezitis NHE. Combination therapy with insulin and sulfonylurea for type II diabetes. Diabetes Care 1990; 13: 687–695.
[15] Franke H, Fuchs H. Ein neues antidiabetisches Prinzip. Ergebnisse klinischer Untersuchungen. Dtsch Med Wochenschr 1955; 1449–1454.
[16] Bertram F, Bendfeldt E, Otto H. Über ein wirksames perorales Antidiabetikum. Dtsch Med Wochenschr 1955; 80: 1455–1459.
[17] Riddle MC. Evening insulin strategy. Diabetes Care 1990; 13: 676–686.
[18] Banerji MA, Lebovitz HE. Insulin-sensitive and insulin-resistant variants in NIDDM. Diabetes 1989; 38: 784–792.
[19] Rossetti L, Giaccari A, De Fronzo RA. Glucose toxicity. Diabetes Care 1990; 13: 610–630.
[20] Ferrannini E, Natali A, Cerri M et al. Hypertension: a metabolic disorder? Diab & Metab 1989; 15: 284–291.
[21] Standl E, Stiegler H, Roth R et al. On the impact of hypertension on the prognosis of NIDDM. Results of the Schwabing GP-Programm. Diab & Metab 1989; 15: 352–358.
[22] Ward WK, La Cara EC, Paquette TL et al. Disproportionate elevation of immuno reactive proinsulin in type 2 (non-insulin-dependent) diabetes mellitus and in experimental insulin resistance. Diabetologia 1987; 30: 698–702.
[23] Temple RC, Carrington CA, Luzio SD et al. Insulin deficiency in non-insulin-dependent diabetes. Lancet 1989; 1: 203–295.
[24] Modan M, Halkin H, Almog S et al. Hyperinsulinemia: a link between hypertension, obesity, and glucose intolerance. J Clin Invest 1985; 809–817.
[25] Ward WK, Bead JC, Halter JB et al. Pathophysiology of insulin secretion in non-insulin-dependent diabetes mellitus. Diabetes Care 1984, 7: 491–502.
[26] Ward WK, Bolgiano DC, McKnight B et al. Diminished secretory response in patients with non insulin dependent diabetes mellitus. J Clin Invest 1984; 74: 1318–1328.
[27] O'Rahilly SO, Turner RC, Matthews DR. Impaired pulsatile secretion of insulin in relatives of patients with non-insulin-dependent diabetes. N Engl J Med 1988; 318: 1225–1230.
[28] Polonsky KS, Given BD, Hirsch LJ et al. Abnormal patterns of insulin secretion in non-insulin-dependent diabetes mellitus. N Engl J Med 1988; 318: 1231–1239.
[29] Calles-Escandon J, Jaspan J, Robbins DC. Postprandial oscillatory patterns of blood glucose and insulin in NIDDM. Abnormal diurnal insulin secretion patterns and glucose homeostasis independent of obesity. Diabetes Care 1989; 12: 709–714.
[30] O'Rahilly S, Nugent Z, Rudenski AS et al. Beta cell dysfunction, rather than insulin insensitivity, is the primary defect in familial type II diabetes. Lancet 1986; 1: 360–363.
[31] Leahy JL, Bonner-Weir S, Weir GC. Abnormal glucose regulation of insulin secretion in models of reduced B-cell mass. Diabetes 1984; 33: 667–673.
[32] Rudenski AS, Hadden DR, Atkinson AB et al. Natural history of pancreatic islet B-cell function in type II diabetes mellitus studies over six years by homeostasis model assessment. Diabetic Med 1988; 5: 35–41.
[33] Clark A, Wells CA, Buley ID et al. Islet amyloid, increased A-cells, reduced B-cells and

exocrine fibrosis: quantitative changes in the pancreas in type II diabetes. Diabetes Res 1988; 9: 151–159.

[34] Schöffling K, Mehnert H, Haupt E. Behandlung mit Sulfonylharnstoffen. In: Mehnert H, Schöffling K (eds) Diabetologie in Klinik und Praxis. Stuttgart, New York: Thieme, 1984; 220–238.

[35] Golay A, Swislocki ALM, Chen YDI et al. Relationship between plasma free fatty acid concentrations, endogenous glucose production, and fasting hyperglycemia in normal and non-insulin-dependent diabetic individuals. Metabolism 1987; 36: 692–696.

[36] Janka HU, Standl E. Hyperinsulinema as a possible risk factor of macrovascular disease in diabetes mellitus. An overview. Diab & Metab 1987; 13: 279–283.

[37] Lebovitz HE, Feinglos MN. Sulfonylurea drugs: mechanisms of antidiabetic action and therapeutic usefulness. Diabetes Care 1978; 1: 189–198.

[38] Bachmann W, Böttger I, Haslbeck M et al. Extrapancreatic action of sulfonylureas: effect of gliquidone on insulin and glucagon binding to rat liver plasma membranes. Eur J Clin Invest 1979; 9: 411–415.

[39] Beck-Nielsen H, Hother-Nielson O, Pedersen O. Mechanisms of action of sulfonylureas with special reference to extrapancreatic effect: an overview. Diabetic Med 1988; 5: 613–620.

[40] Melander A, Bitzen PO, Faber O et al. Sulphonylurea antidiabetic drugs. Drugs 1989; 37: 58–72.

[41] Stout RW. Insulin and atheroma: 20-Yr Perspective. Diabetes Care 1990; 13: 631–654.

[42] Zavaroni I, Bonora E, Pagliara M et al. Risk factors for coronary artery disease in healthy persons with hyperinsulinemia and normal glucose tolerance. N Engl J Med 1989; 320: 702–706.

[43] Pyörälä K, Savolainen E, Kankola S et al. Plasma insulin as coronary heart disease risk factor: relationship to other risk factors and predictive value during 9 1/2 year follow up of the Helsinki Policemen Study population. Acta Med Scand 1985; 701 (Suppl 1): 38–52.

[44] Fontbonne A, Tchobroutsky G, Eschwege E et al. Coronary heart disease mortality risk: plasma insulin level is a more sensitive marker than hypertension or abnormal glucose tolerance in overweight males: the Paris prospective study. Int J Obesity 1988; 12: 557–565.

[45] Hockaday TDR, Phil D. Serum insulin concentrations and anticipatory factors of cardiomyopathy in NIDDM. Diab & Metab 1987; 13: 354–358.

[46] Standl E, Stiegler H, Janka HU et al. Risk profile of macrovascular disease in diabetes mellitus. Diab & Metab 1988; 14: 505–511.

[47] Lardinois CK, Lin GC, Reaven GM. Glyburide in non-insulin dependent diabetes. Its therapeutic effect in patients with disease poorly controlled by insulin alone. Arch Intern Med 1985; 145: 1028–1032.

[48] Allen BT, Feinglos MN, Lebovitz HE. Treatment of poorly regulated non-insulin-dependent diabetes mellitus with combination insulin–sulfonylurea. Arch Intern Med 1985; 145: 1900–1903.

[49] Groop L, Harno K, Nikkilä EA et al. Transient effect of the combination of insulin and sulfonylurea (glicenclamide) on glycemic control in non-insulin dependent diabetics poorly controlled with insulin alone. Acta Med Scand 1985; 217: 33–39.

[50] Gutniak M, Karlander SG, Efendic S. Glyburide decreases insulin requirement, increases B-cell response to mixed meal, and does not affect insulin sensitivity: effect of short- and longterm combined treatment in secondary failure to sulfonylurea. Diabetes Care 1987; 10: 545–554.

[51] Simonson DC, Delprato S, Castellino P et al. Effect of glyburide on glycemic control, insulin requirement, and glucose metabolism in insulin treated diabetic patients. Diabetes 1987; 36: 136–146.

[52] Castillo M, Scheen AJ, Paolisso G et al. The addition of glipizide to insulin therapy in

type II diabetic patients with secondary failure to sulfonylureas is useful only in the presence of a significant residual insulin secretion. Acta Endocrinol 1987; 116: 364–372.
[53] Mauerhoff T, Ketellegers JM, Lambert AE. Effect of glibenclamide in insulin-treated diabetic patients with residual insulin secretion. Diab Metab 1986; 12: 34–38.
[54] Quatraro A, Consoli G, Ceriello A et al. Combined insulin and sulfonylurea therapy in non-insulin-dependent diabetics with secondary failure to oral drugs; a one year follow up. Diab Metab 1986; 12: 315–318.
[55] Reich A, Abraira C, Lawrence AM. Combined glyburide and insulin therapy in type II diabetes. Diab Res 1987; 6: 99–104.
[56] Schade DS, Mitchell WJ, Griego G. Addition of sulfonylurea to insulin treatment in poorly controlled type II diabetes. J Am Med Ass 1987; 257: 2441–2445.
[57] Stenman S, Groop PH, Saloranta C et al. Effects of the combination of insulin and glibenclamide in type 2 (non-insulin-dependent) diabetic patients with secondary failure to oral hypoglycemic agents. Diabetologia 1988; 31: 206–213.
[58] Lundershausen R, Orban S, Pißarek D et al. Langzeiteffekt der Glicenclamid–Insulin–Kombinationsbehandlung beim Sekundärversagen der Sulfonylharnstofftherapie – Ergebnisse einer einjährigen Doppelblindstudie. Wien Klin Wochenschr 1987; 99: 603–608.
[59] Bachman W, Lotz N, Mehnert H et al. Wirksamkeit der Kombinationsbehandlung mit Glibenclamid und Insulin bei Sulfonylharnstoff-Sekundärversagen – Kontrollierte multizentrische doppelblinde klinische Prüfung. Dtsch Med Wochenschr 1988; 113: 631–636.
[60] Lotz N, Bachmann W, Ladik T et al. Die Kombinationstherapie Insulin/Sulfonylharnstoff in der Langzeittherapie des Typ II-Diabetes nach „Sekundärversagen“. Klin Wochenschr 1988; 66: 1079–1084.
[61] Rosak C, Schwarz O, Althoff PH et al. Kombinierte Behandlung von Typ II-Diabetikern mit Insulin und Glibenclamid nach Tablettensekundärversagen. Dtsch Med Wochenschr 1985; 110: 1975–1980.
[62] Osei K, O'Dorisio TM, Falko JM. Concomitant insulin and sulfonylurea therapy in patients with type II diabetes: effects on glycoregulation and lipid metabolism. Am J Med 1984; 77: 1002–1008.
[63] Casner PR. Insulin–glyburide combination therapy for non-insulin-dependent diabetes mellitus: a longterm double blind, placebo-controlled trial. Clin Pharmacol Ther 1988; 44: 594–603.
[64] Lewitt MS, Yu VKF, Rennie GC et al. Effects of combined insulin–sulfonylurea therapy in type II patients. Diabetes Care 1989; 12: 379–383.
[65] Riddle MC, Hart JS, Bonma DJ et al. Efficacy of bedtime NPH insulin with daytime sulfonylurea for a subpopulation of type II diabetic subjects. Diabetes Care 1989; 12: 623–629.
[66] Kinsell LW, Brown FR, Friskey RW et al. Insulin-sparing sulfonamides (Letter). Science 1956; 123: 585.
[67] Stratmann FW. Über Spätversager bei der peroralen Diabetes-Therapie und ihre kombinierte Behandlung Med Klin 1957; 15: 589–591.
[68] Lotz N, Bachmann W, Mehnert H. Combination of sulphonylurea and insulin in the longterm treatment of "secondary failure" in type II diabetes. In: Bachmann W, Lotz N, Mehnert H (eds) Insulin/sulfonylurea combination therapy in type II diabetes. Basel: Karger, 1988; 131–145.
[69] Scheen AJ, Lefebvre PJ. Insulin versus insulin plus sulfonylureas in type 2 diabetic patients with secondary failure to sulfonylureas. Diabetes Res Clin Pract 1989; 6: 33–43.
[70] Hasche H. Combination therapy with different doses of glibenclamide. A double-blind study on 36 patients with secondary failure. In: Bachmann W, Lotz N, Mehnert H (eds) Insulin/sulfonylurea combination therapy in type II diabetes. Basel: Karger, 1988; 25–32.
[71] Taskinen MR, Sane T, Helve E et al. Bedtime insulin for suppression of overnight free-fatty acid, blood glucose, and glucose production in NIDDM. Diabetes 1989; 38: 580–588.

[72] Berger M, Bott U, Grüßer M et al. Behandlungs- und Schulungsprogramm für Typ II-Diabetiker, die Insulin spritzen. Köln: Deutscher Ärzte-Verlag, 1990.
[73] Klip A, Leiter LA. Cellular mechanism of action of metformin. Diabetes Care 1990; 13: 696–704.
[74] Wu MS, Johnston P, Shen WHH et al. Effect of Metformin on carbohydrate and lipoprotein metabolism in NIDDM patients. Diabetes Care 1990: 13: 1–8.
[75] Müller L, Puls W. Pharmacology of α-glucosidase inhibitors. In: Caspary WF (ed) Structure and function of the small intestine. Diabetes Forum Series I. Amsterdam: Excerpta Medica, 1987; 281–300.
[76] Fölsch UR, Lembcke B. The clinical use of α-glucosidase inhibitors. In: Caspary WF (ed) Structure and function of the small intestine. Diabetes Forum Series I. Amsterdam: Excerpta Medica, 1987; 301–420.
[77] Bachmann W, Sieger C, Haslbeck M et al. Combination of insulin and glicenclamide in the treatment of adult-onset diabetes (type 2). Diabetologia 1981; 21: 245.

Management of hyperlipidaemia in the diabetic patient

D. J. Betteridge

Introduction

The most important cause of morbidity and mortality in diabetic patients remains premature and extensive atherosclerotic vascular disease. Information on the prevalence of atherosclerosis-related disease comes both from post-mortem studies and cross-sectional and prospective studies of diabetic populations [1]. In terms of prevention of atherosclerosis within the diabetic population it is important to note that high rates of vascular disease may not be an inevitable consequence of the diabetic state. In populations, e.g. the Japanese and Hong Kong Chinese, where the prevalence of atherosclerosis-related disease is low in the general population the prevalence in diabetics is also low, albeit at a higher level than the non-diabetic [2]. These epidemiological considerations suggest that the huge toll of atherosclerosis-related disease, particularly coronary heart disease (CHD) and peripheral vascular disease, may be reduced in Western populations by attention to risk factors other than the glucose/insulin disorder itself. There is no doubt that the major risk factors for CHD well delineated in non-diabetic populations, have a similar impact on risk within diabetic populations. Stamler and colleagues were able to analyse the six-year CHD mortality in the 5,245 diabetic men screened for the MRFIT Study in the USA. It was possible to compare prospectively the risk of CHD mortality in this large group of diabetic men to the CHD mortality risk in 350,997 non-diabetics [3]. The principal risk factors, serum cholesterol, cigarette smoking and hypertension had a similar impact in terms of increasing vascular risk in the diabetics as seen in the non-diabetics. However, within the diabetic group CHD mortality was 3-fold higher for each given risk factor. A further interesting point to emerge from this study was that in the absence of the three major risk factors there was still an increased risk for diabetes suggesting additional mechanisms of atherosclerosis [3]. Important candidates to explain the increased risk of the diabetic state *per se* would include hyperinsulinaemia, hyperglycaemia, abnormalities of coagulation factors, particularly fibrinogen, enhanced platelet

Table 1 Optimal lipid and lipoprotein levels [4, 5]

Total plasma cholesterol	< 5.2 mmol/l
LDL cholesterol	< 3.5 mmol/l
Total plasma triglyceride	< 2.3 mmol/l
HDL cholesterol	> 0.9 mmol/l

reactivity and obesity. It is obvious that many factors may influence the development of accelerated atherosclerosis in diabetes. However, the lipid and lipoprotein abnormalities may have particular relevance as they are open to therapeutic intervention.

In recent years there has been a wealth of new information relating lipid and lipoprotein abnormalities to vascular risk. This information has been reviewed by two important consensus conferences on each side of the Atlantic and it has been concluded that there is sufficient evidence to attribute a causal role to plasma cholesterol, and particularly low density lipoprotein (LDL) cholesterol in the development of atherosclerosis [4, 5]. On the basis of these consensus conference reports, guidelines for lipid and lipoprotein levels for the general population have been published (see Table 1). It is of interest that the European NIDDM Policy Group have accepted these recommendations as targets for metabolic control in the treatment of non-insulin-dependent diabetes [6]. Furthermore, the American Diabetes Association Consensus Panel on the Role of Cardiovascular Risk Factors in the Prevention of and Treatment of Macrovascular Disease in Diabetes has published a recent statement giving goals of therapy in relation to lipid abnormalities, hypertension and other factors [7].

It is therefore an opportune time to consider the identification and therapy of dyslipoproteinaemia within the diabetic population. In this chapter lipid and lipoprotein abnormalities which occur in the diabetic state will be described briefly together with how they should be managed in some detail.

Lipids, lipoproteins and vascular disease

It is the level of plasma LDL that accounts for the relationship between plasma cholesterol and CHD. LDL is the major cholesterol-rich lipoprotein and carries about 70% of plasma cholesterol. Much is now known about the metabolism of this important lipoprotein, mainly through the work of the Nobel Laureates, Brown and Goldstein, who discovered the LDL receptor and the crucial role that this plays in the regulation of plasma LDL levels in the 1970s.

LDL cholesterol serves to transport cholesterol from the liver to the periphery for utilisation in membrane renewal and, in certain tissues, hormone production. Cells acquire LDL following binding of LDL to a specific, high affinity cell surface receptor, the LDL receptor, which recognises LDL apoprotein B. Following binding to the receptor LDL is internalised through a process of endocytosis. The endocytotic vesicle fuses with cellular lysosomes where acid hydrolases hydrolyse the lipoprotein cholesterol ester to free cholesterol, which gains access to the cytoplasm. The increasing cellular cholesterol concentration has important regulating roles in cellular cholesterol homeostasis, inhibiting cholesterol synthesis and stimulating its own re-esterification to cholesterol ester. The expression of LDL receptors is also decreased. Excess LDL is removed from the circulation via hepatic LDL receptors. It is the activity of these receptors which govern plasma LDL levels so that in the monogenic familial disorder of cholesterol metabolism, familial hypercholesterolaemia, there is a defective gene for the LDL receptor, which results in a marked increase in plasma LDL levels and prolongation of the half time in the circulation [8].

Recently there have been important advances in the understanding of how LDL interacts with cells to produce the fatty streak, the early lesion of atherosclerosis. Studies in experimental atherosclerotic animals have implicated the circulating blood monocyte for a central role in the formation of the foam cell, typical of the fatty streak. The adhesion of circulating blood monocytes to arterial endothelium is the first identifiable lesion in cholesterol-fed animals. At a later stage monocytes penetrate into the subendothelial space and take on the characteristics of macrophages and become lipid-laden foam cells. At this stage the accumulation of macrophages appears to be toxic to the overlying endothelium which is disrupted allowing platelet adhesion and aggregation and subsequent progression of the fatty streak to the fibro-fatty plaque of atherosclerosis [9]. It was Brown and Goldstein who showed that native LDL incubated with monocytes does not lead to foam cell formation. However if the LDL is modified chemically, such as by acetylation, then LDL is avidly taken up by monocytes leading to foam cell formation [10]. More recently, principally through the work of Steinberg and his colleagues, it has become clear that a possible physiological modification of LDL is lipid peroxidation. When LDL is incubated with cultured endothelial cells it is modified in such a way that it is recognised by a specific receptor on monocyte/macrophages, which has subsequently been termed the acetyl LDL or scavenger receptor. This modification of LDL by endothelial cells appears to be a lipid peroxidation and can be prevented by antioxidants. The possible role of endothelial cell-modified LDL in the development of atherosclerosis has been reviewed recently by Steinberg and his colleagues[11] and the scavenger receptor has been fully elucidated [12].

The other principal cholesterol-rich lipoprotein in plasma is high density lipoprotein (HDL). HDL, like LDL, is strongly related to the development of vascular disease, but unlike LDL the relationship between HDL and vascular disease is inverse. High levels of HDL appear to protect against atherosclerosis, whereas low levels of HDL are an important risk factor [13]. The mechanism or mechanisms by which HDL influences atherogenesis remain to be fully determined [14]. However, HDL does appear to be involved in the process of reverse cholesterol transport, returning cholesterol from the periphery back to the liver, which is the major site of cholesterol excretion. However, HDL may be involved in other ways, possibly through interactions with arterial wall prostacyclin production and platelet aggregation. It is also important to remember that a major proportion of HDL in the plasma comes from the surface components of triglyceride-rich particles when they are broken down. Therefore high plasma HDL levels may reflect the rate of catabolism of triglyceride-rich lipoproteins.

The role of triglyceride in the development of coronary heart disease remains controversial. Many studies have shown that plasma triglyceride levels are associated with vascular disease, both in cross-sectional studies and in prospective studies. However this relationship does not appear to be independent of other risk factors, such as plasma cholesterol, HDL cholesterol and obesity [15]. However recently there has been renewed interest in the role of plasma triglyceride. Analysis of the results of the Framingham study indicates that triglyceride is an independent risk factor in women and in men with low HDL levels [16]. Support for this comes from the Paris prospective study [17]. It is of interest that in studies of the diabetic population triglyceride often comes out more strongly in relation to vascular disease than cholesterol [18]. This has been shown prospectively in the Paris study [19]. Perhaps before the issue of triglycerides is fully clarified there will have to be simple measures for the individual triglyceride-rich particles. Certainly remnant particles of chylomicron and VLDL catabolism are known to be highly atherogenic in that they accumulate in type 3 hyperlipidaemia which is associated with premature and extensive atherosclerosis [20]. There is evidence that the hypertriglyceridaemia so commonly seen in non-insulin-dependent diabetes may also reflect an increase in these remnant particles [21, 22].

Lipid and lipoprotein abnormalities in diabetes mellitus

In the individual diabetic patient the extent of lipid and lipoprotein abnormalities depends on several factors, particularly the extent of insulin resistance, the degree of hyperglycaemia, concurrent obesity, the presence of albuminuria and dietary intake. Of course primary disorders of lipid metabolism can occur in patients with diabetes and also other secondary causes may coexist. It is not possible here to give a detailed review of the pathophysiology of lipoprotein abnormalities in diabetes. This subject has been extensively reviewed [23, 24]. In the insulin-dependent diabetic lipid and lipoprotein abnormalities will show considerable correlation with glycaemic control and patients with near normoglycaemia tend to have normal lipid and lipoprotein levels. However if control is not optimum then triglyceride levels may be raised through both increased production and decreased clearance of VLDL. LDL may also be raised in these circumstances. In addition to the increased production of LDL from VLDL, LDL clearance may be reduced through decreased binding to the LDL receptor caused by post-transciptional modification of LDL apoprotein B through glycation. Furthermore, insulin is important for normal expression of cellular LDL receptors. HDL tends to be normal or even slightly increased in insulin-dependent diabetics.

Lipid and lipoprotein abnormalities tend to be more common in non-insulin-dependent diabetes, particularly the combination of hypertriglyceridaemia and low HDL levels. An important mechanism for the hypertriglyceridaemia is increased production of VLDL by the liver associated with insulin resistance. In some patients there appears to be a decreased VLDL catabolism as well. It is well known that insulin is important for the normal activity of lipoprotein lipase which plays a crucial role in the catabolism of triglyceride-rich particles. HDL levels tend to be low in non-insulin-dependent diabetes. A possible mechanism here is the reduced clearance of triglyceride-rich particles in these diabetics.

It is becoming increasingly apparent that in addition to quantitative abnormalities in lipid and lipoprotein levels there are qualitative differences in lipoproteins associated with the diabetic state and more work is needed in this area.

Screening for lipid abnormalities in the diabetic clinic

As hypertriglyceridaemia is so common in the diabetic population it is the author's opinion that a fasting blood sample should be obtained for lipid

$$\text{LDL cholesterol} = \text{total cholesterol} - \left(\text{(HDL cholesterol} + \frac{\text{triglyceride)}}{2.19}\right)$$

Fig. 1 Friedewald formula [25]

Table 2 Secondary hyperlipidaemias

	Main lipid obnormality	Chylo-microns	Lipoprotein changes		
			VLDL	LDL	HDL
Excess alcohol	Triglyceride ↑	↑	↑		
Hypothyroidism	Cholesterol ↑			↑	
Chronic renal failure	Triglyceride ↑		↑	↑→	
Nephrotic syndrome	Cholesterol ↑ and Triglyceride ↑		↑	↑	
Cholestasis	Cholesterol ↑			↑	↓

analysis in diabetic patients. The logistics of obtaining a fasting sample have not proved to be a problem in the author's experience. For usual clinical care it is sufficient to obtain a fasting total triglyceride, total cholesterol and an HDL cholesterol. HDL cholesterol is an important measure in its own right and also enables the calculation of LDL cholesterol using the Friedewald calculation which is valid so long as the total triglyceride is below 4.5 mmol/l (Fig.1) [25]. The fasting lipid profile should be performed as part of the annual assessment of all diabetic patients. If the lipid profile is satisfactory, along the guidelines recommended (see Table 1), then a further measurement can be obtained in a year's time. If lipid and lipoprotein levels are not satisfactory then it is important to exclude secondary causes of hyperlipidaemia (see Table 2) and also consider the possibility of a coexistent primary hyperlipidaemia (Table 3). An algorithm detailing an approach to the identification and treatment of hyperlidaemia in diabetes is shown in Fig. 2.

Treatment of hyperlipidaemia

The management of dyslipidaemia in the diabetic patient should be part of a general modification of important risk factors for coronary heart disease. This should include anti-smoking advice, reduction of obesity, appropriate

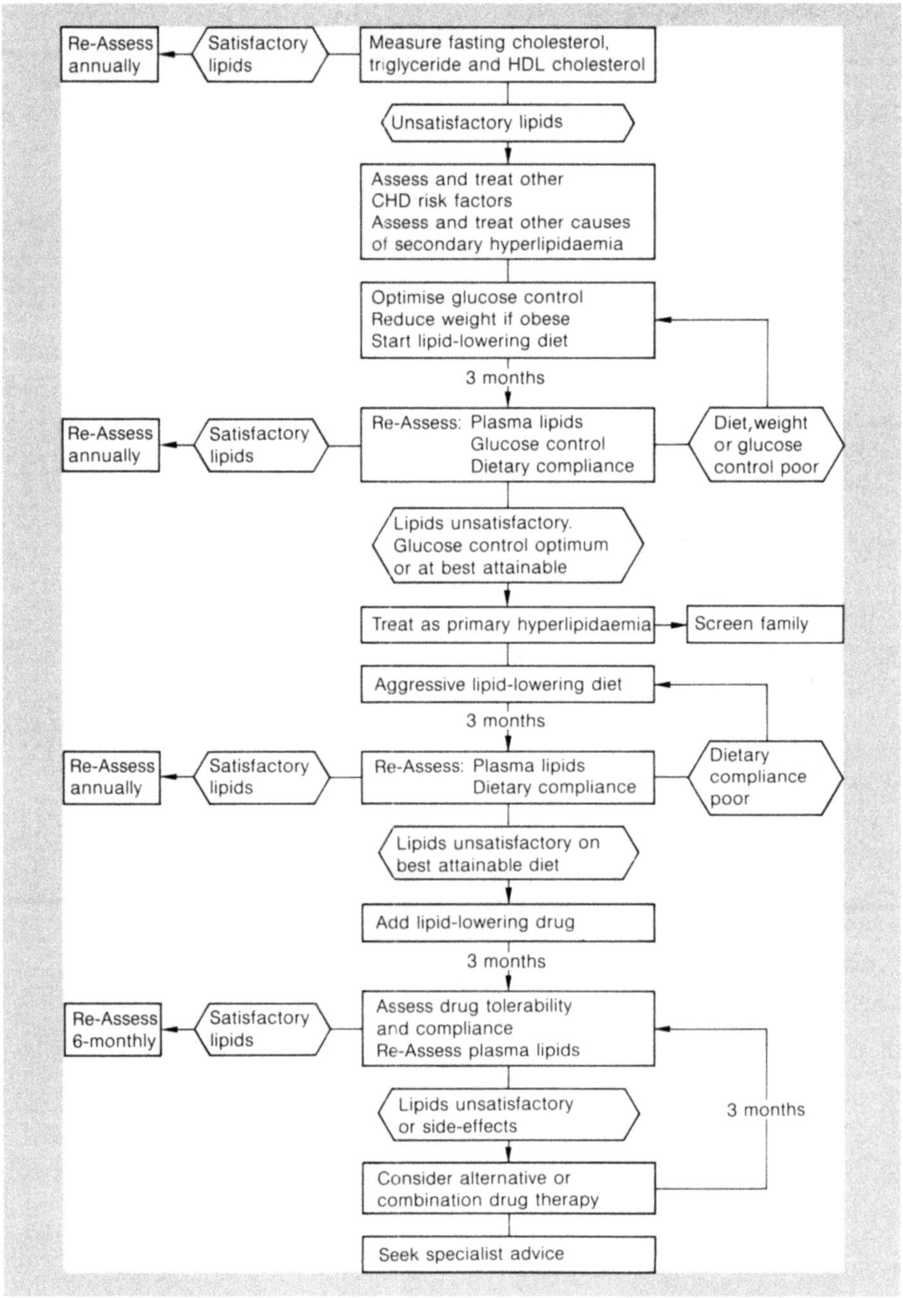

Fig. 2 An aproach to the identification and treatment of hyperlidaemia in diabetes

Table 3 Primary hyperlipidaemias

	Frederickson lipoprotein phenotype	Typical lipid levels (mmol/l)	Lipo-pro-teins	CHD risk	Pan-creatitis	Clinical signs
Polygenic hyper-cholesterolaemia	IIa	Cholesterol 6.5–9 Triglyceride < 2.3	LDL ↑ HDL →↓	+	–	Xanthelasma, corneal arcus
Familial combined (mixed) hyperlipidaemia	IIa, IIb IV	Cholesterol 6.5–10 Triglyceride 2.5–12	V- ↑→ LDL ↑→ LDL →↓ HDL	+ +	–	Corneal arcus, xanthelasma
Familial hyper-cholesterolaemia	IIa or IIb	Cholesterol 7.5–16 Triglyceride < 5.0	LDL ↑ V- →↑ LDL →↓ HDL	+ + +	–	Tendon xanthomata corneal arcus, xanthelasma
Remnant particle disease (dysbetalipoproteinaemia	III	Cholesterol 9–14 Triglyceride 9–14	IDL ↑ HDL →↓	+ + +	+	Palmar, tuberous and occasional tendon xanthomata
Chylomicronaemia syndrome liproprotein lipase deficiency, apoprotein C-II deficiency	I	Triglyceride 10–30 Cholesterol < 6.5	Chylo-microns ↑	–	+ + +	Eruptive xanthomata Lipaemia retinalis Hepatosplenomegaly
Familial hypertriglyceridaemia	IV–V	Triglyceride 10–30 Cholesterol 6.5–12	VLDL ↑ Chylo-microns →↑	?	+ +	Eruptive xanthomata Lipaemia retinalis Hepatosplenomegaly
HDL abnormalities						
Hypoalphalipoproteinaemia	–	HDL cholesterol < 0.9	HDL ↓	+ +	–	–
Hyperalphalipoproteinaemia	–	HDL cholesterol > 2.0	HDL ↑	–	–	–

treatment of hypertension and the encouragement of appropriate exercise. Some of these other risk factors have important interrelations with lipid abnormalities. Obesity predisposes to dyslipidaemia, particularly hypertriglyceridaemia and low HDL levels and some drugs used for the treatment of hypertension, particularly non-selective beta-blockers and thiazide diuretics may adversely affect lipid and lipoprotein levels. Smoking tends to be associated with low HDL concentrations. Best endeavours should be undertaken to improve glycaemic control with insulin or hypoglycaemic agents as appropriate. There is no doubt that improved glycaemic control is associated with improvement of diabetic dyslipidaemia.

Nutritional counselling

The cornerstone of management of dyslipidaemia in the diabetic patient is nutritional counselling. Weight reduction should be pursued in the overweight patient. Success is more likely with frequent consultations and agreed target weights with the dietician. A slow reduction in weight should be aimed for as rapid reduction in weight associated with very low energy diets reduces lean body mass. Appropriate exercise programmes are beneficial in achieving weight loss and also have a beneficial effect on lipid and lipoprotein levels. Advice on exercise has to be tailored to the individual patient and must take account of the presence of diabetic complications.

In addition to attempts to reduce overweight the diet is modified with particular emphasis on reduction of calories from fat, particularly saturated fat. The general principles of the fat modified diet are shown in Table 4. An important feature in relation to dietary measures is the reduction of excess alcohol intake as this can stimulate lipoprotein production in the liver. Various national Diabetic Associations have adopted the recommendations outlined in the Table for diabetic patients, however there is dispute concerning the amount of dietary carbohydrate that should be advised, particularly for non-

Table 4 Principles of a lipid lowering diet

- Reduce total fat and particularly saturated fat (10% daily calories)
- Moderately increase mono- and polyunsaturated fat (10% calories each)
- Decrease dietary cholesterol (< 300 mg/day)
- Increase high protein, low saturated fat foods
- Increase complex carbohydrate, fruit, vegetables
- Decrease sodium intake

insulin-dependent diabetics. The concern is whether high carbohydrate diets will exacerbate the elevated plasma triglycerides and low HDL levels seen in these patients [26]. The question of the amount of carbohydrate that is appropriate for these patients remains to be clarified.

An alternative to the high carbohydrate diet (50 – 60% of total energy) is to replace some of the calories from carbohydrate with monounsaturated fat. This has been studied by Grundy's group who have found that a diet high in monounsaturates leads to improved glycaemic control and reduction in plasma triglyceride levels and an increase in HDL cholesterol levels compared to the higher carbohydrate diet in non-insulin-dependent diabetics [27]. Certainly this provides an alternative approach and will be more palatable for some patients.

There has been a lot of interest in the role of omega-3 fatty acids derived from marine fish in recent years. There is no doubt that high intake of these unsaturated fatty acids under metabolic ward conditions in non-diabetics is associated with reduced hepatic production of VLDL [28]. However, when these fatty acids are taken as a dietary supplement in diabetics deleterious effects on glycaemic control have been observed and furthermore increased plasma LDL levels have occurred [29, 30]. Therefore omega-3 supplements cannot be advocated in diabetes although the intake of fish itself need not be curtailed.

It is clear that further work needs to be done to determine the optimum diet for the hyperlipidaemic diabetic patient. More recent findings suggest that not all saturated fatty acids for affect plasma cholesterol levels. Stearic acid appears to be as effective as oleic acid in lowering plasma cholesterol and LDL cholesterol in normal subjects [31]. This sort of work may lead to the development of more palatable diets in the future.

Drug therapy

It is only after measures to improve glycaemic control, to reduce overweight and the prescription of a fat-modified diet have failed to achieve acceptable lipid and lipoprotein concentrations that drug therapy is considered. For each individual the risk/benefit ratio in terms of the prescription of lipid-lowering drugs has to be considered. The currently available classes of hypolipidaemic agents will be discussed in turn. Drug therapy for dyslipidaemia in diabetes has been recently reviewed [32 – 34].

Fibric acid derivatives

Fibric acid derivatives are known to act on lipoprotein metabolism at several points. They reduce hepatic synthesis of VLDL and in addition appear to stimulate activity of the enzyme lipoprotein lipase which results in increased clearance of triglyceride-rich particles. They also reduce cholesterol synthesis through non-specific inhibition of HMG CoA reductase, the rate-determining enzyme of cholesterol synthesis. As a result of these various effects on lipoprotein metabolism, plasma cholesterol and triglyceride are reduced through a reduction in VLDL, IDL and LDL. HDL cholesterol on the other hand tends to increase with fibrate treatment, possibly related to the effects of fibrates on the clearance of triglyceride-rich particles.

Of the currently available fibric acid derivatives bezafibrate and gemfibrozil have been used most extensively in both insulin-dependent and non-insulin-dependent diabetic patients, and they are useful preparations in the treatment of diabetic dyslipoproteinaemia, which is often of mixed type associated with low HDL levels. Reductions of up to 20% in total serum cholesterol and up to 50% in total serum triglyceride can be expected. When serum HDL cholesterol concentrations are low then increases of approximately 15% can be expected.

Fibric acid derivatives are generally well tolerated and side effects are few. Untoward effects include gastrointestinal upset, a reversible myopathy and impotence. Clofibrate, the first of this class of drugs, increases the lithogenicity of bile and in two largescale studies with this agent an increased incidence of gallstones was reported. Furthermore in one of the trials an increased incidence of gastrointestinal neoplasms was observed. This compound has now been largely superceded by the newer fibrates. Gemfibrozil was the drug chosen for the Helsinki Heart Study, a long term primary prevention trial in middle aged men [35]. In this study gemfibrozil treatment was associated with a reduction in ischaemic heart disease and the long-term safety profile appeared advantageous. Fibric acid derivatives may have additional beneficial effects in diabetes. Some fibrates have been shown to improve blood glucose control. Furthermore, fibrinogen, an additional vascular risk factor, often raised in diabetes, may be lowered by these agents.

Fibric acid derivatives are useful in the treatment of mixed hyperlipidaemia in diabetic subjects and may have additional benefits as outlined above. If satisfactory cholesterol levels are not obtained with a fibrate alone, then a resin drug may be added to the fibrate treatment. Currently it is not possible to recommend the combination of a fibric acid derivative and a HMG CoA reductase inhibitor until further work has been done on the safety of this combination, as there have been preliminary reports of severe myositis in non-diabetic patients receiving a combination of fibrate and an HMG CoA reductase inhibitor [36]. In isolated hypertriglyceridaemia associated with diabetes fibrate treatment may be associated with an increase in serum LDL cholesterol when initial cholesterol levels are low. In this situation it is important to monitor LDL levels during therapy.

Bile acid binding resins

Drugs of this class, e.g.colestipol and cholestyramine, when given in appropriate doses can lead to a reduction in LDL cholesterol of up to 30%. They bind intestinal bile acids, thus interrupting the enterohepatic circulation. As a result hepatic synthesis of bile acids from cholesterol is stimulated and this leads to an increased expression of hepatic LDL receptors and increased plasma LDL catabolism. A major advantage of the resins is that they are not absorbed from the intestinal tract but compliance is a problem because of a high frequency of gastrointestinal side effects, including a bloating sensation, nausea and constipation. To some extent these side effects can be overcome by starting resin treatment in low dosage.

Cholestyramine was the drug chosen for the Lipid Research Clinic Primary Prevention Trial in hypercholesterolaemic men and was associated with a reduction in coronary heart disease events [37]. Furthermore cholestyramine appeared safe in long-term usage. However there are certain properties of the resins that make this very useful class of drugs in the non-diabetic less useful in the diabetic population. Resin therapy may be associated with an increase in plasma triglyceride levels due to increased hepatic synthesis secondary to the removal of an inhibitory effect of bile salts. This may be a particular problem for the use of a resin in non-insulin-dependent diabetes where hepatic production of VLDL is already one of the major mechanisms of hyperlipidaemia. Furthermore, resin therapy is difficult when patients have to take other medications as resins can interfere with the absorption of various drugs. However, there is no doubt that resins may be effective in a small group of diabetic patients with isolated hypercholesterolaemia and normal triglyceride concentrations, particularly those with a coexistent familial hypercholesterolaemia.

Probucol

Probucol produces a modest reduction in total plasma cholesterol. It not only reduces plasma LDL cholesterol but also HDL cholesterol. For this reason probucol has remained a second or third line agent for the treatment of isolated hypercholesterolaemia. It has no effect on plasma triglyceride levels. The mechanism of action of the drug is not fully understood but it appears to reduce LDL cholesterol by increasing LDL clearance independent of the LDL receptor. It is possible that the incorporation of probucol to the lipid core of LDL leads to modification of LDL and subsequent increased removal by the liver through a receptor independent pathway. Despite the fact that probucol lowers HDL there are several reports suggesting that probucol therapy is associated with mobilisation of tissue and tendon deposits of cholesterol. Furthermore, probucol has potent antioxidant activities and has been shown to inhibit the oxidative modification of LDL and subsequently its interaction with monocyte macrophages. There is preliminary evidence in experimental animals that probucol, through this antioxidant effect, may have potential as an antiatherogenic agent [38]. However this needs to be confirmed. For the time being probucol cannot be considered a firstline agent for the treatment of the dyslipidaemia associated with diabetes but its antioxidant role needs to be further pursued and if this is confirmed then this drug and similar agents may have a potential beneficial effect in the prevention of atherosclerosis associated with diabetes.

Nicotinic acid and nicotinic acid derivatives

In high doses nicotinic acid effectively reduces plasma LDL and increases HDL levels through actions unrelated to its role as a vitamin. Nicotinic acid acts at several points in lipid and lipoprotein metabolism. It is antilipolytic inhibiting the release of free fatty acids from adipose tissue and consequently substrate flow for hepatic triglyceride synthesis. Hepatic production of VLDL is reduced with consequent reduction of plasma LDL. The inhibition of lipolysis no doubt contributes to the decreased hepatic VLDL production but additional possibilities include a direct effect on the production of apoprotein B in the liver and also decreased esterification of triglycerides. Nicotinic acid is considered a first line agent for the treatment of hyperlipidaemia, particularly in the United States, and if tolerated can produce reductions in plasma LDL cholesterol of up to 40% with an increase in HDL cholesterol of up to 20%. However large doses of nicotinic acid (3–6g) are needed for these effects to be seen and compliance is a problem because of troublesome side effects, particularly cutaneous flushing and gastrointestinal effects. There is a certain degree of tachyphylaxis to the flushing and aspirin may be effective in inhibiting the flush which appears to be mediated by prostaglandins. In addition to these side effects abnormalities of liver function may be observed together with an increase in uric acid and the precipitation of clinical gout. Nicotinic acid therapy may exacerbate peptic ulceration. However, nicotinic acid has shown favourable results in long-term prospective studies. In the Coronary Drug Project nicotinic acid therapy was associated with a decrease in the recurrence of myocardial infarction [39]. Furthermore in the 15-year follow-up of this study there was also a reduction in total mortality in those treated with nicotinic acid [40]. In combination with the resin colestipol nicotinic acid has been shown to have a beneficial effect on angiographically demonstrable atheroma plaques in patients following coronary artery bypass grafting [41].

Although useful in the treatment of primary hyperlipidaemia for the reasons stated, nicotinic acid cannot be recommended as firstline treatment in the diabetic population. Nicotinic acid therapy in non-insulin-dependent diabetes has been associated with a worsening of glycaemic control [42, 43]. The precise mechanism for this has yet to be fully worked out but may be related to increased insulin resistance. A nicotinic acid derivative, acipimox, does not lead to deterioration of glycaemic control in non-insulin-dependent diabetes and may be useful in the treatment of dyslipidaemia within the diabetic population.

Hydroxymethylglutaryl coenzyme A reductase inhibitors

The HMG-CoA reductase inhibitors are a new exciting class of hypolipidaemic agents. The first of this class of drugs, lovostatin, has been available in the United States for over two years and clinical experience is available for over 7 years. Other reductase inhibitors are becoming available worldwide including simvastatin and pravastatin. Drugs of this class are specific competitive inhibitors of HMG CoA reductase which is the rate-determining step in cholesterol synthesis. By reducing cholesterol synthesis LDL receptor expression is increased and therefore catabolism of LDL is increased, particularly via the liver. The catabolism of remnant particles is also increased. Slight increases in HDL cholesterol are seen with these agents, the mechanism of which remains obscure and often a mild to moderate effect in reducing plasma triglyceride is observed. There is no doubt that this class of drugs is highly effective and LDL cholesterol reductions of 40% are commonly observed. Generally the drugs are well tolerated and only minor side effects are observed including gastrointestinal upsets, mild and reversible changes in liver function tests, sleep disturbance, headache and skin rashes. The most serious problem to date with the reductase inhibitors has been a drug induced myopathy, occasionally resulting in rhabdomyolysis, myoglobinuria and acute renal failure. With monotherapy this complication is rare, and most of the cases of severe myopathy have been when the drugs have occurred used with other medications including cyclosporine, gemfibrozil and nicotinic acid or in patients with liver dysfunction [36].

These drugs may be particularly useful in diabetes and indeed are reported to produce substantial effects on LDL cholesterol, LDL apoprotein B and VLDL cholesterol in controlled clinical trials in non-insulin-dependent diabetes [44, 45]. HDL cholesterol was not altered in the studies reported so far in diabetes. Of particular relevance to the treatment of the non-insulin-dependent diabetic is that the reductase inhibitors have the potential to reduce the concentration of remnant particles. There does not appear to be any deleterious effect on glycaemic control thus far observed. An important subgroup of diabetics may derive particular benefit from reductase inhibitors and that is diabetics with hyperlipidaemia associated with proteinuria, either with full blown nephrotic syndrome or more chronic renal impairment. The use of fibrates in these patients is relatively contraindicated as they are renally excreted. On the other hand reductase inhibitors are principally excreted by the liver. They have been used in patients with nephrotic syndrome and moderate renal impairment in the non-diabetic population with safety and they should be of similar use in the diabetic population. Of course this group is particularly at high risk of premature vascular disease.

Summary and conclusions

The lipid and lipoprotein abnormalities associated with diabetes provide potential for effective therapeutic intervention designed to reduce the toll of cardiovascular disease in this population at particular high risk. Although primary prevention trials of lipid lowering are not available in the diabetic population the evidence is so overwhelming from studies in the non-diabetic population that attempts should be made by improved glycaemic control, nutritional counselling and where appropriate, hypolipidaemic drug therapy, to reduce lipid and lipoprotein levels within the diabetic patient towards optimum levels.

References

[1] Pyörala K, Laakso M, Uusitupa M. Diabetes and atherosclerosis: an epidemiologic view. Diabetes/Metabolism Rev 1987; 3: 463–524.

[2] Keen H, Jarrett RJ. The WHO Multinational Study of Vascular Disease in Diabetes: 2. Macrovascular disease prevalence. Diabetes Care 1979; 2: 187–195.

[3] Stamler J. Personal Communication. In Consensus Statement. Role of Cardiovascular Risk Factors in Prevention and Treatment of Macrovascular Disease in Diabetes. Diabetes Care 1989; 12: 573–579.
[4] Consensus Conference: Lowering blood cholesterol to prevent heart disease. J Am Med Assoc 1985; 253: 2080–2086.
[5] Study Group of the European Atherosclerosis Society. Strategies for the prevention of coronary heart disease, a policy statement of the European Atherosclerosis Society. Eur Heart J 1987; 8: 77–88.
[6] Alberti KGMM, Gries FA. Management of non-insulin-dependent diabetes mellitus in Europe: A consensus view. Diabetic Medicine 1988; 5: 275–281.
[7] Consensus Statement: Role of cardiovascular risk factors in prevention and treatment of macrovascular disease in diabetes. Diabetes Care 1989; 12: 573–579.
[8] Brown MS, Goldstein JL. Receptor-mediated control of cholesterol metabolism. Science 1976; 191: 150–154.
[9] Ross R. The pathogenesis of atherosclerosis – an update. N Engl J Med 1986; 314: 488–500.
[10] Goldstein JL, Ho YK, Basu SK et al. Binding site on macrophages that mediates uptake and degradation of acetylated low density lipoprotein producing massive cholesterol deposition. Proc Natl Acad Sci 1979; 76: 333–337.
[11] Steinberg D, Parthasarathy S, Carew TE et al. Beyond cholesterol. Modifications of low density lipoprotein that increase its atherogenicity. N Engl J Med 1989; 320: 915–924.
[12] Kodama T, Freeman M, Rohner L et al. Type 1 macrophage scavenger receptor contains α-helical and collagen-like coils. Nature 1990; 343: 531–535.
[13] Miller NE. High density lipoprotein: a major risk factor for coronary atherosclerosis. In: Shepherd J, ed. Lipoprotein Metabolism. Clinical Endocrinology and Metabolism, vol 1 no.3. London: Bailliere, Tindall, 1987; 603–622.
[14] Betteridge DJ. High density lipoprotein and coronary heart disease. Br Med J 1989; 298: 974–975.
[15] Hulley SB, Rosenman RH, Bawal RD et al. Epidemiology as a guide to clinical decisions. The association between triglyceride and coronary heart disease. N Engl J Med 1980; 302: 1383–1389.
[16] Castelli WP. The triglyceride issue: a view from Framingham. Am Heart J 1986; 12: 432–437.
[17] Cambien F, Jacqueson A, Richard JL et al. Is the level of serum triglyceride a significant predictor of coronary death in 'normocholesterolaemic' subjects? The Paris Prospective Study. Am J of Epidemiol 1986; 124: 624–632.
[18] West KM, Ahuja MMS, Bennett PH et al. The role of circulating glucose and triglyceride concentrations, and their interactions with other 'risk factors' as determinants of arterial disease in nine diabetic population samples from the WHO Multinational Study.
[19] Fontbonne A, Eschwege E, Cambien F et al. Hypertriglyceridaemia as a risk factor of coronary heart disease mortality in subjects with impaired glucose tolerance or diabetes. Results from the 11-year follow-up of the Paris Prospective Study. Diabetologia 1989; 32: 300–304.
[20] Morganroth J, Levy RI, Frederickson DS. The biochemical, clinical and genetic features of type III hyperlipidaemia. Ann Intern Med 1975; 82: 158–174.
[21] Weisweiler P, Drosner M, Schwandt P. Dietary effects on very low density lipoprotein in Type 2 (non-insulin-dependent) diabetes mellitus. Diabetologia 1982; 23: 101–104.
[22] Pietri AO, Dunn FL, Grundy SM et al. The effect of continuous subcutaneous insulin infusion on very low density lipoprotein triglyceride metabolism in type 1 diabetes mellitus. Diabetes 1983; 32: 75–81.
[23] Howard BV. Lipoprotein metabolism in diabetes mellitus. J Lipid Res 1987; 28: 613–628.

[24] Betteridge DJ. Lipids, diabetes and vascular disease: the time to act. Diabetic Medicine 1989; 6: 195–218.
[25] Friedewald WT, Levy RI, Frederickson DS. Estimation of the concentration of low density lipoprotein cholesterol in plasma without use of the preparative ultracentrifuge. Clin Chem 1972; 18: 499–502.
[26] Hollenbeck CB, Coulston AM. Effect of variation in diet on lipoprotein metabolism in patients with diabetes mellitus. Diabetes/Metabolism Reviews 1987; 3 (no. 3): 669–689.
[27] Garg A, Bonanome A, Grundy SM et al. Comparison of a high-carbohydrate diet with a high monounsaturated fat diet in patients with non-insulin dependent diabetes mellitus. N Engl J Ned 1988; 319: 829–834.
[28] Phillipson Be, Rothrock DW, Connor WE et al. Reduction of plasma lipids, lipoproteins and apoproteins by dietary fish oils in patients with hypertriglyceridaemia. N Engl J Med 1985; 312: 1210–1216.
[29] Glauber H, Wallace P, Griver K et al. Adverse metabolic effects of omega-3 fatty acids in non-insulin-dependent diabetes mellitus. Ann Intern Med 1988; 108: 663–668.
[30] Haines AP, Sanders TAB, Imeson JD et al. Effects of a fish oil supplement on platelet function, haemostatic variables and albuminurias in insulin-dependent diabetics. Thrombosis Res 1986; 43: 643–655.
[31] Bonanome A, Grundy SM. Effect of dietary stearic acid on plasma cholesterol and lipoprotein levels. N Engl J Med 1988; 318: 1244–1248.
[32] Lopes-Virella MF, Colwell JA. Pharmacological treatment of lipid disorders in diabetes mellitus. Diabetes/Metabolism Reviews 1987; 3 (no. 3): 691–722.
[33] Garg A, Grundy SM. Management of dyslipidaemia in NIDDM. Diabetes Care 1990; 13: 153–158.
[34] Winocour PH, Laker MF. Drug therapy for diabetic dyslipoproteinaemia: a practical approach. Diabetic Medicine 1990; 7: 292–298.
[35] Frick MH, Elo O, Haapa K et al. Helsinki Heart Study: primary prevention trial with gemfibrozil in middle aged men with dyslipidaemia. N Engl J Med 1987; 317: 1237–1245.
[36] Tobert JA. Efficacy and long-term adverse effect pattern of lovastatin. Am J Cardiol 1988; 62: 28J-34J.
[37] Lipid Research Clinics Programme. The Lipid Research Coronary Primary Prevention Trial. Results I and II. J Am Med Assoc 1984; 1251: 351–374.
[38] Carew TE, Schwenke DC, Steinberg D. Anti-atherogenic effect of probucol unrelated to its hypocholesterolaemic effect: evidence that antioxidants in vivo can selectively inhibit low density lipoprotein degradation in macrophage-rich fatty streaks and slow the progression of atherosclerosis in the Watanabe heritable hyperlipidaemic rabbit. Proc Natl Acad Sci USA 1987; 84: 7725–7729.
[39] Coronary Drug Project Research Group: Clofibrate and niacin in coronary heart disease. JAmA 1975; 231: 360–381.
[40] Canner PL, Berge KG, Wenger NK et al. Fifteen year mortality in coronary drug project patients: long term benefit with niacin. J Am Coll Cardiol 1986; 8: 1245–1255.
[41] Blankenhorn DH, Nessum SA, Johnson RL. Beneficial effects of combined cholesterol-niacin therapy on coronary atherosclerosis and coronary bypass grafts. J Am Med Assoc 1987; 257: 3233–3240.
[42] Miettinen TA, Taskinen M-R, Pelkonen R et al. Glucose tolerance and plasma insulin in man during acute and chronic administration of nicotinic acid. Acta Med Scand 1969; 186: 247–253.
[43] Molnar ED, Berge Ke, Rosevear JW et al. The effect of nicotinic acid in diabetes mellitus. Metabolism 1964; 13: 181–189.
[44] Garg A, Grundy SM. Lovastatin for lowering cholesterol levels in non-insulin-dependent diabetes mellitus. N Engl J Med 1988; 318: 81–86.
[45] Garg A, Grundy SM. Gemfibrozil alone and in combination with lovastatin for treatment of hypertriglyceridaemia in NIDDM. Diabetes 1989; 38: 364–372.

Fish oil administration in diabetes

T. Jensen

Introduction

In the late-1970s Dyerberg et al. observed that Greenland Eskimos with a traditionally high consumption of seal and other seafoods have a low prevalence of atherosclerosis and a low mortality of myocardial infarction [1]. They suggested that dietary fish had some properties that could potentially prevent coronary artery disease, and they claimed that the long-chain n-3 polyunsaturated fatty acids eicosapentaenoic acid (C 20:5 n-3) and docosahexaenoic acid (C 22:6 n-3) were the active components of fish. Their findings stimulated a number of experimental and clinical studies revealing that n-3 fatty acids have potentially antiatheromatous effects [2, 3], and recently, epidemiological and intervention studies have shown an inverse dose-response relation between fish consumption and death from coronary heart disease [4, 5].

Since atherosclerotic vascular disease is a major cause of morbidity and mortality in patients with diabetes mellitus [6–8], the effects of fish oil on cardiovascular risk factors have recently been evaluated in these patients [9, 10]. Although it seems clear that some of the beneficial effects of fish oil are the same in diabetic patients as in nondiabetic subjects, the close relationship between lipid and glucose metabolism and the possible different pathophysiological mechanisms involved in atherogenesis in diabetic patients as compared with nondiabetic subjects preclude extrapolation of all findings in the nondiabetic population to patients with diabetes mellitus [11, 12]. Moreover, the effects of n-3 fatty acids are apparently different in patients with insulin-dependent or non-insulin-dependent diabetes mellitus and in patients with or without microvascular complications.

The purpose of this chapter is to discuss the perspectives of n-3 fatty acids in the prevention and treatment of atherosclerotic vascular disease in diabetic patients. The present knowledge of the beneficial and potentially deleterious effects of n-3 fatty acids will be described and attempts to identify subgroups of patients in whom dietary fish most safely may be recommended will be proposed.

The effects of n-3 polyunsaturated fatty acids

Mechanisms of action

Marine phytoplankton and zooplankton are able to elongate and desaturate the polyunsaturated fatty acid alpha-linolenic acid to eicosapentaenoic acid (Fig. 1). The fatty acids enter the food chain and cold water fish such as mackerel and herring are the main sources of these polyunsaturated fatty acids.

A number of established and hypothetical cardiovascular risk factors are affected by n-3 fatty acids. In most studies they reduce plasma triglyceride and very low density lipoprotein (VLDL) cholesterol [3, 13]. In contrast, the effects of fish oil consumption on low density lipoprotein (LDL) cholesterol

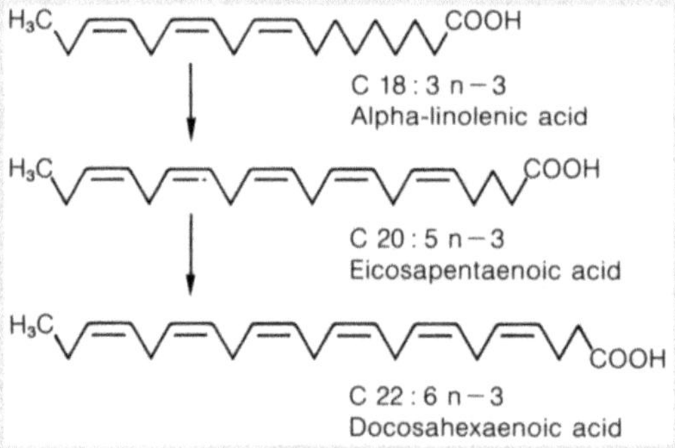

Fig. 1 Structure and synthesis of n-3 polyunsaturated fatty acids. The synthesis of eicosapentaenoic acid from alpha-linolenic acid. As an example, in eicosapentaenoic acid C 20 indicates the number of carbon atoms, 5 indicates the number of carbon-carbon double bonds and n-3 denotes the number of carbon atoms from the methyl end to the first double bond.

and high density lipoprotein (HDL) cholesterol have been inconsistent, possibly reflecting differences in the characteristics of the patients studied and in the various brands and dosages of fish oil used. However, in at least three separate studies a paradoxical elevation of LDL cholesterol levels were noted [9, 14, 15] and Thiery et al. recently reported that supplementation with fish oil resulted in enhancement of atherosclerosis in rabbits [16]. In all of these studies, a whole-fish-oil concentrate with a relatively high proportion of saturated fatty acids was used.

Eicosapentaenoic acid is both a substrate and an inhibitor of the cyclo-oxygenase pathway [17] which metabolites arachidonic acid to prostaglandins and thromboxane A_2. It thereby reduces the production of the platelet aggregating thromboxane A_2 and increases the production of the vasodilatory prostaglandin I_3 [18, 19]. The net result is a change in hemodynamic balance towards a more vasodilatory state, with less platelet aggregation. These effects together with reduced blood viscosity [20], reduced vasospastic response to catecholamines and angiotensin [21], and increased activity of endothelium-derived relaxation factor [22], may all explain the antihypertensive action of fish oil observed in most studies [23, 24]. The n-3 fatty acids are also incorporated in cell membrane phospholipids and may modify receptors, transport pathways and enzymes related to cell surfaces [25].

Possible prevention of atherosclerosis

A number of animal studies have provided considerable evidence that fish oil prevents atherosclerosis. Weiner et al. found that dietary supplementation with 30 ml cod liver oil daily for 8 months in a hyperlipidemic swine model markedly retarded progression of coronary atherosclerosis [2]. The protective effect of cod liver oil was unrelated to changes in plasma concentration of lipoproteins, but associated with platelet arachidonic acid content and serum thromboxane B_2. They hypothesized that n-3 fatty acids mainly inhibit platelet-endothelial cell interaction or have a direct protective effect on the vascular wall. Similar preventive effect of fish oil on the progression of atherosclerosis have been described in dogs [26] and monkeys [27]. With the increasing evidence that atherosclerosis starts with damage to the endothelium with subsequent platelet activation and release of chemoattractants and growth factors, efforts to intervene against these early steps in atherosclerosis seem attractive [28].

In a retrospective epidemiologic study, Kromhout et al. found a strong inverse relation between fish consumption during a 20-year period and coronary artery disease [4]. Other studies have found similar inverse relations between intake of fish and cardiovascular mortality [29, 30]. Interestingly, in the study by Kromhout et al., the relation between intake of fish and coronary artery disease was apparent even with the consumption of small amounts of n-3 fatty acids, suggesting that the intake of 100–150 g fish per week over long periods has beneficial biological effects. Recently, Burr et al., in a 2-year prospective intervention study found that the intake of 200–400 g fish per week significantly reduced the overall mortality in men who had recovered from myocardial infarction [5].

Diabetes mellitus and n-3 fatty acids

Beneficial and potential deleterious effects

In 1986 Haines et al. published the first detailed study of the effects of fish oil supplementation in 41 insulin-dependent diabetic patients [9]. They gave 19 patients 15 g fish oil (MaxEpa) daily and 22 patients 0.6 g olive oil daily for six weeks and found a significant reduction in platelet thromboxane production and a significant increase in LDL cholesterol during fish oil supplementation compared with olive oil supplementation. No changes were noted in blood pressure or glycosylated hemoglobin in that study. The increase in LDL cholesterol was unexpected and the authors proposed that fish oil supplementation might hasten the conversion of VLDL cholesterol to LDL cholesterol [31], or alternatively it could be the saturated fat (approximately 30%) in MaxEpa that was responsible for the rise in LDL cholesterol. Also, Tilvis et al. found reduced platelet thromboxane production during fish oil supplementation in insulin-dependent diabetic women [32]. In a smaller study of insulin-dependent diabetic patients, Miller et al. found no changes in LDL cholesterol, fasting blood glucose or glycosylated hemoglobin during dietary supplementation with 20 g MaxEpa daily for eight weeks [33]. Recently, in a double-blind crossover study from the Steno Memorial Hospital, it was found that dietary supplementation with cod-liver oil significantly reduced the blood pressure from 146/90 mmHg to 139/85 mmHg in albuminuric insulin-dependent diabetic patients [34]. During cod-liver oil supplementation the HDL cholesterol increased and thc VLDL cholesterol and triglyceride decreased. No changes were observed in glomerular filtration rate, degree of albuminuria or glycosylated hemoglobin during supplementation with cod-liver oil.

Non-insulin dependent diabetes mellitus is often associated with hypertriglyceridemia [35] suggesting a close relationship between hypertriglyceridemia and insulin resistance [36] and between glucose and lipid metabolism [37]. Since reduction in plasma triglyceride and VLDL cholesterol concentration has been observed in most fish oil trials [3, 13], the metabolic effects of dietary n-3 fatty acid supplementation has also been studied in non-insulin-dependent diabetes mellitus. The triglyceride-lowering effect of 8 – 15 g fish oil capsules daily was confirmed in three separate studies [38 – 40], whereas in one study n-3 fatty acid decreased serum triglyceride only in patients with hypertriglyceridemia [10]. However, in two studies the serum apoprotein B concentration significantly increased after fish oil supplementation [10, 38]. The mechanism of the paradoxical increase in apoprotein B concentration is unknown, but the finding may represent modification in the VLDL composition facilitating VLDL conversion to LDL. However, because LDL apoprotein B levels correlate directly with the presence of coronary artery disease, these elevations may be unfavorable regardless of the underlying mechanisms [41]. Other adverse metabolic effects of n-3 fatty acids have been found in non-insulin-dependent diabetes mellitus. In a detailed study, Glauber et al. found elevated basal hepatic glucose output and impaired insulin secretion but unchanged peripheral glucose disposal in six non-insulin-dependent diabetic men after the intake of 18 g fish oil concentrate daily for one month [39]. Similarly, Friday et al. found impaired glucose hemostasis after fish oil supplementation in patients with non-insulin-dependent diabetes mellitus [40]. Thus, although uncontrolled, these reports have stressed the importance of more studies to clarify whether n-3 fatty acid supplementation will have any place in the prevention of vascular complications in non-insulin-dependent diabetes mellitus.

Future perspectives and recommendations of n-3 fatty acids in diabetes mellitus

Not all diabetic patients are at same the risk of cardiovascular disease. The increased mortality of cardiovascular disease is for the most part explained by an exremely high mortality in the subgroup of patients developing clinical nephropathy [42, 43]. These patients have a number of established cardiovascular risk factors such as atherogenic changes in plasma lipoproteins [44] and elevated blood pressure [45]. They also have signs of vascular vulnerability. The permeability of the whole vascular bed is clearly elevated in patients with incipient and clinical nephropathy [46], and recently, elevated plasma levels of von Willebrand factor and impaired fibrinolytic response to exercise have been demonstrated in these patients, suggesting that they have endothelial cell dysfunction or damage (Fig. 2) [47]. Apart from beneficial effects on blood pressure and plasma concentrations of lipoproteins, cod-liver oil intake also resulted in partial normalization of the elevated vascular permeability in albuminuric patients [34]. In support of a direct protective

	Risk factor	
Arterial lumen	Elevated blood pressure	(*)
	Atherogenic changes in plasma concentrations of lipids and lipoproteins	(*)
	Platelet hyperreactivity	(*)
	Increased blood viscosity	(*)
Endothelial cells	Increased permeability	(*)
	Reduced fibrinolytic capacity	
	Increased release of von Willebrand factor	

Fig. 2 Established and hypothetical cardiovascular risk factors in the arterial lumen or the endothelial cells in insulin-dependent diabetic patients with albuminuria. Risk factors modifiable by omega-3 fatty acids are marked with an asterisk.

effect of dietary fish on the vascular wall, Wahlquist et al. recently reported that diabetic fish eaters have higher arterial compliance compared with diabetic non-fish eaters [48]. Thus, although the many diverse effects of n-3 fatty acids are far from clarified in insulin-dependent diabetic patients with albuminuria, the intervention on several clustered risk factors in these high risk patients is very attractive. However, only future studies can settle whether long-term intake of n-3 fatty acids will be effective in prevention of atherosclerosis.

In contrast, it still seems premature to start long-term intervention studies of dietary fish oil supplementation in non-insulin-dependent diabetes mellitus. Most deleterious effects of n-3 fatty acids have been found in such patients and before long-term studies can be initiated we need to know more about the biochemical and metabolic consequences of increased intake of fish oil in non-insulin-dependent diabetes mellitus.

In the future, more studies of the effects of n-3 fatty acids on the development of microvascular complications are expected. Recent animal studies have suggested that fish oils may have protective effects on the development of diabetic cardiomyopathy [49] and on the progression of renal disease [50]. However, it is still preliminary to say whether such effects can be extrapolated to humans.

In conclusion, the effects of dietary supplementation with fish oils are different in diabetic patients as compared with non-diabetic subjects. Most beneficial effects are seen in insulin-dependent diabetic patients with albuminuria; in contrast most deleterious effects are seen in non-insulin-dependent patients. Insulin-dependent diabetic patients with albuminuria have a number of established and hypothetical cardiovascular risk factors and constitute a high risk group for early cardiovascular death. Therefore, long-term fish oil studies, intervening on several clustered risk factors seem attractive in such patients.

References

[1] Dyerberg J, Bang HO. Hemostatic function and platelet polyunsaturated fatty acids in Eskimos. Lancet 1979; 2: 433–435.
[2] Weiner BH, Ockene IS, Levine PH et al. Inhibition of atherosclerosis by cod liver oil in a hyperlipidemic swine model. N Engl J Med 1986; 315: 841–846.
[3] Phillipson BE, Rotherock DW, Connor WE et al. Reduction of plasma lipids, lipoproteins, and apoproteins by dietary fish oils in patients with hypertriglyceridemia. N Engl J Med 1985; 312: 1210–1216.
[4] Kromhout D, Bosschieter ED, de Lezenne Coulander C. The inverse relation between fish consumption and 20-year mortality from coronary heart disease. N Engl J Med 1985; 312: 1205–1209.
[5] Burr ML, Fehily AM, Gilbert JF et al. Effects of changes in fat, fish, and fibre intakes on death and myocardial reinfarction: Diet and Reinfarction Trial (DART). Lancet 1989; 2: 757–761.
[6] Kannel WB, McGee DL. Diabetes and vascular disease. The Framingham Study. JAMA 1979; 241: 2035–2038.
[7] Jarrett RJ, McCartney P, Keen H. The Bedford Survey: Ten years mortality rates in newly diagnosed diabetics, borderline diabetics and normoglycaemic controls and risk indices for coronary heart disease in borderline diabetics. Diabetologia 1982; 22: 79–84.
[8] Fuller JH, Shipley MJ, Rose G et al. Mortality from coronary heart disease and stroke in relation to degree of glycaemia: The Whitehall Study. Br Med J 1983; 287: 867–870.
[9] Haines AP, Sanders TAB, Imeson JD et al. Effects of a fish oil supplement on platelet function, haemostatic variables and albuminuria in insulin-dependent diabetics. Thromb Res 1986; 43: 643–655.
[10] Kasim SE, Stern B, Khilnani S et al. Effects of omega-3 fish oils on lipid metabolism, glycaemic control, and blood pressure in type II diabetic patients. J Clin Endocrinol Metab 1988; 67: 1–5.
[11] Sorisky A, Robbins DC. Fish oil and diabetes. The net effect. Diabetes Care 1989; 12: 302–304.
[12] Axelrod L. Omega-3 fatty acids in diabetes mellitus. Gift from the sea? Diabetes 1989; 38: 539–543.
[13] Mehta JL, Lopez LM, Lawson D et al. Dietary supplementation with omega-3 polyunsaturated fatty acids in patients with stable coronary heart disease: effects on indices of platelet and neutrophil function and exercise performance. Am J Med 1988; 84: 45–52.
[14] Demke DM, Peters GR, Linet OI et al. Effects of a fish oil concentrate in patients with hypercholesterolemia. Atherosclerosis 1988; 70: 73–80.
[15] Sullivan DR, Sanders TA, Trayner IM et al. Paradoxical elevation of LDL apoprotein B levels in hypertriglyceridemic patients and normal subjects ingesting fish oil. Atherosclerosis 1986; 61: 129–134.
[16] Thiery J, Seidel D. Fish oil feeding results in an enhancement of cholesterol-induced atherosclerosis in rabbits. Atherosclerosis 1987; 63: 53–56.
[17] Needleman P, Raz A, Minkes MS et al. Triene prostaglandins: prostaglandin and thromboxane biosynthesis and unique biological properties. Proc Natl Acad Sci 1979; 76: 944–948.
[18] Siess W, Roth P, Scherer B et al. Platelet-membrane fatty acids, platelet aggregation, and thromboxane formation during a mackerel diet. Lancet 1980; 1: 441–444.

[19] Fischer S, Weber PC. Prostaglandin I_3 is formed in vivo in man after dietary eicosapentaenoic acid. Nature 1984; 307: 165–168.
[20] Popp-Snijders C, Schouten JA, van der Meer J et al. Fatty fish-induced changes in membrane lipid composition and viscosity of human erythrocyte suspensions. Scand J Clin Lab Invest 1986; 46: 253–258.
[21] Lorenz R, Spengler U, Fischer S et al. Platelet function, thromboxane formation and blood pressure control during supplementation of the Western diet with cod liver oil. Circulation 1983; 67: 504–511.
[22] Shimokawa H, Lam JY, Chesebro JH et al. Effects of dietary supplementation with cod-liver oil on endothelium-dependent responses in porcine coronary arteries. Circulation 1987; 76: 898–905.
[23] Mortensen JZ, Schmidt EB, Nielsen AH et al. The effects of n-6 and n-3 polyunsaturated fatty acids on hemostasis, blood lipids and blood pressure. Thromb Haemost 1983; 50: 543–546.
[24] Norris PG, Jones CH, Weston MJ. Effect of dietary supplementation with fish oil on systolic blood pressure in mild essential hypertension. Br Med J 1986; 293: 104–105.
[25] Leaf A, Weber PC. Cardiovascular effects of n-3 fatty acids. N Engl J Med 1988; 318: 549–557.
[26] Landymore RW, MacAulay M, Sheridan B et al. Comparison of cod-liver oil and aspirin-dipyridamole for the prevention of intimal hyperplasia in autologous vein grafts. Ann Thorac Surg 1986; 41: 54–57.
[27] Davis HR, Bridenstine RT, Vesselinovitch D et al. Fish oil inhibits development of atherosclerosis in rhesus monkeys. Atherosclerosis 1987; 7: 441–449.
[28] Ross R. The pathogenesis of atherosclerosis: an update. N Engl J Med 1986; 314: 488–500.
[29] Shekelle RB, Missell LV, Paul O et al. Fish consumption and mortality from coronary heart disease. N Engl J Med 1985; 313: 820.
[30] Norell SE, Ahlbom A, Feychting M et al. Fish consumption and mortality from coronary heart disease. Br Med J 1986; 293: 426.
[31] Rose HG, Haft GK, Juliano J. Clofibrate-induced low density lipoprotein elevation. Therapeutic implications and treatment by cholestipol resin. Atherosclerosis 1976; 23: 413–427.
[32] Telvis RS, Rasi V, Viinikka L et al. Effects of purified fish oil on platelet lipids and function in diabetic women. Clin Chim Acta 1987; 164: 315–322.
[33] Miller ME, Anagnostou AA, Ley B et al. Effects of fish oil concentrates on hemorheological and hemostatic aspects of diabetes mellitus: A preliminary study. Thromb Res 1987; 47: 201–214.
[34] Jensen T, Stender S, Goldstein K et al. Partial normalization by dietary cod-liver oil of increased microvascular albumin leakage in patients with insulin-dependent diabetes and albuminuria. N Engl J Med 1989; 321: 1572–1577.
[35] Goldberg RB. Lipid disorders in diabetes. Diabetes Care 1981; 4: 561–572.
[36] Steiner G, Morita S, Vranic M. Resistance to insulin but not to glucagon in lean human hypertriglyceridemics. Diabetes 1980; 29: 899–905.
[37] Lillioja S, Bogardus C, Mott DM et al. Relationship between insulin-mediated glucose disposal and lipid metabolism in man. J Clin Invest 1985; 75: 1106–1115.
[38] Schectman G, Kaul S, Kissebah AH. Effect of fish oil concentrate on lipoprotein composition in NIDDM. Diabetes 1988; 37: 1567–1573.
[39] Glauber H, Wallace P, Griver K et al. Adverse metabolic effect of omega-3 fatty acids in non-insulin-dependent diabetes mellitus. Ann Intern Med 1988; 108: 663–668.
[40] Friday KE, Childs MT, Tsunehara CH et al. Elevated plasma glucose and lowered triglyceride levels from omega-3 fatty acid supplementation in type II diabetes. Diabetes Care 1989; 12: 276–281.
[41] Avogaro P, Bon GB, Cassolato G et al. Are apolipoproteins better determinators than lipid for atherosclerosis? Lancet 1979; 1: 901–903.

[42] Borch-Johnsen K, Kreiner S. Proteinuria: value as predictor of cardiovascular mortality in insulin-dependent diabetes mellitus. Br Med J 1987; 294: 1651–1654.
[43] Jensen T, Borch-Johnsen K, Kofoed-Enevoldsen A et al. Coronary heart disease in young type 1 (insulin-dependent) diabetic patients with and without diabetic nephropathy: Incidence and risk factors. Diabetologia 1987; 30: 144–148.
[44] Jensen T, Stender S, Deckert T. Abnormalities in plasma concentrations of lipoproteins and fibrinogen in type 1 (insulin-dependent) diabetic patients with increased urinary albumin excretion. Diabetologia 1988; 31: 142–145.
[45] Feldt-Rasmussen B, Borch-Johnsen K, Mathiesen ER. Hypertension in diabetes as related to nephropathy. Early blood pressure changes. Hypertension 1985; 7(suppl II): 18–20.
[46] Feldt-Rasmussen B. Increased transcapillary escape rate of albumin in type 1 (insulin-dependent) diabetic patients with microalbuminuria. Diabetologia 1986; 29: 282–286.
[47] Jensen T, Bjerre-Knudsen J, Feldt-Rasmussen B et al. Features of endothelial dysfunction in early diabetic nephropathy. Lancet 1989; 1: 461–463.
[48] Wahlqvist ML, Lo CS, Myers KA. Fish intake and arterial wall characteristics in healthy people and diabetic patients. Lancet 1989; 1: 944–946.
[49] Black SC, Katz S, McNeill JH. Cardiac performance and plasma lipids of omega-3 fatty acid-treated streptozocin-induced diabetic rats. Diabetes 1989; 38: 969–974.
[50] Ito Y, Barcelli U, Yamashita W et al. Fish oil has beneficial effects on lipids and renal disease in nephrotic rats. Metabolism 1988; 37: 352–357.

The pharmacological treatment of obesity and diabetes mellitus

S. C. Bain, P. M. Dodson

Introduction

The plethora of articles on dieting in the popular press bears testament to the importance that the general public attach to weight reduction. Although the motivation for this interest is more likely to be social than scientific there are good medical reasons for prevention and treatment of obesity.

The desirable range of weight for height in adults, defined by the body mass index, is 20 – 25 kg/m^2 [weight/height^2] [1]. A body mass index (BMI) over 28.5 kg/m^2 is a marker for coronary risk factors, such as raised serum cholesterol and hypertension [2]. As the BMI increases above this level all-cause mortality in men shows a progressive rise [3]. Obesity may also precipitate or aggravate many disorders, including hypertension, osteoarthritis, hiatus hernia, diabetes and hyperlipidaemia [4].

Obesity is associated with insulin resistance in the non-diabetic population and many newly presenting non-insulin-dependent diabetics are overweight [5]. In our clinic 64% of patients referred for management of non-insulin-dependent diabetes (NIDDM) have a BMI greater than 28 kg/m^2. Dietary modification has a key role in the treatment of patients with both insulin-dependent diabetes (IDDM) and NIDDM. For a large proportion of NIDDM patients, dietary change is sufficient to control the major metabolic abnormalities associated with the condition. This is especially the case for obese NIDDM subjects in whom weight reduction alone may normalise carbohydrate tolerance.

In the overweight diabetic the initial aim is to achieve weight loss by energy restriction. Dietary recall histories are often used to assess the energy intake at presentation and a deduction of 500 kcal from this figure determines the recommended energy intake. The aim is to promote weight loss of 1 – 2 kg/month. Unfortunately, this method consistently underestimates daily energy intake (by as much as 800 kcals) and this leads to recommendations that are unrealistic. This may account for poor dietary compliance in some patients.

It is possible to calculate the energy intake of a weight-stable individual using a nomogram, in which age, sex, exercise status and body mass are taken into account [6]. A realistic weight-reducing diet aims for an energy deficit of not more than 500 kcal from this calculated intake.

When placed on a low energy diet in a controlled environment all obese patients lose weight. In the clinical setting, despite realistic dietary targets, a substantial proportion of obese diabetics do not achieve weight reduction. This presumably reflects poor compliance with dietary advice, however the fact remains that the obese diabetic is at high risk of premature cardiovascular disease. The attainment of ideal body weight (IBW) should remain a major aim of therapy in those in whom diet has failed and this group should not be denied other treatments.

In those patients who are regarded as dietary failures second line therapy may be tried as an adjunct to continued attempts at low energy intake. These include behavioural therapy, surgical techniques and pharmacologic agents. Behaviour therapy is aimed at the identification and avoidance of cues that promote eating. Excellent results have been achieved but at great cost in time to both therapist and patients [7]. Surgical procedures include jaw wiring, tying nylon cord around the patients waist, partial gastroplasty and ileo-jejunal bypass [8]. None of these techniques are widely used and ileo-jejunal surgery has fallen into disrepute due to the mechanical and metabolic complications that may ensue.

Although the general public are keen to take medication which might aid their pursuit of thinness the medical profession has been slow to acquiesce to this demand. There are various reasons for this. Firstly, many appetite suppressants are central nervous stimulants, related to amphetamine. The addictive properties of this drug, and others in the group, have rightly caused concern amongst medical practitioners. Secondly, evidence that weight reduction achieved by any method, including drug therapy, reduces mortality is not yet available. Assessment of a risk to benefit ratio for anorectic agents is therefore impossible. Finally there is the stigma of obesity. Many perceive the obese to be lazy, lacking willpower, and suffering from a self-inflicted condition. The use of potentially addictive drugs in such circumstances meets with resistance.

As a consequence, the demands made of anorectic agents have been more stringent than has been the case with other medications. Plateauing of weight loss after a period of treatment is termed 'tolerance' whilst the regaining of lost weight after cessation of therapy is regarded as an indication of treatment failure. Both oral hypoglycaemic drugs and antihypertensive agents have these same "failings" and yet both are widely prescribed. Perhaps a major hurdle, yet to be overcome, is the acceptance of obesity as a chronic condition requiring long-term (perhaps lifelong) therapy. Indeed, the British National Formularly (BNF) still recommends that anorectic preparations should not be given for more than a 3–6 month period [9].

There is undoubtedly a resurgence of interest in anorectic agents and clinicians will be under increasing pressure from both patients and pharmaceutical companies to prescribe these drugs. This will especially be the case in conditions such as diabetes where weight regulation is such an important aspect of treatment. This chapter will deal with the agents that are currently used in the treatment of obesity and those which have a theoretical role in therapy. Reference will be made to studies that have been performed in diabetic patients. Further discussion will consider the effect that drugs used in the treatment of diabetes may have on body mass.

Agents used for the treatment of obesity that may be used in diabetics

Drugs which act on the central nervous system

Drugs acting on catecholamine receptors: Most centrally acting anorectic agents are derivatives of phenylethylamine (eg. phenteramine, diethylpropion), the exception being mazindol, an imidazoisoindole. These drugs have sympathomimetic effects and belong to the same category as amphetamine. The Food and Drug Administration reviewed the effectiveness of 'amphetamine-like drugs' in 1975, analysing 105 studies [10] . Drug-treated patients lost an average of 0.25kg per week more than those taking placebo and were nearly twice as likely to achieve a weight reduction of 0.45kg per week. There were no significant differences between any of the active drugs under consideration.

With regard to safety, experiments in primates have examined the reinforcing properties of intravenous preparations of these agents and compared them with the reduction in food intake [11]. The ratio of anorexiant dose to reinforcing dose has been used as a measure of abuse potential. These studies confirm the clinical impression that phenteramine and fenfluramine are rarely addictive but suggest that diethylpropion should have a high abuse potential. This has not proved to be the case in clinical practice, although addiction has been reported [12].

In the U.K. three sympathomimetic agents (diethylpropion, mazindol, and phenteramine) are marketed for use in the treatment of obesity. The BNF states that their use "is not justified as any possible benefits are outweighed by the risks involved" [9].

Agents acting on the serotonin (5HT) receptor: A number of compounds are available whose net effect is to facilitate 5HT synaptic activity. These include fenfluramine, fluoxetine, and femoxatine. There appears to be a link between serotonin and weight regulation [13]. Serotonergic systems occupy a strategic anatomical location in the brain, projecting to and passing through the hypothalamus, and they are also widely distributed in the gut. These compounds have been shown to inhibit food consumption, an effect consistent with the hypothesis that enhancing central serotoninergic transmission causes anorexia.

Fenfluramine has been shown to release serotonin from nerve endings and inhibit reuptake into the neurone. Compounds which interfere with the synthesis of 5-HT or its synaptic transmission inhibit fenfluramine's anorexic action. Despite its sedative effects fenfluramine was, until recently, grouped with the central nervous stimulants because of its structural similarity to phenylethylamine. However, in laboratory animals the anorexic effect of fenfluramine can be dissociated from that of amphetamine, implying a separate mechanism [14].

The characteristic effect of fenfluramine in laboratory animals is a reduction in food intake without change in activity status [13]. In particular the drug appears to prolong the state of satiety and activate a system which brings feeding to a close. Fluoxetine, a more specific inhibitor of serotonin reuptake, has been shown to have similar effects. In addition to an effect on total food intake it has been suggested that 5-HT also plays a role in the selection of macronutrients, particularly protein and carbohydrate. In experimental conditions both fenfluramine and fenoxetine have been shown to suppress food intake whilst sparing protein consumption [15].

The presence of 5-HT receptors in the gut invites the suggestion that part of the reduction in food consumption may be due to a peripheral effect. The contribution made by alterations in gut 5-HT have not been extensively studied but it appears that fenfluramine slows gastric emptying in human subjects [16].

Fenfluramine has been shown to be effective in obese subjects in placebo-controlled clinical trials, although these have tended to be of short duration. In one study, fenfluramine was administered to 176 patients for 12 months and compared with diet alone [17]. Subjects were then followed for a further year on no therapy. A plateau of weight loss occurred between the eighth and 12th month and weight remained 10–11 kg lower for the remainder of the year. When treatment was stopped the patients regained weight over the following twelve months. Similarly fluoxetine, marketed as an antidepressant, has been shown to produce weight loss in depressed and non-depressed obese subjects [18].

Unfortunately fenfluramine may cause a number of unpleasant side- effects [19]. These include dry mouth, abdominal pain and diarrhoea. Alopecia has been reported and drowsiness is common. Some patients feel generally unwell and may complain of a feeling of depression or a sensation of unreality. Nightmares may occur and withdrawal of the drug can cause depression which is most marked after four days. Abuse has been reported in established drug addicts. Despite this lengthy list the number of dropouts reported from clinical studies of fenfluramine is usually low and not significantly different from placebo.

There are important pharmacological differences between the sterioisomers of fenfluramine. The dextro (d) isomer appears to contain most, if not all, of the appetite-suppressing effects of the racemic (d,l) mixture. A recent large, randomised, placebo- controlled, double-blind study has confirmed that dexfenfluramine (dF) is an effective anorectic agent [20]. Unfortunately tiredness, diarrhoea, dry mouth, polyuria and drowsiness affected significantly more patients on dF than on placebo. The number of withdrawals at 12 months was high in both groups (dF 37%, placebo 45%).

There have been a number of studies assessing the effects of fenfluramine in patients with NIDDM [21 – 25]. Treatment of twenty five NIDDM patients with diet and fenfluramine resulted in improved mean glucose tolerance and random blood sugar levels compared with a longitudinal control group treated with diet alone [24]. The improvement was seen in both obese and non-obese patients and multiple regression analysis suggested that this was only partly due to weight loss. The effect of fenfluramine on carbohydrate tolerance was compared with placebo in a double-blind, crossover study of 59 obese NIDDM subjects [23]. Seventeen were already receiving sulphonylureas and twenty five were taking biguanides. Patients received fenfluramine (60 mg/day) or placebo for three months and then crossed over to the alternative therapy. In thirty eight patients who completed the study fenfluramine resulted in a significant improvement in glucose tolerance as assessed by a 50 g oral 2-hour glucose tolerance test. This improvement did not correlate with any change in body weight or insulin secretion. The change in glucose tolerance was greatest in patients on sulphonylurea and diet therapy and least in patients on diet alone. Nine patients dropped out whilst taking fenfluramine compared with 11 who were on the placebo limb of the study.

A more recent study examined the effect of fenfluramine on insulin action and insulin secretion in healthy subjects and NIDDM patients using intravenous glucose tolerance tests [25]. In eight healthy individuals short-term fenfluramine treatment (60 mg/day for three days) produced no change in insulin secretion or whole-body insulin sensitivity compared with placebo. Nine patients (4 men, 5 women) with NIDDM were then studied in a double-blind crossover fashion. They were aged 44–74 years and had inadequate glycaemic control (mean HbA1C 9.6%, normal $< 6.6\%$), despite moderate to maximal doses of glyburide (glibenclamide). In this group there was a significant fall in fasting blood glucose after treatment with fenfluramine compared with baseline levels (13 ± 1.2 vs. 8.4 ± 0.89 mmol/l), but no change in serum insulin or C-peptide concentrations. During euglycaemic-hyperinsulinaemic clamp studies there was a significant increase in insulin action after fenfluramine treatment even though clamp insulin levels were lower. The insulin secretory response to arginine was unchanged.

To summarise, these studies indicate that fenfluramine produces a significant improvement in glucose tolerance in both obese and non-obese NIDDM patients. Insulin-sensitivity appears to increase since there is no change in insulin secretion and the effects are independent of changes in body weight. Fenfluramine may, therefore, prove to be a useful adjunct to diet therapy in the obese maturity-onset diabetic and in those patients poorly controlled on oral hypoglycaemic agents.

Drugs affecting the gastrointestinal tract

1. Agents which alter taste: Benzocaine is a topical anaesthetic for the mouth and upper respiratory tract. When taken in lozenge form it will 'numb the taste buds' and may reduce food intake. Data is very limited and there is a risk of trauma to the mouth during glutition. Sensitisation to this agent can also occur. Quinine, added to food, reduces intake in experimental animals but has not been tested in humans.

2. Bulk-forming agents: Methylcellulose is a hydrophilic colloid which after ingestion swells into a soft gel of uniform consistency that is not absorbed. It is the most commonly used bulk-forming drug and is claimed to reduce food intake by producing gastrointestinal distension and hence feelings of satiety. There is little evidence to support the claim that these effects produce weight loss. Side-effects include flatulence and intestinal obstruction. Mucilage, another bulking agent, has been subjected to a double- blind crossover trial in obese patients but numbers were small and the dropout rate was high [26]. No studies have been performed in diabetics.

3. Sucrose polyester: Sucrose polyester (SPE) is a non-absorbable fat produced by esterifying sucrose and fatty acids. It has the same characteristics as normal cooking oil and can be used as a substitute in many common foods. It is therefore, a means of reducing the energy available from a food source without decreasing intake. Cholesterol levels are also lowered since a portion of both dietary and entero-hepatic cholesterol is retained in the non-absorbed lipophilic phase. This agent has been studied in obese hypercholesterolaemic patients but not in diabetics [27,28] . Significant weight reduction was noted in five patients with familial hypercholesterolaemia when SPE was used as a fat substitute but not in a study comparing SPE with both a conventional low fat diet and a 'normal' diet in obese patients with primary hypercholesterolaemia. Significant reductions in low density lipoprotein cholesterol levels were seen in both studies and SPE was said to provide "the lubricity and organoleptic benefits of authentic foods" [28].

4. Drugs that limit absorption of fat: Agents that inhibit fat absorption or digestion are of theoretical benefit in the treatment of obesity. Neomycin, an antibiotic, causes an increase in the faecal excretion of fat but induces changes in the intestinal mucosa that make it unacceptable for long term use.

Cholestyramine, a resin which remains within the bowel lumen, binds bile salts leading to their excretion. This action leads to a significant reduction in serum cholesterol levels but when given to obese patients it has not been found to increase fat loss to a significant extent.

Tetrahydrolipostatin, an inhibitor of intestinal lipases, has been shown to reduce body mass in animals but studies in man are not yet available.

5. Opiate antagonists: Endogenous opioid peptides may be involved in the regulation of feeding behaviour. In the mid-1970's there were reports that endogenous opiate antagonists such as naloxone and naltrexone curtailed eating behaviour. This prompted a randomised parallel double-blind placebo-controlled trial of naltrexone in obese patients [29]. In this study there was no beneficial effect of the drug and some patients developed abnormal liver function tests whilst on naltrexone.

6. Thermogenic agents: Abnormalities in the regulation of thermogenesis may be involved in the pathogenesis of obesity. In particular, defective diet-induced thermogenesis could account for the adaptation to a low energy diet seen in some obese patients.

Catecholamines have a thermogenic effect which is mediated via the beta-1 receptor and the effects of ephedrine on weight loss in obese patients have been assessed. Ephedrine is a synthetic adrenergic drug having both alpha- and beta-agonist activity. In unselected obese adults three months treatment with two different doses of this agent produced no additional weight loss over placebo [30]. However, in a group of ten obese women selected for their adaptation to a low-energy intake, two months treatment with ephedrine produced a significant weight reduction [31]. Although the latter study reported no clinically important side-effects, ephedrine may increase blood pressure, heart rate and peripheral vascular resistance. Central nervous stimulation may also occur resulting in insomnia and nervousness.

In animal experiments, beta-adrenergic agonists have been found to decrease body weight and fat content without reducing food intake. This suggests that they act by increasing energy expenditure. Selective beta-agonists would be expected to cause fewer cardiovascular side-effects but so far an effective anorectic agent of this type is not available.

Unfortunately it is unlikely that agents which exert their effects via beta-receptor stimulation will be suitable for use in diabetic patients. Beta-agonists currently available, such as salbutamol, are well known to raise plasma glucose and ketone bodies in subjects with impaired glucose tolerance and this would probably contraindicate their use [32, 33].

Thyroxine (T_4) is another agent which produces an increase in metabolic expenditure. However, pharmacological doses promote osteoporosis, increased breakdown of protein and a rise in cardiovascular mortality. In spite of this there has been interest in the use of triiodothyronine (T_3) and T_4 in combination with very low carbohydrate diets. One of the major problems with these diets is an early fall in resting metabolic rate which reduces the rate of weight loss. Attempts have been made to arrest this fall by administration of thyroid hormones but with only limited success [34]. At present, thyroid hormones have no place in the management of obesity except in hypothyroid patients.

Growth hormone is also calorigenic and has been shown to reduce protein loss during low calorie dieting [35]. This drug can only be administered parenterally and remains an experimental tool. Since growth hormone is a gluconeogenic hormone it is unlikely that it will ever have a role in the treatment of obesity in diabetes.

Agents used in the treatment of diabetes and their effects on obesity

In contrast to the situation in insulin-dependent diabetes (IDDM) there are various pharmacological options for the treatment of NIDDM. Following dietary failure the physician can choose to treat a patient with oral hypoglycaemic agents (a sulphonylurea or biguanide) or insulin. Unfortunately, a logical approach to the treatment of NIDDM is hampered by the lack of understanding of the aetiology and pathogenesis of the condition. Indeed, there are still doubts as to whether improvement in parameters of metabolic control produces a beneficial effect on progression of large vessel disease and mortality. In this setting the effect on body weight of the various hypoglycaemic agents may be of major importance. Not only does weight gain have a deleterious effect on carbohydrate tolerance, but it may also adversely affect blood pressure and lipid levels.

Sulphonylureas

Sulphonylureas have been available since the mid-1950's and are often the first line of drug therapy following diet failure in NIDDM. Despite widespread use the precise mechanism of action has yet to be fully clarified [36]. The beta-cells of the pancreatic islets appear to have specific receptors for sulphonylureas and stimulation of these leads to insulin secretion. Other 'extra-pancreatic effects' of these agents may simply be a manifestation of improved glycaemic control. All sulphonylureas appear to share a common mode of action and the 'second generation agents' differ from first generation ones simply in terms of potency.

The effects of sulphonylurea therapy on body mass are well known, with most patients gaining weight after starting treatment [37]. The mechanism may be the reduction in caloric loss due to correction of glycosuria in combination with the anabolic effect of increased insulin secretion [38]. In one trial, sixty-one non-obese patients were treated with chlorpropamide or metformin in a crossover fashion (37 on metformin first) for twelve months [39]. Whilst taking the sulphonylurea, subjects gained a mean of 4.6 kg and this contrasted with a slight loss (mean 1.5 kg) during metformin treatment. The UK Prospective Study of Therapies of Maturity-Onset Diabetes has reported on the effects of diet, sulphonylurea, insulin and biguanide therapy on body weight [40]. Two hundred and eighty-six patients were documented after one year, of which 59 were given chlorpropamide or glibenclamide alone following diet failure. Twenty-one of these patients were obese (> 20% over ideal body weight) at randomisation. Compared with the patients who remained on diet alone, both sulphonylurea- treated groups gained a significant amount of weight (median 2 kg) after 12 months. Obese and non-obese patients fared much the same in this regard.

It is unclear whether the 'second generation' sulphonylureas have a less detrimental effect on body weight. A study comparing the effect of diet and glipizide therapy with diet alone reported similar weight loss in the two groups after one month [41]. However, only 20 patients were studied, they consumed an entirely liquid formula diet and the mean weight loss was very high (6.5 ± 0.5 kg).

More studies are available assessing the effects of gliclazide on weight. A multicentre study involving 17 French hospitals evaluated changes in body weight in 347 patients [42]. Many of these had been treated with sulphonylureas and/or biguanides prior to entry but some were diet failures. Two-hundred and sixteen were considered to be obese (> 110% ideal body weight) before gliclazide therapy and 131 patients had normal body weight. After treatment for a mean of 5.7 months the obese group lost a significant amount of weight (77.4 + 1.5 kg falling to 74.07 + 1.4 kg) whilst the non-obese showed a slight, non- significant gain of 0.4 kg. Another study assessed weight changes in thirty NIDDM patients treated for 12 months on diet and gliclazide [43]. Thirteen patients were newly diagnosed and seventeen were poorly controlled on other sulphonylureas. Patients were frequently assessed (monthly and then at three month intervals) for measurement of weight and other metabolic parameters. There was a significant fall in weight over the study period (mean 4.82 kg) irrespective of previous therapy. Unfortunately both of these studies used poorly controlled patients as a baseline and did not include control subjects on other agents or placebo. Therefore they did not address the possibility that dietary reinforcement and intensive follow-up may have produced the marked improvement in body weight (and also metabolic control).

Other studies suggest that the dramatic weight losses described above may not be typical. Changes in body weight were described in 44 NIDDM patients treated with gliclazide for up to 51 months [range 1 – 51] [44]. In the twelve patients who received the agent for 30 months or more, the mean change in weight from baseline was -0.7 kg (not significant). A multicentre trial, conducted in Britain, reported on the effects of gliclazide on weight in 193 patients treated for three months only [45]. There was a mean overall weight loss for the whole group of 0.62 kg ($p < 0.05$) with 112 patients losing weight, 75 patients gaining weight and six unchanged. Weight loss was most marked in those patients who had previously been poorly controlled on other oral hypoglycaemic agents. Patients with a body mass index greater than 30 kg/m^2 were said to lose more weight than 'the less overweight subjects'. However, patients who were more than 120% of IBW were excluded from the study. Zuro Hernandez studied the effects of gliclazide in 50 NIDDM patients (mean body weight 119% IBW) treated for 36 months [46]. There was a significant decrease in body weight from 68.2 ± 1.7 to 64.0 ± 1.4 kg over the study period although, again a suitable control group was not studied.

One study has compared the effects of gliclazide on weight with other sulphonylureas in a parallel study [47]. After 12 months therapy, patients given gliclazide had no significant change in body weight, compared with a gain of 2 kg in those receiving glibenclamide. However, this finding must be tempered by the fact that patients receiving glipizide and chlorpropamide also did not gain weight over the study period.

Biguanides

The biguanides include buformin, phenformin and metformin. None of these agents are available in the USA following the withdrawal of phenformin because of the occurrence of lactic acidosis. Metformin is widely used in Europe and Canada. In patients with NIDDM, metformin has beneficial weight-reducing (and lipid-lowering) effects. The mechanism of weight loss is unknown [48]. Anorexia may be involved, and a direct effect on the satiety centre has been proposed. Weight reduction is not related to the improvement in glycaemic control.

In the UK Prospective Study, referred to earlier, 11 obese NIDDM patients were treated with metformin and diet only [40]. These subjects did not gain weight in comparison with those given sulphonylureas or insulin. Sixty one NIDDM patients treated with metformin for 12 months recorded a mean weight loss of 1.5 kg compared with a gain of 4.5 kg when the same group received a sulphonylurea [39].

Insulin

Exogenous insulin therapy often leads to weight gain in patients with NIDDM. Of 54 sulphonylurea treatment failures given insulin for six months nearly three-quarters gained weight [49]. The mean increase was 4.2 kg, with a maximum of 13 kg. Interestingly patients gained weight even when the transfer from tablets to insulin resulted in a deterioration of glycaemic control. The 42 diet-failures who received insulin in the UK Prospective Study showed a less dramatic rise after 12 months treatment [40] . The median gain of 2 kg was similar to that seen with sulphonylurea therapy. Another study has shown that insulin-treated diabetics are less likely to lose weight on a very-low-calorie diet than those not receiving insulin [50].

Weight gain during insulin therapy is usually attributed to a reduced loss of energy due to the correction of glycosuria. Insulin also has antilipolytic, antiglycogenolytic and protein conserving actions which may be important. Inhibition of distal tubular sodium excretion leads to fluid and sodium retention and this might retard initial weight loss in patients on very-low-calorie diets.

Although patients with IDDM have an absolute requirement for insulin, there are a variety of treatment regimens available. Intensive insulin therapy, with insulin-delivery devices or multiple daily injections, is being used increasingly to achieve near normoglycaemia which may slow the development and progression of microvascular complications. Evidence from the Diabetes Control and Complications Trial shows that subjects randomised to intensive treatment gained significantly more weight (5.1 ± 4.6 kg) than the standard treatment group (2.4 ± 3.7 kg) during the first year of therapy [51]. There was no relationship between change in weight and the reported caloric intake or exercise level. Higher baseline glycosylated haemoglobin (HbA_1C) levels and greater decrements in HbA_1C during intensive therapy were both associated with greater weight increase. The benefits of intensive insulin therapy may, therefore, be counteracted by the adverse consequences of excessive weight gain.

Guar gum

The American and British Diabetic associations both recommend that a diet high in fibre derived from leguminous, cereal or tuberous sources should be prescribed for diabetic patients. Viscous fibre, when intimately mixed with food, has been shown to delay carbohydrate absorption and this may account for the improvement in glycaemic control seen in both IDDM and NIDDM patients on this diet. Increasing the fibre content of a diet is usually accompanied by other changes, such as an alteration in the amount and source of carbohydrate and a reduction in total energy intake. These alterations could also produce favourable changes in blood glucose and promote weight loss.

Guar gum is a natural vegetable fibre extracted from the Indian Cluster bean that has been promoted for use in diabetes mellitus. Its polysaccharide component, galactomannan, forms a non-absorbable viscous gum when mixed with water and this has various effects on bowel function. Guar delays the absorption of sugars and oligosaccharides from the gut so reducing post-prandial glucose levels. The mechanisms by which this is achieved remain unclear but there are reports of delayed gastric emptying, slower transit of food through the small intestine and reduction in stimulatory gut hormones, all of which may be involved [52]. Unfortunately the effects tend to be small and there is still debate over whether guar confers a significant therapeutic benefit in patients adhering to the standard diabetic diet [53].

The benefits of this preparation as regards weight reduction are also doubtful. A comparison of a low fibre diabetic diet with one supplemented by guar in obese newly diagnosed diabetics showed no difference in weight loss after 20 weeks [54]. There was, however, a higher prevalence of abdominal discomfort and flatulence in the guar-treated group. This study has been criticised since the method and timing of administration of guar, which can affect its efficacy, was not described [55]. Also, the high starting dose of guar used may have been responsible for the high incidence of side-effects. However, it is of note that other studies in NIDDM have shown no significant weight reduction [57].

Alpha-glucosidase inhibitors

Alpha-glucosidase inhibitors, such as acarbose and miglitol, are a relatively new group of agents that may have a place in the treatment of NIDDM and IDDM [58]. Their action is limited to the lumen of the bowel and they are not systemically absorbed. The drugs inhibit enzymatic activity in the brush border of the small intestine and so delay carbohydrate breakdown and absorption. This leads to a lowering of post-prandial glucose peaks, with subsequent improvement in glycaemic control, but without alteration in fasting blood glucose levels [59]. It was originally hoped that these agents would be especially helpful in the treatment of obese NIDDM's since they appeared to provide a means of inducing 'malabsorption' and hence a reduction in energy intake. Unfortunately the overspill of carbohydrates into the large bowel leads to an increase in bacterial fermentation producing the painful condition of meteorism and induction of flatulence. Furthermore, the short chain fatty acids produced by fermentation can be absorbed by the colon, leading to continued energy absorption which takes place during transit of the undigested carbohydrate. It is now clear that in doses tolerated by man, energy loss is not significant and weight reduction not attained.

Conclusions

The prevention and treatment of obesity is an important aspect in the management of patients with diabetes mellitus. In obese subjects with NIDDM, weight reduction alone may normalise glucose tolerance. In both IDDM and NIDDM, obesity may worsen blood pressure and cholesterol levels, thus increasing the risk of premature cardiovascular morbidity and mortality. Unfortunately many diabetics are unable to lose weight despite sensible advice on reduction of energy intake. Second line therapy may be appropriate for this group of patients. Currently, behavioural therapy is the favoured mode of treatment, however there remains a role for pharmacological agents. These can no longer be dismissed on the grounds that they are unsafe or lack efficacy. At present there are no strict recommendations concerning which patients should be offered drug treatment. Factors such as the degree of obesity, the presence of other coronary risk factors and the existance of those medical conditions aggravated by obesity may guide the physician. A previous history of drug abuse will remain a contraindication to therapy with centrally acting agents. It must be stressed that anorectic agents should not be considered until dietary measures have failed and even then they are not a substitute for continued attempts at low energy intake.

The most widely studied anorectic agent is fenfluramine. This is an effective drug with negligible abuse potential but side-effects may be troublesome. In patients with NIDDM, fenfluramine increases tissue sensitivity to insulin, leading to improved glycaemic control. This effect is independent of weight change and is clinically significant. Fenfluramine should not be given in short courses but for a prolonged period. Plateauing of weight loss should be anticipated and explained to the patient before treatment is commenced. Weight is likely to be regained when therapy is withdrawn. Dexfenfluramine may be useful in diabetes but its side-effect profile does not seem to confer any major advantage. Fluoxetine is currently marketed only as an antidepressant.

Central nervous stimulants may be used in those patients who are unable to tolerate 5-HT agonists. SPE may be of value but studies in diabetics are awaited. Thermogenic drugs, opiate antagonists, bulk-forming agents and drugs which inhibit fat absorption have no current role in the treatment of obesity in diabetes.

The presence of obesity may influence the choice of hypoglycaemic therapy in patients with NIDDM. Following diet failure, patients in whom weight reduction is necessary should receive a biguanide. If this does not achieve adequate glycaemic control or the agent is not tolerated, then treatment with a sulphonylurea or insulin must be considered. First generation sulphonylurea drugs will cause weight gain in most patients with NIDDM. Second generation agents may have a less detrimental effect but the evidence for this is not substantial. The use of a sulphonylurea and a biguanide in combination is acceptable but may lead to problems with compliance.

Insulin also promotes weight gain in patients with NIDDM. This may occur even when there is no improvement in glycaemic control. The effect on body mass is especially important in the elderly NIDDM patient since there is no evidence that alteration in glycaemic control has any effect on life expectancy [60]. Even in IDDM patients the effects of insulin therapy on body weight may be important. The postulated benefits of intensive therapy aimed at near-normoglycaemia may be offset by the complications of obesity. Excessive weight-gain may also reduce patient compliance with these regimes and subjects should be warned that rigid adherence to the recommended energy intake will still be necessary.

Finally, it is of interest that although the beneficial effects of fenfluramine on glucose levels were reported in the early 1970's the use of this agent in NIDDM is not widespread. Indeed, the Concensus View of management of NIDDM in Europe, published in 1988, made no mention of any anorectic agents [61]. Perhaps in the 1990's obesity will become established as a target for pharmacologic intervention in the same way that hypercholesterolaemia and hypertension have in the past two decades.

References

[1] Royal College of Physicians. Report of a working party on obesity. J R Coll Physicians Lond 1983; 17: 5–65.

[2] Tuomilehto J, Salonen JT, Marti B et al. Body weight and risk of myocardial infarction and death in the adult population of eastern Finland. Br Med J 1987; 295: 623–627.

[3] Wannamethee G, Shaper AG. Body Weight and Mortality in Middle Aged British Men: Impact of Smoking. Br Med J 1989; 299: 1497–1502.

[4] Managing Obesity Successfully. Drug and Therapeutics Bulletin 1989; 27: 33–36.

[5] Truglia JA, Livingston DVM, Lockwood DH. Insulin resistance: Receptor and post-binding defects in human obesity and non-insulin-dependent diabetes mellitus. Am J Med 1985; 979(suppl 2B): 13–22.

[6] Lean MEJ, James WPT. Prescription of Diabetic Diets in the 1980's. Lancet 1986; I: 723–725.

[7] Wing RR. Behavioral strategies for weight reduction in obese Type II diabetic patients. Diabetes Care 1989; 12: 139–144.

[8] Bray GA, Gray DS. Treatment of obesity: An overview. Diabetes/Metabolism Reviews 1988; 4: 653–679.

[9] Section 4.5 Appetite suppressants. British National Formulary 1989; 18: 167–168.

[10] Weintraub M, Bray GA. Drug treatment of obesity. Medical Clinics of North America 1989; 73: 237–249.

[11] Griffiths RR, Brady JV and Bradford LD. Predicting the abuse liability of drugs with animal drug self-administration procedures: Psychomotor stimulants and hallucinogens. Adv Behav Pharmacol 1979; 2: 163–208.

[12] Levi A. Abuse of fenfluramine. Br Med J 1973; II: 49.

[13] Blundell JE. Serotonin and appetite. Neuropharmacology 1984; 23: 1537–1551.

[14] Blundell JE, Latham CJ, Moniz E et al. Structural analysis of the actions of amphetamine and fenfluramine on food intake and feeding behaviour in animals and in man. Curr Med Res Opin 1979; 6 (suppl 1): 34–52.

[15] Blundell JE, Rogers PJ. Effects of anorexic drugs on food intake, food selection and preferences and hunger motivation and subjective experiences. Appetite 1980; 1: 151–165.

[16] Horowitz M, Collins PJ, Tuckwell V et al. Fenfluramine Delays Gastric Emptying of Solid Food. Br J Clin Pharmac. 1985; 19: 849–851.
[17] Hudson K D. The anorectic and hypotensive effect of fenfluramine in obesity. J Royal coll Gen Pract 1977; 27: 497–501.
[18] Ferguson JM and Feighner JP. Fluoxetine-induced weight loss in overweight non-depressed humans. Int J Obes 1987; 11 (suppl 3): 163–170.
[19] Munro JF. The management of obesity. Br J Hosp Med 1973; 10: 8–14.
[20] Guy-Grand B, Crepaldi G, Lefebvre P et al. International Trial of Long-term Dexfenfluramine in Obesity. Lancet 1989; II: 1142–1145.
[21] Dykes JRW. The Effect of a Low-calorie Diet with and without Fenfluramine on the Glucose Tolerance and Insulin Secretion of Obese Maturity Onset Diabetics. Post Grad Med J 1973; 49: 318–324.
[22] Turtle JR and Burgess JA. Hypoglycaemic Action of Fenfluramine in Diabetes Mellitus. Diabetes 1973; 22: 858–867.
[23] Wales JK. The Effect of Fenfluramine on Obese, Maturity-Onset Diabetic Patients. Curr Med Res Opin 1979; 6 (suppl. 1): 226–235.
[24] Doar JWH, Thompson ME, Wilde CE et al. The Influence of Fenfluramine on Oral Glucose Tolerance Tests, Plasma Sugar and Insulin Levels in Newly Diagnosed Late- Onset Diabetic Patients. Curr Med Res Opin 1979; 6 (suppl. 1): 247–254.
[25] Pestell RG, Crock PA, Ward GM et al. Fenfluramine Increases Insulin Action in Patients with NIDDM. Diabetes Care 1989; 12: 252–258.
[26] Enzi G, Inelmen EM and Crepaldi G. Effect of a hydrophilic mucilage in the treatment of obese patients. Pharmatherapeutica 1980; 2: 421–426.
[27] Gluek CJ, Jandacek R, Hogg E et al. Sucrose Polyester: Substitution for Dietary Fats in Hypocaloric Diets in the Treatment of Familial Hypercholesterolaemia. Am J Clin Nutr 1983; 37: 347–354.
[28] Mellies MJ, Vitale C, Jandacek RJ et al. The Substitution of Sucrose Polyester for Dietary Fat in Obese, Hypercholesterolaemic Outpatients. Am J Clin Nutr 1985; 41: 1–12.
[29] Malcolm R, O'Neil PM, Sexauer JD et al. A Controlled Trial of Naltexone in Obese Humans. Int J Obes 1985; 9: 347–353.
[30] Pasquali R, Baraldi G, Cesari MP et al. A controlled trial using ephedrine in the treatment of obesity. Int J Obes 1985; 9: 93–98.
[31] Pasquali R, Cesari MP, Melchionda N et al. Does Ephedrine promote weight loss in low-energy-adapted obese women? Int J Obes 1987; 11: 163–168.
[32] Gundogdu AS, Brown PM, Juul S et al. Comparison of hormonal and metabolic effects of salbutamol infusion in normal subjects and insulin-requiring diabetics. Lancet 1979; II: 1317–1321.
[33] Lulich KM, Goldie RG, Ryan G et al. Adverse reactions to beta-2 agonist bronchodilators. Medical Toxicology 1986; I: 286–299.
[34] Welle SL and Campbell RG. Decrease in resting metabolic rate during rapid weight loss is reversed by low dose thyroid hormone treatment. Metabolism 1986; 35: 289–291.
[35] Clemmons DR, Snyder DK, Williams R et al. Growth-hormone administration conserves lean body mass during dietary restriction in obese subjects. J Clin Endocrinol Metab 1987; 64: 878–883.
[36] Gerich JE. Oral hypoglycaemic agents. NEJM 1989; 321: 1231- 1245.
[37] Clarke BF and Duncan LJP. Comparison of chlorpropamide and metformin treatment on weight and blood-glucose response of uncontrolled obese diabetics. Lancet 1968; I: 123–126.
[38] Welle S, Nair KS and Lockwood D. Effect of a sulphonylurea and insulin on energy expenditure in Type II diabetes mellitus. J Clin Endocrin Metabolism 1987; 66: 593–597.
[39] Clarke BF and Campbell IW. Comparison of metformin and chlorpropamide in non-obese, maturity-onset diabetics uncontrolled by diet. Br J Med 1977; 2: 1576–1578.

[40] Multi-centre study. UK prospective study of therapies of maturity-onset diabetes. 1.Effect of diet, sulphonylurea, insulin or biguanide therapy on fasting plasma glucose and body weight over one year. Diabetologia 1983; 24: 404–411.
[41] Liu GC, Coulston AM, Lardinois CK et al. Moderate weight loss and sulphonylurea treatment of non-insulin-dependent diabetes mellitus. Arch Intern Med 1985; 145: 665–669.
[42] Charbonnel B. Clinical and metabolic effects of the treatment of diabetic patients with gliclazide. In: Keen H, Caldwell ADS, Murphy M et al., eds. Gliclazide and the treatment of diabetes. Royal Society of Medicine International Congress and Symposium series 1980; 20: 123–127.
[43] Donnet JP. Metabolic and weight assessment of long-term efficacy of Diamicron in the non insulin-dependent diabetic. La Vie Medicale 1982; 10: 725–728.
[44] Robb GH and Lowe SM. Lack of weight gain with gliclazide treatment for 30 months in Type II diabetes. Curr Med Res Opin 1984; 9: 7–9.
[45] Shaw KM, Wheeley MStG, Lowe SM et al. Gliclazide: A UK hospital multicentre study. Diabetic Med 1985; 2: 484–490.
[46] Zurro Hernandez J, Lavielle R. Is sulphoylurea therapy effective long term? A 3-year study with gliclazide. Curr Med Res Opin 1986; 10: 351–358.
[47] Harrower A. Comparison of diabetic control in Type 2 (non- insulin dependent) diabetic patients treated with different sulphonylureas. Curr Med Res Opin 1985; 9: 676–680.
[48] Vigneri R and Goldfine ID. Role of metformin in treatment of diabetes mellitus. Diabetes Care 1987; 10: 118–122.
[49] Peacock I, Tattersall RB. The difficult choice of treatment for poorly controlled maturity onset diabetes: tablets or insulin? Br Med J 1984; 288: 1956–1959.
[50] Harris MD, Davidson MB, Bush MA. Exogenous insulin therapy slows weight loss in type 2 diabetic patients. Int J Obes 1988; 12: 149–155.
[51] The DCCT research group. Weight gain associated with intensive therapy in the Diabetes Control and Complications Trial. Diabetes Care 1988; 11: 567–573.
[52] Guar gum. Of help to diabetics? Drug and Therapeutics Bulletin 1987; 25: 65–67.
[53] Baker P. Placebo-controlled trial of guar in poorly controlled Type II diabetes. Practical Diabetes 1988; 5: 36–38.
[54] Beattie VA, Edwards CA, Hosker JP et al. Does adding fibre to a low energy, high carbohydrate, low fat diet confer any benefit to the management of newly diagnosed overweight type II diabetics? Br Med J 1988; 296: 1147–1149.
[55] Lakhdar A, Farish E, McLaren EH. Fibre and patients with diabetes (letter). Br Med J 1988; 296: 1471.
[56] Bloom SR. Fibre and patients with diabetes (letter). Br Med J 1988; 296: 1471.
[57] Najemnik C, Kritz H, Irsigler K et al. Guar and its effects on metabolic control in Type II diabetic subjects. Diabetes Care 1984; 7: 215–219.
[58] McCulloch DK, Tattersall RB. 'Pharmacological Fibre' – Alpha-glucosidase inhibition in the management of diabetes. Diabetes Med 1984; 2: 189–190.
[59] Baron AD, Eckel RH, Schmeiser L et al. The effect of short-term alpha-glucosidase inhibition on carbohydrate and lipid metabolism in type II (noninsulin-dependent) diabetics. Metabolism 1987; 36: 409–415.
[60] Panzram G. Mortality and survival in Type II (non-insulin-dependent) diabetes mellitus. Diabetologia 1987; 30: 123–131.
[61] Alberti KGMM, Gries FA. Management of non-insulin-dependent diabetes mellitus in Europe: a concensus view. Diabetes Med 1988; 5: 275–281.

General aspects of aldose reductase inhibition

M. P. Cohen

Introduction

Importance

The identification of aldose reductase activity in tissues in which complications of diabetes occur has led both to mechanistic theories regarding the pathogenesis of diabetic complications as well as to the search for inhibitors of aldose reductase that are nontoxic, effective *in vivo,* and exert a salutary influence on the development or progression of these complications. During the past decade, the medical literature has been inundated with reports of studies describing activation of the polyol pathway by hyperglycemia or galactosemia in numerous experimental models and tissues, and examining the metabolic and potential pathophysiologic consequences of this activation. Several clinical trials with compounds that inhibit aldose reductase activity also have been mounted. Given the dearth of therapeutic options for the morbid and mortal complications of diabetes, this work has received considerable attention from both professional and lay communities. The fire of interest is further fueled by the fact that, despite years of research, the exact mechanisms responsible for the pathogenesis of diabetic complications have eluded satisfactory description. Thus, the concept that activation of the polyol pathway in diabetes has deleterious effects leading to compromised function in involved organs, and the notion that blocking the pathway by inhibiting the responsible enzyme could forestall the evolution of tissue damage in patients with diabetes, are quite attractive. However, the bright horizon for aldose reductase inhibitors in the clinical arena seems to be fading. Nevertheless, aldose reductase inhibitors remain important investigative tools, and continue to hold promise for unravelling the possible links between increased polyol pathway activity and the structure-function lesions characterizing chronic complications of diabetes mellitus.

Aldose reductase

Aldose reductase is a member of the aldo-keto reductase enzyme family that is ubiquitous in mammalian tissues. It catalyzes the first of two consecutive reactions that comprise the polyol pathway. Aldose reductase reduces free glucose to sorbitol, which is oxidized to fructose by sorbitol dehydrogenase. Both aldose reductase and sorbitol dehydrogenase have broad substrate specificities, including glucose and galactose for the former enzyme, and xylitol and ribitol for the latter. Notably, however, sorbitol dehydrogenase has limited ability to further metabolize galactitol, the sugar alcohol formed from galactose. This feature has been exploited experimentally with the use of galactose-fed models to probe the consequences of polyol accumulation in various tissues.

Under normal conditions, aldose reductase has a very low affinity for glucose and is operative at low catalytic rates. When glucose concentration is in the physiologic range, other enzymes responsible for glucose metabolism, such as hexokinases, have much higher affinities for glucose. When glucose concentration is elevated and hexokinase is saturated, aldose reductase activity increases, causing increased formation of sorbitol. Due to its limited ability to penetrate cell membranes, intracellular accumulation of sorbitol occurs, creating an osmotic effect. This sequence led to the theory that the tissue hydration accompanying the osmotic effects that arise from sorbitol accumulation as a result of hyperglycemia-induced activation of the polyol pathway was instrumental in the development of certain complications of diabetes [2, 3]. This theory is discussed more fully in later sections of this chapter.

Aldose reductase inhibitors

A variety of structurally unrelated, heterocyclic substances possess aldose reductase-inhibiting properties. Compounds capable of inhibiting the enzyme include spirohydantoins, quinolones, isoxazolidines, xanthines, flavinoids, and quercitrins. A common feature is the presence of a chromone ring system. Trade names of some agents, such as Sorbinil and Tolrestat, have appeared in the literature for years and are by now familiar. Others, such as the compounds developed by ICI (Statil), Ono, Senju, or Alcon, have emerged more recently [4–10]. Most of these inhibitors act through non-competitive inhibition, indicating that they do not compete with either the substrate or the nucleotide cofactor (NADPH) site; they appear to interact at another site, called the inhibitor site, on the aldose reductase enzyme [11].

In a recent review, Hararti correctly pointed out several factors that must be taken into account in evaluating clinical and experimental effects of aldose reductase inhibitors, and in intrepreting the results with respect to their possible ramifications for understanding the pathogenesis or for treatment of diabetic complications [12]. First, aldose reductase is present in many tissues not involved with diabetic complications; second, the long term effects of aldose reductase inhibition in such tissues is unknown. Third, there is evidence for immunologically distinct aldose reductases in different species and different tissues. Further, differences in susceptibility of the enzyme in different tissues have been identified [13]. Such considerations suggest that extrapolation of data from animal studies to human disease, or from one tissue to another, is not justified.

Pathophysiologic considerations

Overview

The paradigm for the participation of aldose reductase in the pathogenesis of a complication of diabetes is the ocular lens, the first tissue in which an association between excess sorbitol formation and a pathologic change was described [2, 14]. Subsequent studies in different tissues, including peripheral nerve, retina, and the renal glomerulus, and in several experimental animal models have demonstrated that a triad of metabolic changes accompanying activation of the polyol pathway and originally described in the lens also occurred in these tissues. These changes consist of sorbitol accumulation, myo-inositol depletion, and decreased Na/K-ATPase activity [2, 3, 15–19]. Further, treatment with aldose reductase inhibitors, insulin, or myo-inositol supplementation can prevent the metabolic changes, thereby linking them to hyperglycemia-induced activation of the polyol pathway. Other experiments have shown that similar treatments will prevent or ameliorate certain functional changes classically associated with complications of diabetes, such as reduced motor nerve conduction velocity, acute increases in the glomerular filtration rate, and proteinuria, in these tissues in experimental models [20–23]. Most recent experiments have probed a putative relationship between glucose-induced changes in cell myo-inositol and impairment of fundamental regulatory mechanisms involving phosphoinositide turnover [24–26]. They also address the *"black box"* that lies between polyol pathway-related metabolic changes and the structure-function changes traditionally associated with complications in various tissues, such as basement membrane thickening, increased collagen synthesis, glomerular expansion, nerve fiber pathology, and retinal cell dropout. It is in this area that aldose reductase inhibitors may prove most valuable, for they allow probing of specific questions concerning causal links between enhanced polyol pathway activity and defined biochemical, pathologic and functional parameters that are pathophysiologically associated with diabetic complications.

Diabetic neuropathy

Although several pathogenetic mechanisms may contribute to the pathogenesis of diabetic neuropathy, the metabolic abnormalities associated with hyperglycemia-induced activation of the polyol pathway in the peripheral nerve perhaps have received the most attention in recent years. In part this reflects the contributions of insightful investigators to a better understanding of the structural, functional and biochemical abnormalities that underlie the neuropathic syndromes, and in part the pervasive publicity that surrounded clinical trials of aldose reductase inhibitors for treatment of diabetic neuropathy.

Sorbitol and fructose are present in high concentration in normal peripheral nerve, and accumulate further in the nerves of animals with experimental diabetes and of human diabetic patients. The elevated levels of sorbitol and fructose fall significantly with insulin treatment, confirming that hyperglycemia underlies their increase. Aldose reductase is found in the cytoplasm of the Schwann cell but not in the axon, fixing the locus of origin of at least some of the aldose reductase-related metabolic abnormalities to this cell body.

An early explanation for nerve damage secondary to sorbitol accumulation invoked an increased intracellular osmotic effect leading to tissue overhydration. In this construct, sorbitol-induced edema of the Schwann cell would cause cell lysis and, eventually, demyelination due to loss of the myelin-sustaining role of these cells. However, Schwann cell edema has not been demonstrated consistently in human or experimental diabetes. Further, the sorbitol concentration in diabetic nerve, although greater than in nondiabetic nerve, probably is too low to exert a significant osmotic effect. Other, more promising explanations for polyol pathway-related nerve damage have come to light from the diligent work of several investigators.

This work has identified a sequence of metabolic abnormalities triggered by activation of the polyol pathway and involving depletion of myo-inositol and reduction of Na/K-ATPase activity [24, 27]. The changes in myo-inositol content and Na/K-ATPase, like those in sorbitol concentration, are prevented by aldose reductase inhibitors, and are associated with slowing of nerve conduction velocity in diabetic animals. Insulin and myo-inositol supplementation also restore nerve myo-inositol levels and improve Na/K-ATPase activity and nerve conduction. Decreased nerve Na/K-ATPase activity is believed to lead to decreased energy utilization and intracellular accumulation of sodium, decreasing the ability of the nerve to generate action potential. Myo-inositol depletion is believed to compromise nerve phosphoinositide turnover and phosphoinositide-mediated regulation of Na/K-ATPase, contributing to the increase in intra-axonal sodium concentration. A protein kinase C-dependent mechanism linking defects in phosphoinositide metabolism and Na/K-ATPase activity ascribed to myo-inositol depletion has been proposed [28]. This cascade of interrelated metabolic abnormalities, intimately associated with changes in relevant electro-physiologic events and function in the peripheral nerve in experimental diabetes, offers a logical pathophysiologic explanation for acute diabetic neuropathy and for potential benefits of aldose reductase inhibitors in the treatment of this disorder. Recent evidence also has implicated this sequence of metabolic abnormalities to structural and morphologic lesions characteristic of chronic diabetic peripheral nerve disease, namely swelling of large myelinated fibers at the node of Ranvier, axo-glial dysjunction, and axonal degeneration and deformity of nerve fibers. These studies have shown that aldose reductase inhibition reverses paranodal swelling, the antecedent of axo-glial dysjunction, in sural nerves of the diabetic BB rat, and can increase the number of regenerating myelinated nerve fibers in patients with established diabetic neuropathy [29–31].

Diabetic retinopathy

As in other complications of diabetes, consideration of a potential role for polyol pathway activation in the pathogenesis of diabetic retinopathy must take into account the relevant pathologic and physiologic features of the retinal microvasculature in diabetes. The retinal capillaries contain endothelial cells, which line the capillary lumen and form a permeability (blood-retinal) barrier, and pericytes (mural cells), which are enveloped by a basement membrane produced by the two cell types. Intramural pericytes are selectively lost early in the course of diabetic retinopathy, leaving a ghost-like pouch of surrounding basement membrane. Breakdown of the blood-retinal barrier is another early feature. Dilatation and endothelial cell proliferation occur in the capillaries in which there is a loss of mural cells, while adjacent capillaries have diminished perfusion and eventually become acellular tubes consisting solely of basement membrane, which becomes thickened in diabetic retinas. Dilated capillaries develop microaneurysmal outpouchings, leak intravascular fluid, and may eventually give use to growth and proliferation of new capillaries (neovascularization).

The mural cell contains aldose reductase and accumulates sorbitol in experimental hyperglycemia and galactosemia [32–35]. Mural cells maintained in high glucose medium undergo degenerative changes and show decreased cell multiplication and mitotic rates, suggesting participation of the polyol pathway in mural cell dropout. Such an interpretation is supported by the finding that aldose reductase inhibition prevents pericyte loss in rats and dogs fed high galactose diets [36, 37].

Other experimental evidence lending credence to the hypothesis that increased aldose reductase activity contributes to the pathogenesis of diabetic retinopathy includes prevention of retinal capillary basement membrane thickening, and of microaneurysms, by aldose reductase inhibitors in galactosemic rats [36, 38, 39], and the development of diabetic-like microaneurysms in galactosemic dogs [40]. Aldose reductase inhibitors also reportedly prevent retinopathic changes in streptozotocin-diabetic and fructose-fed rats [41, 42]. It is curious, however, that the increased collagen synthesis (presumably reflecting basement membrane synthesis) by retinal pericytes grown in high glucose media is not corrected with aldose reductase inhibition [43, 44].

Whether polyol accumulation *per se,* or a sequence of associated metabolic abnormalities analogous to that described in peripheral nerve, is instrumental in the development of retinopathic changes is not clear. The overall absolute level of sorbitol that accumulates in the retinas of diabetic rats is insufficient to be of osmotic significance, but sequestering of sorbitol in specific cellular locations could create a significant osmotic force in individual cells. On the other hand, increase retinal sorbitol in alloxan diabetic rabbits is associated with myo-inositol depletion and reduced Na/K-ATPase activity [17]. These changes are prevented by aldose reductase inhibition, and are associated with a reduction in the electroretinogram C wave that also corrects with aldose reductase inhibition or with myo-inositol supplementation [45]. The relationships between mural cell dropout, basement membrane thickening, and endothelial cell proliferation and the metabolic abnormalities of myo-inositol depletion, decreased Na/K-ATPase activity, and altered phosphoinositide metabolism found in retinal microvessels of diabetic animals need to be delineated. Studies examining these questions are proceeding in conjuction with experiments seeking to unravel analogous relationship that may exist in other tissues subject to diabetic complications.

Diabetic nephropathy

Aldose reductase is present in glomerular epithelial and mesangial cells, and its activity is increased with hyperglycemia or galactosemia [46, 47]. In most but not all experimental studies, the triad of changes associated with polyol pathway activation (sorbitol accumulation, myo-inositol depletion, decreased Na/K-ATPase activity) has been found in renal glomeruli, the characteristic site of the nephropathic lesions of diabetes [18, 19, 48, 49]. These metabolic changes can be partially or completely normalized by treatment with an aldose reductase inhibitor. Glomerular hyperperfusion in acute streptozotocin diabetes can be prevented by the aldose reductase inhibitor sorbinil; increased albumin excretion in experimental diabetes also can be prevented with aldose reductase inhibition [22, 23, 50]. The single study that failed to find correction of hyperperfusion and albuminuria with an aldose reductase inhibitor employed a compound which penetrates the ocular lens but for which there is no evidence of entry or efficacy in glomerular cells [9]. The increased glomerular filtration rate and proteinuria are ameliorated with dietary myo-inositol supplementation [21, 51]. The latter findings imply a relationship between polyol pathway induced myo-inositol depletion and the early hemodynamic and filtration abnormalities of diabetes.

Compromised phosphoinositide turnover resulting from myo-inositol deficiency has been invoked as the possible mediator of hemodynamic changes, perhaps by impairing signal transduction of vasoactive hormones that act through products of phosphoinositide hydrolysis to promote smooth muscle contraction [52, 53]. However, diabetes and high glucose have been reported to enhance glomerular protein kinase C activation and phosphoinositide turnover [54], a finding that opens alternative mechanistic avenues to explain early glomerular abnormalities in diabetes, including protein kinase mediated stimulation of cell growth and of vasodilatory prostaglandins.

Other work in experimental animals has not found a link between polyol pathway activation and some of the biochemical lesions characteristic of diabetic nephropathy. For example, aldose reductase inhibition does not influence the increased nonenzymatic glycation of glomerular basement membrane, even though an effect might be anticipated through reduction of fructose production [55, 56]. Aldose reductase inhibition also does not influence the decreased sulfation of the heparan sulfate proteoglycans of glomerular basement membrane that occurs in experimental diabetes, an abnormality believed to compromise the function of the glomerular filtation barrier [56, 57]. Future studies undoubtedly will explore possible links between polyol pathway-induced metabolic alterations and other biochemical, morphologic, and functional abnormalities that characterize the nephropathic lesion in diabetes.

Clinical considerations

Clinical studies examining the effect of aldose reductase inhibitors on symptoms and signs of diabetic neuropathy in human patients have been conducted for the past several years. Scattered reports of anecdotal and small scale studies have appeared in the literature, but results from large scale clinical trials have not been published. Several pharmaceutical houses have been engaged in clinical trials evaluating the safety and efficacy of their respective agents, but aside from interim presentations, abstracts, and comments offered at professional meetings or special conferences sponsored by the involved pharmaceutical concern, the coordinated findings of multicenter cooperative clinical trials are not yet available for review. Ongoing studies for some compounds include parameters for retinopathy and nephopathy as well as neuropathy. Summaries of various clinical studies and the information derived to date appear in other relevant chapters of this book (Mogensen, Kohner, Greene).

The fundamental question is whether these agents will have a meaningful role in the treatment of complications of diabetes. This question encompasses several important issues, including efficacy, side-effects, risks (as yet unknown) of long-term therapy, tissue specificity (e.g. can a single compound be used for different complications in different tissues), use for prevention versus established disease, and the prospects for other pharmacologic agents that address alternative putative pathogenetic factors contributory to the development or progression of diabetic complications. These issues are of obvious concern to those pharmaceutical houses that are engaged in the development and testing of various aldose reductase inhibitors. At least one compound (sorbinil) has fallen by the wayside because of an unacceptable side-effect profile. Studies with another (ICI's Statil licensed to Merck for codevelopment) recently have been abandoned because of poor efficacy. However, Dr. Greene's view, quoted in the April 15, 1990 issue of Medical Advertising News, might prevail: *"The general feeling is that this reflects the compounds used by these two companies. They were bad. It does not mean the ARI field is closing down. They do have a future"*. And, it is hoped, the future will resolve the outstanding issues mentioned above.

References

[1] Cogan DG, Kinoshita JH, Kador PF et al. Aldose reductase and complications of diabetes. Ann Intern Med 1984; 101: 82.
[2] Kinoshita JH. Cataracts in galactosemia. Invest Ophthalmol 1965; 4: 786.
[3] Kinoshita JH. Mechanisms initiating cataract formation. Proctor Lecture. Invest Ophthalmol 1974; 13: 713.
[4] Peterson MJ, Sarges R, Aldinger CE et al. CP-45,634: A novel aldose reductase inhibitor that inhibits polyol pathway activity in diabetic and galactosemic rats. Metabolism 1979; 28: 456.
[5] Dvornik D, Simard-Duquesne N, Kraml M et al. Polyol accumulation in galactosemic and diabetic rats: Control by an aldose reductase inhibitor. Science 1973; 182: 1146.
[6] Kador PF, Sharpless NE. Sturcture-activity studies of aldose reductase inhibitors containing the 4−0X0−4H-chromen ring system. Biophys Chem 1978; 8: 81.
[7] Low MF, Dickerson JE, Chandler ML et al. The prevention of biochemical changes in lens, retina and nerve of galactosemic dogs by the aldose reductase inhibitor AL 01576. J Ocular Pharmacol 1989; 5: 233.
[8] Matsuda M, Awata T, Ohashi Y et al. The effects of aldose reductase inhibitor on the corneal endothelial morphology in diabetic rats. Curr Eye Res 1987; 6: 391.
[9] Daniels B, Hostetter T. Aldose reductase inhibitors and glomerular abnormalities in diabetic rats. Diabetes 1989; 38: 981.
[10] Kakuta H, Hotta H, Fukasawa N et al. Long-term clinical study of the effect of an aldose reductase inhibitor, ONO-2235, on diabetic neuropathy. in: Current Status of Prevention and Treatment of Diabetic Complications. Elsevier, Excerpta Medica, 1990; 483.
[11] Kador PF, Sharpless NE. Pharmacophor requirements of the aldose reductase inhibitor site. Molec Pharmacol 1983;24: 521.
[12] Hararti Y. Diabetic peripheral neuropathies. Ann Int Med 1987; 107: 546.
[13] Kador PF, Kinoskita JH, Tung WH et al. Differences in the susceptibility of aldose reductase to inhibition. Invest Ophthalmol Vis Sci 1980; 19: 980.
[14] Van Heyningen R. Metabolism of xylose by the lens. Rat lens *in vivo* and *in vitro*. Biochem J 1959; 73: 197.
[15] Finegold D, Lattimer SA, Nolle S et al. Polyol pathway activity and myo-inositol metabolism. A suggested relationship in the pathogenesis of diabetic neuropathy. Diabetes 1983; 32: 988.
[16] Greene DA, Lattimer SA. Impaired rat nerve sodium-potassium adenosine triphosphatase activity in acute streptozotocin diabetes and its correction by dietary myo-inositol supplementation. J Clin Invest 1983; 72: 1058.
[17] MacGregor LC, Rosecan LR, Laties AM et al. Altered retinal metabolism in diabetes. I. Microanalysis of lipid, glucose, sorbitol and myo-inositol in the choroid and the individual layers of the rabbit retina. J Biol Chem 1986; 261: 4046.
[18] Beyer Mears A, Ku L, Cohen MP. Glomerular polyol accumulation in diabetes and its prevention by oral sorbinil. Diabetes 1984; 33: 604.
[19] Cohen MP, Dasmahapatra A, Shapiro E. Reduced glomerular sodium/potassium adenosine triphosphatase activity in acute streptozotocin diabetes and its prevention by oral sorbinil. Diabetes 1985; 34: 1071.
[20] Greene DA, DeJesus PV, Winegrad AI. Effects of insulin and dietary myo-inositol on impaired peripheral motor nerve conduction velocity in acute streptozotocin diabetes. J Clin Invest 1975; 55: 1326.
[21] Goldfarb SA, Simmons DA, Kern E. Amelioration of glomerular hyperfiltration in acute experimental diabetes by dietary myo-inositol and by an aldose reductase inhibitor. Trans Assoc Am Physicians 1986; 86: 67.

[22] Bank N, Mower P, Aynedjian H et al. Sorbinil prevents glomerular hyperperfusion in diabetic rats. Am J Physiol 1989; 256: F1000.
[23] Beyer Mears A, Murray FT, Del Val M et al. Reversal of proteinuria by sorbinil, an aldose reductase inhibitor in spontaneously diabetic (BB) rats. Pharmacology 1988; 36: 112.
[24] Greene DA, Lattimer SA, Sima AA. Sorbitol, phosphoinositides, and sodium potassium ATPase in the pathogenesis of diabetic complications. N Engl of Med 1987; 316: 599.
[25] Simmons DA, Kern EF, Winegrad AI et al. Basal phosphatidylinositol turnover controls aortic Na/K-ATPase activity. J Clin Invest 1986; 77: 503.
[26] Winegrad AI. Does a common mechanism induce the diverse complications of diabetes? Diabetes 1987; 36: 396.
[27] Greene DA, Lattimer S, Ulbrecht J et al. Glucose-induced alterations in nerve metabolism: current perspective on the pathogenesis of diabetic neurophathy and future directions for research and therapy. Diabetes Care 1985; 8: 290.
[28] Lattimer SA, Sima AF, Green DA: In vitro correction of impaired Na^+-K^+-ATPase in diabetic nerve by protein kinase C agonists. Amer J Physiol 1989 256: E264.
[29] Sima AF, Lattimer SA, Yagihashi S et al. Axo-glial dysjunction. A novel structural lesion that accounts for poorly-reversible conduction slowing in the spontaneously-diabetic Bio-breeding rat. J Clin Invest 1986; 77: 474.
[30] Greene DA, Chakrabarti S, Lattimer SA et al. Role of sorbitol accumulation and myo-inositol depletion in paranodal swelling of large myelinated nerve fibers in the insulin-deficient spontaneously diabetic Bio-breeding rat. J Clin Invest 1987; 79: 1479.
[31] Sima AF, Bril V, Nathaniel V et al. Regeneration and repair of myelinated fibers in sural-nerve biopsy specimens from patients with neuropathy treated with sorbinil. N Engl J Med 1988; 319: 548.
[32] Gabbay KH. Purification and immunological identification of bovine retinal aldose reductase. Isr J Med Sci 1972; 8: 1626.
[33] Buzney SM, Frank RN, Varma SD et al. Aldose reductase in retinal mural cells. Invest Ophthalmol Vis Sci 1977; 16: 392.
[34] Kern TS, Engerman RL. Hexitol production by canine retinal microvessels. Invest Ophthalmol Vis Sci 1985; 26: 382.
[35] Akagi Y, Terubayashi H, Millen J et al. Aldose reductase localization in dog retinal mural cells. Curr Eye Res 1986; 5: 883.
[36] Robison WG, Nagata M, Laver W et al. Diabetic-like retinopathy in rats prevented with an aldose reductase inhibitor. Invest. Ophthalmol Vis Sci 1989; 30: 2285
[37] Kador PF, Akagi Y, Terubayashi H et al. Prevention of pericyte ghost formation in retinal capillaries of galactose-fed dogs by aldose reductase inhibitors. Arch Ophthalmol 1988; 106: 1099.
[38] Robison WG, Kador PF, Kinoshita JH. Retinal capillaries: Basement membrane thickening by galactosemia prevented with aldose reductase inhibitor. Science 1983; 221: 1177.
[39] Robison WG, Kador PF, Akagi Y et al. Prevention of basement membrane thickening in retinal capillaries by a novel inhibitor of aldose reductase, Tolrestat. Diabetes 1986; 35: 295.
[40] Engerman RL, Kern TS. Experimental galactosemia produces diabetic-like retinopathy. Diabetes 1984; 33: 97.
[41] Kojima K, Matsubara H, Harada T et al. Effects of aldose reductase inhibitor on retinal microanagiopathy in streptozotocon-diabetic rats. Jpn J Ophthalmol 1985; 29: 99.
[42] Hotta N, Kakuta H, Fukasawa H et al. Aldose reductase inhibitor and fructose-rich diet: Its effect on the development of diabetic retinopathy. Diabetes 1984; 33: 199A.
[43] Li W, Shen S Khatami M et al. Stimulation of retinal capillary pericyte protein and collagen synthesis in culture by high-glucose concentration. Diabetes 1984; 33: 785.
[44] Li W, Khatami M, Rockey JH. The effects of glucose and an aldose reductase inhibitor on the sorbitol content and collagen synthesis of bovine retinal capillary pericytes in culture. Exp Eye Res 1985; 40: 439.

[45] MacGregor LC, Matschinsky FM. Treatment with aldose reductase inhibitor or with myo-inositol arrests deterioration of the electroretinogram of diabetic rats. J Clin Invest 1985; 76: 887.
[46] Ludvigson MA, Sorenson RL. Immunohistochemical localization of aldose reductase. Diabetes 1980; 29: 450.
[47] Kikkawa R, Umemura K, Haneda M et al. Evidence for existence of polyol pathway in cultured rat mesangial cells. Diabetes 1987; 36: 240.
[48] Hutton JC, Schofield PJ, Williams JF et al. The localization of sorbitol pathway activity in the rat renal cortex and its relationship to the pathogenesis of the renal complications of diabetes mellitus. Aust J Exp Biol Med Sci 1975; 53: 49.
[49] Cohen MP. Aldose reductase, glomerular metabolism and diabetic nephropathy. Metabolism 1986; 35: 55.
[50] Williamson JR, Chang K, Tilton RG et al. Increased vascular permeability in spontaneously diabetic BB/W rats and in rats with mild versus severe streptozotocin-induced diabetes: prevention by aldose reductase inhibitors and castration. Diabetes 1987; 36: 813.
[51] Pugliese G, Tilton RG, Speedy A et al. Modulation of hemodynamic and vascular filtration changes in diabetic rats by dietary myo-inositol. Diabetes 1990; 39: 312.
[52] Griendling KK, Beck BC, Ganz P et al. Angiotension II stimulation of vascular smooth muscle phosphoinositide metabolism. Hypertension Dallas 1987; 9: 5181.
[53] Troyer DA, Schwertz DW, Kreisberg JI et al. Inositol phospholipid metabolism in the kidney. Annu Rev Physiol 1986; 48: 51.
[54] Craven P, DeRubertis, R. Protein kinase C is activated in glomeruli from streptozotocin diabetic rats. Possible mediation by glucose. J Clin Invest 1989; 83: 1667.
[55] Cohen MP. Diabetic nephropathy and the polyol pathway. in: Current Status of Prevention and Treatment of Diabetic Complications. Elsevier, Excerpta Medica, 1990; 206.
[56] McPherson JD, Shilton BH, Walton DJ. Role of fructose in glycation and cross linking of proteins. Biochemistry 1988; 27: 1901.
[57] Cohen MP, Klepser H, Wu VY. Undersulfation of heparan sulfate of glomerular basement membrane in experimental diabetes and lack of correction with aldose reductase inhibition. Diabetes 1988; 37: 1324.

Platelet-active drugs in diabetes mellitus*

J. A. Colwell

Introduction

Accelerated atherosclerosis is the most common contributor to morbidity, mortality, and high costs of hospitalization in patients with diabetes mellitus in the United States [1]. It has been reliably estimated that people with diabetes in the U.S. and many other countries have at least a two to four fold risk for coronary artery and peripheral vascular disease when compared to control subjects [2]. Recognition of these facts has increased in recent years, and a number of review articles have considered their implications [3–8].

Concomitant with this recognition of the wide scope and impact of macrovascular disease as a complication of diabetes have been observations on the pathogenesis of atherosclerosis in people with diabetes mellitus. While it is recognized that atherosclerosis is a very complicated process and that the presence of the heterogenous disease which characterizes diabetes mellitus adds to the complexity, it is also widely accepted that platelets may play an important role in this process. Accordingly, in this chapter we will review the evidence of altered platelet function in diabetes and how this may affect the process of accelerated atherosclerosis in that disorder. Large scale clinial studies in diabetic and nondiabetic subjects have now progressed to the stage where definitive recommendations may be made regarding the use of specific antiplatelet agents as primary or secondary prevention strategies. Further, there are many smaller clinical studies of agents which affect platelet function which may prove to be useful as adjunctive therapeutic approaches in diabetes. It is the purpose of this chapter to provide an updated review of this subject.

Pathophysiology

Atherosclerosis

The response to injury view of the pathogenesis of atherosclerosis ascribes a role of the platelet in the process [9–11]. According to this view, endothelial

* Supported by Veterans Administration Research Funds

Table 1 Alterations of platelet function in diabetes

In Vitro	In Vivo
↑ Adhesiveness	↑ Turnover
↑ Aggregability	↓ Suvival
↑ Thromboxane release	↑ Betathromboglobulin
Platelet-plasma interactions	↑ Plasma factor 4
vWF Fibrinogen	↑ Platelet-derived growth factor
Immune complexes	↑ Circulating platelet aggregates
Glycosylated LDL	

damage is followed by adherence of monocyte-derived macrophages to the site of injury. Platelets may also adhere, aggregate to form white thrombi, release procoagulant materials, and synthesize and release a variety of arachidonic acid metabolites. One of these, thromboxane, is a potent vasoconstrictor and stimulator of platelet aggregation. Platelet-plasma interactions with lipoproteins, immune complexes, and other materials may occur. Growth factors may be released by monocytes, platelets, and endothelial cells and these may contribute to cellular proliferation in the area of injury. Altered metabolism of lipoproteins in diabetes often occurs and may exaggerate the process, and evidence is accumulating that glycation of circulating and vascular wall proteins is also contributing to the process.

Many studies have been directed at the issue of altered platelet function in diabetes. Table 1 lists many of the alterations that have been found, both in type I and type II diabetic subjects. Such findings are generally most prominent in patients with existing vascular complications. However, studies in animal models and in insulin-dependent diabetic patients who are of short duration and free from clinically obvious vascular disease suggest that altered platelet function not only occurs as a result of established vascular disease, but may also occur secondary to the metabolic state of diabetes mellitus.

Recognition of the possible role for platelets in the pathogenesis of accelerated atherosclerosis has led to controlled clinical trials in nondiabetic and in diabetic subjects. The agent which has received the most attention is aspirin.

Pharmacology of aspirin

Aspirin has been the primary agent of choice in the majority of trials in which antiplatelet agents have been used [12]. The thrombotic effects of aspirin are thought to be primarily to its platelet-inhibitory action. Aspirin causes irreversible acetylation of platelet cyclo-oxygenase, the enzyme which catalyses the conversion by platelets of arachidonic acid-derived endoperoxides into thromboxane. A single 325 mg aspirin tablet or long term administration of very low doses of aspirin (such as 20 mg/day) will depress platelet thromboxane synthesis by at least 90% [12]. Thus, because of a low toxic-therapeutic ratio, aspirin has been an attractive choice in clinical trials, in order to prevent vascular thrombosis.

Platelet cyclo-oxygenase is very sensitive to inhibition by aspirin in nondiabetic and in diabetic individuals. Megakaryocyte cyclo-oxygenase is also inhibited by aspirin. Since platelets cannot synthesize new cyclo-oxygenase, thus inhibition lasts for the lifetime of that platelet population. However, platelet turnover may be accelerated in diabetic patients, and platelet survival may be shortened (Table 1). This is particularly found in patients with established vascular disease. Thus, newly- formed platelets may enter the circulation at a more rapid rate than in nondiabetic subjects, and platelet thromboxane production may then follow because non-acetylated cyclo-oxygenase has been formed from megakaryocyte synthesis in the presence of lowered aspirin levels. There is therefore a rationale for either frequent administration of aspirin in diabetes or, preferably, for the use of sustained release preparations to provide consistent blood levels.

A second issue with aspirin therapy in diabetes is inhibition by aspirin of the synthesis of prostacyclin, a potent vasodilator and platelet de-aggregating prostanoid. However, the vascular endothelium has the capacity to synthesize cyclo-oxygenase as the aspirin level falls, so this issue can be handled by once a day dosing with aspirin or by using very low dose schedules, which have less of an effect to inhibit prostacyclin formation. In any event, there are now many studies in which high doses of aspirin have been used, and none of them show that aspirin has a thrombotic potential. Thus, the concern about prostacyclin inhibition may not be relevant to clinical use of aspirin in thrombotic disorders.

There are other actions of aspirin which may have relevance to its use as an antiplatelet agent. Arachidonic acid is metabolized via a lipoxygenase enzyme system, in addition to the cyclo-oxygenase pathways. Leukotrienes are formed, and these compounds may have influences in vascular responses and on platelet function. In addition, aspirin may have antithrombotic effects by virtue of inhibition of release of platelet factors 3 and 4 (PF3+4). PF3 promotes viscous metamorphosis of platelets and PF4 enhances the reaction between thrombin and fibrinogen. Inhibition of PF3 will occur with 500 mg of aspirin and of PF4 with 200 mg of aspirin (with intravenous administration). Finally, there is some diminution in the activities of factors II, VII, IX, and X, probably due to vitamin K inhibition, when a higher dose of aspirin (2000 mg) is given intravenously.

Thus, when high doses of aspirin are used in clinical trials, it is possible that some effects noted may be due to activities distinct from its well studied actions to inhibit platelet cyclo-oxygenase.

An additional consideration regarding aspirin which may be relevant to clinical trial results is that there are certain aspects of platelet function which could be involved in atherosclerosis and/or thrombosis, but which are not affected by aspirin therapy. The primary wave of platelet aggregation after ADP or collagen is not affected by aspirin. High doses of thrombin or collagen will produce platelet aggregation in platelets in which cyclo-oxygenase is blocked by aspirin. Finally, platelet adhesion, as differentiated from platelet aggregation, is not affected by aspirin therapy. While the precise roles for these functions in atherosclerosis are not known, it must be recognized that there are alternative pathways of platelet function which are not affected by aspirin therapy.

Survey of clinical trials

Secondary prevention: nondiabetic individuals

There have been many trials of antiplatelet agents, primarily in nondiabetic subjects who had previously suffered from a myocardial infarction, strokes, transient ischemic attack, or unstable angina. Generally, diabetic subjects have constituted a minority (less than 10%) of patients in these trials. Many of these secondary prevention trials have reported trends which have suggested an effect of antiplatelet therapy to reduce subsequent major vascular events. However, it has recently been recognized by Antiplatelet Trialists' Collaboration group [13] that an overview which addressed results from all major antiplatelet trials in which inhibitors of platelet aggregation were used would provide suitable numbers of patients and events to make definitive recommendations. While such a meta-analysis may be subject to certain statistical concerns, it nevertheless provides excellent guidelines to clinicians who need an informed analysis in order to know how to proceed with patients who have suffered a major vascular event.

Unfortunately, there are limited data available on the diabetic subjects who were included in most of these trials. Therefore, it is also important to review those trials which have been done in diabetic individuals to see if the generalizations which can be made from trials in nondiabetic individuals also apply to people with diabetes. The situation, therefore, may appear to be analogous to the case regarding treatment of hypertension and hyperlipidemia in diabetes, where extrapolation from trials in nondiabetic subjects is necessary because of very limited data in diabetes. Actually, there are more trials of antiplatelet agents in diabetes than there are of antihypertensive or hypolipidemic agents, so definitive recommendations can be made.

The meta-analysis reviewed results from 25 large scale trials in which antiplatelet agents were used after a transient ischemic attack, occlusive stroke, unstable angina, or myocardial infarction. In all, there were 3.000 deaths among a total of 29.000 patients reviewed. A disappointing finding was that antiplatelet therapy had no effect on total mortality. However, allocation to antiplatelet treatment reduced vascular mortality by 15% (SD: 4%) and nonfatal vascular events (stroke, myocardial infarction) by 30% (SD: 4%). There were no differences between different types of antiplatelet therapy tested. Doses of aspirin ranged from 325 to 1500 mg daily; dipyridamole (75 mg tid) was sometimes used in addition; sulfinpyrazone or ticlopidine were used in some trials. There was very limited information in very low doses of aspirin (such as, 100 mg/day). Thus, a daily dose of 325 mg of aspirin was recommended as a secondary prevention strategy. In discussion, the authors emphasized the important point of considering reduction of absolute as well as relative risk. Thus, a patient with established vascular disease might have about a 6% risk of vascular death and a 6% risk of a nonfatal vascular event in 2 years. Antiplatelet treatment should lower this risk to about 5% and 4%, respectively. However, if a patient has had a recent myocardial infarction, the two year risk for vascular death is about 12% and for a nonfatal vascular event is 9%. Antiplatelet therapy should reduce this to 10% and 6%, respectively, and therefore, could be viewed as more effective in this group. The reported data did not allow definitive recommendations about duration of therapy.

One very large study, the Second International Study of Infarct Survival (ISIS-2) was reported too late to be included in this meta-analysis. Results from this trial in which aspirin's role in evolving myocardial infarction was determined in 17.187 participants, were also supportive of a protective role for aspirin [14]. There was a 49% reduction in nonfatal myocardial infarction, and a 23% reduction in cardiovascular death, after 5 weeks in the aspirin group. All these reductions were statistically significant.

Thus, the evidence is strong that aspirin therapy is indicated as a secondary prevention strategy in survivors of myocardial infarction and stroke, in patients with transient ischemic attacks or unstable angina, and in those with an evolving heart attack.

Primary prevention: nondiabetic individuals

Results of primary prevention trials may have particular relevance to patients with diabetes mellitus for several reasons. First, as already indicated, altered platelet function and increased thromboxane production by platelets can be demonstrated very early in animal models of diabetes and in IDDM patients shortly after diagnosis. Thus, if platelets are involved in the genesis of diabetic vascular disease, it may be critical to start therapy before there are recognized vascular events. Secondly, it is well known that diabetic patients may have silent myocardial ischemia and/or silent myocardial infarctions. Therefore, major macrovascular disease may not be clinically apparent in diabetic patients, so a policy of "primary prevention" (before vascular disease is recognized) could be a good strategy.

Fortunately, there now are two primary prevention trials in nondiabetic individuals which can provide some guidance. Both of these trials have been done in male physicians, so generalizations must be limited. Between 1978–1984, a 6-year randomized trial was done in 5.139 apparently healthy male physicians in Great Britain [15]. Two-thirds of these took 300 to 500 mg of aspirin daily and 1/3 were asked to avoid aspirin preparations. About 25% gave up aspirin in the treatment group and 9% started aspirin in the control group. Total mortality was 10% lower, nonvascular deaths were 15% lower, and vascular deaths were 6% lower in the treated group when compared to controls; however, these were not significantly different. There was a close to 50% reduction in transient ischemic attacks. Fatal or nonfatal myocardial infarction incidence was not affected. The authors concluded that this was a negative study, in spite of the trends reported.

More promising results were reported from the Physicians Health Study in the U.S. [16]. In this study, 11.037 physicians received 325 mg of aspirin every other day and an equal number received an aspirin placebo. After 5 years of follow-up, the Data Monitoring Board recommended early termination of the aspirin component of the study primarily because of significant reduction (44%) in the risk of total myocardial infarction in the aspirin group. There were 139 myocardial infarctions among those assigned to aspirin and 239 in those assigned to the placebo group. This risk reduction was apparent in those aged 50 or over. There was a significant reduction in deaths from acute myocardial infarctions in the aspirin group, but no reduction in total cardiovascular mortality, primarily because sudden deaths were more prevalent in the aspirin group. When a combined endpoint of nonfatal myocardial infarction, nonfatal stroke, and cardiovascular death was used, there were 307 important vascular events in the aspirin and 370 in the placebo group. This was a statistically significant (P = .01) 18% reduction in important vascular events in the aspirin group.

There was an increased risk of bleeding (bruising, GI bleeding, epistaxis, etc.) in the aspirin group, but overall rates were quite low in both groups, perhaps due to the low dose of aspirin used. There was an apparent, but not statistically significant (P = .06) increase in hemorrhagic stroke in those assigned to aspirin therapy. Overall, there were 119 ischemic and hemorrhagic strokes in the aspirin group and 98 in the placebo group (N.S.). Clearly, resolution of this issue requires another randomized trial with a sample size large enough to determine the relative risks and benefits of aspirin therapy for primary prevention of stroke.

There are several other issues of concern in this trial. First, the absolute rate of cardiovascular events was very low, leading to an absolute risk reduction of nonfatal myocardial infarction of only two events per thousand per year. However, myocardial infarction rates were consistently higher in those with risk factors than in those without. Thus, the absolute impact of antiplatelet therapy would be greatest in such high risk groups. As would be expected, the subgroup with diabetes had about a 5-fold increase in coronary events. This issue will be considered in more detail when the antiplatelet trials in diabetic subjects are reviewed (below).

These primary prevention trials suggest that low dose aspirin therapy may prevent myocardial infarction in men over age 50 who have not had a major vascular event. This therapy is best viewed as adjunctive to other measures directed at vascular risk factors. Long-term data are needed to properly assess benefits and risks of continued, long-term therapy.

Secondary prevention: diabetic individuals

Macrovascular disease: There is one large scale VA Cooperative Study which has explored the effect of aspirin plus dipyridamole vs. placebo on macrovascular events in 231 diabetic men who had already had amputation for diabetic gangrene or active gangrene [17]. The study's combined primary endpoints was death from atherosclerotic vascular disease plus amputation of the opposite extremity for gangrene. There were 24 atherosclerotic deaths in the drug group (21.8%) and 23 in the placebo group (19.0%). There were 22 patients in the drug treatment group (20.0%) and 29 patients in the placebo group (24.0%) with opposite-side amputations. Survival curve analyses revealed little difference between these groups for the major vascular endpoints, total mortality, all amputations, or myocardial infarctions. There was a difference for cerebrovascular endpoints (strokes and transient ischemic attacks), with an incidence of 8.2% (9 patients) in the drug treatment group and 19.0% (23 patients) in the placebo group.

Thus, antiplatelet agents had no effect on the primary vasacular endpoints of vascular death and amputation of the opposite extremity in this population. No effects were seen on secondary vascular endpoints, except for a suggestion of protection against strokes and transient ischemic attacks. However, since this was found only after multiple analyses of the data in a secondary endpoint group, caution was advised in its interpretation. Several explanations for the negative conclusions from this study were entertained: 1) Event rates were lower than predicted (36.4% vs. 60%) decreasing the power of the study. 2) Vascular disease was too far advanced. This view is supported by studies cited above in nondiabetic individuals, in which antiplatelet therapy may have an effect as a primary preention strategy, or if it is started soon after a myocardial infarction. 3) A high dose of aspirin (325 mg tid) was used in the study, so prostacyclin inhibition was likely. However, aspirin may potentiate dipyridamole's action in diabetic animal models of platelet thrombosis [18], and this effect may be independent of prostacyclin production. Further, other secondary prevention trials in nondiabetic individuals (cited above) revealed no thrombotic effects of high dose aspirin therapy, so this explanation appears unlikely.

There is a second study of aspirin alone (325 mg tid) or aspirin plus dipyridamole (75 mg tid) therapy vs. placebo in 475 IDDM and NIDDM men and women [19]. Primary endpoint in this study was progression of retinopathy, as assessed by microaneurysm counting. This study is considered in more detail below, in the section on microangiopathy. During the 3-year study period, there were 4 deaths in the aspirin-treated groups and 4 deaths in the placebo group, and no difference was apparent in vascular vs. non-vascular causes of death.

There is one secondary preventive trial (AICLA Study) in which a relatively large complement of diabetic patients was enrolled, making subgroup analysis more meaningful [20, 28]. In this study, there were 129 diabetic patients enrolled, out of the 604 in the total sample (21%). Patients were enrolled who either had previously had a thrombotic stroke (84%) or transient ischemic attacks (TIA) (16%). Whereas 10 of 49 diabetic subjects randomized to placebo had a subsequent cerebrovascular event in 3 years (20%), only 5 of the 90 patients randomized to aspirin (325 mg tid) or to aspirin plus dipyridamole (75 mg tid) had a subsequent stroke or TIA (5.5%, $P < .01$).

These secondary prevention trials in large groups of diabetic subjects suggest that antiplatelet therapy may offer protection against subsequent thrombotic stroke and transient ischemic attacks. However, prevention from other macrovascular events has not been shown.

Microvascular disease: A. Retinopathy. There are two major large scale clinical trials which have studied the effects of aspirin (or aspirin plus dipyridamole), vs. placebo on diabetic retinopathy. The protocol for the first of these, the DAMAD Study [19], was described above. The major microvascular endpoint was the mean yearly increase in progression of retinal microaneurysms, as assessed by fluoroscein angiograms over a three year period. Mean yearly increase in microaneurysms was significantly less (P = .02) in the aspirin-treated group (0.69 ± 5.1 SD, n = 145) and in the aspirin plus dipyridamole group (0.34 ± 3.0, n = 142) than in the placebo group (1.44 ± 4.5, n = 133). There was a clear relationship between the deterioration in ophthalmological signs (exudates, cotton-wool spots, macular lesions, neovascularization, etc.) and the increase in yearly microaneurysms (Stable, 0.38 ± 3.96, n = 293 vs. Deteriorating, 1.79 ± 4.89, n = 127, P = .002). These studies indicate that aspirin alone and in combination with dipyridamole significantly slow the progression of microaneurysm evolution in early diabetic retinopathy.

Recently, preliminary results from the landmark Early Treatment Diabetic Retinopathy Study (ETDRS, 21) have become available [22, 23]. In this study, 3.711 IDDM and NIDDM patients with mild non-proliferative through early proliferative diabetic retinopathy were followed for up to 10 years. Although the primary goal of the study was to determine the effects of various approaches of laser therapy to different forms of diabetic retinopathy, there was also an aspirin (650 mg once daily) vs. placebo randomization process in the trial. The rationale was that such a large sample size could not only give information on the safety and efficacy of aspirin in preventing progression of retinal vascular disease, but that it could also provide informaton on aspirin's value in the prevention of macrovascular endpoints. Like the DAMAD Study, this trial is viewed as a secondary prevention trial regarding microvascular endpoints, but can be viewed as a primary prevention trial regarding macrovascular disease, since diabetic patients with clinically apparent macrovascular disease were generally excluded from the trial.

In contrast to the DAMAD Study, this trial showed no effect of aspirin on progression of diabetic retinopathy in persons with mild non-proliferative though early proliferative retinopathy. The major endpoints chosen for this trial was the development of high risk retinopathy, as opposed to the more subtle endpoint of progression of microaneurysms used in the DAMAD Study. A second endpoint, visual acuity, also showed no effect of aspirin.

An important finding in this study was that aspirin therapy was not associated with an increased risk of vitreous hemorrhage in these diabetic patients. This had been a concern at the inception of the trial, and like the DAMAD Study, aspirin use was not associated with this potentially serious complication in a group of patients with diabetic retinopathy. Thus, diabetic patients do not need to avoid taking aspirin because of the fear of visual damage.

B. Nephropathy. There is one study of antiplatelet therapy in IDDM patients with biopsy-proven diabetic glomerulosclerosis [24]. This was a small selective study, and was not performed in a double-blind fashion. However, there were promising results in a subgroup of patients studied. There were 28 IDDM patients with diabetic nephropathy who were placed on aspirin 325 mg tid, plus dipyridamole 75 mg tid. All patients had urinary protein in excess of 0.4 grams/24 hours, and had normal to impaired renal function, but not renal failure. Seven of the 28 patients (25%) had no progression of diabetic nephropathy over the follow-up time of 4 – 10 years (mean 6.6 years). This subgroup had a stable glomerular filtration rate and a significant decrease in proteinuria during the study. In contrast, the other 21 patients (75%) showed the expected progression of renal impairment, and all 7 deaths were seen in this group. The changes in GFR and proteinuria were similar to those reported in other small, uncontrolled studies using antihypertensive agents in diabetic patients with nephropathy.

While this is not a large-scale prospective randomized trial, it is a study which gives support to the concept that altered platelet function and/or renal eicosanoid metabolism may play a role in diabetic nephropathy in some patients [25, 26]. Although the study group was not large enough to do statistically meaningful subgroup analyses, the patients who appeared to respond to antiplatelet therapy were those with the least degree of renal impairment upon entry into the study. This suggests that antiplatelet therapy may be most effective when started early in the course of renal vascular disease. This concept is supported by a report which indicates that microalbuminuria (albumin excretion rates of 20 – 200 µg/min) is reduced to normal by the thromboxane synthetase inhibitor UK 38.485 in IDDM patients with otherwise normal renal function [27]. This possibility may also explain the results in the two studies on retinopathy, since the patients in the DAMAD Study appeared to have retinopathy which was milder than that in the patients enrolled in the ETDRS.

Primary prevention trials: diabetic individuals

There is one large-scale randomized trial, the ETDRS [21 – 23], which can be looked upon as a primary prevention trial, as far as macrovascular disease is concerned. However, as noted above, this is a secondary prevention trial of the effect of aspirin on diabetic retinopathy, since all patients had retinopathy upon entry. Results comparing aspirin to placebo regarding major cardiovascular events from this large scale trial are awaited with great interest, and are currently under analysis.

There are two other studies in diabetic subjects whieh may be viewed as primary prevention trials. In all cases, subgroup analyses are necessary, so conclusions must be taken with caution. The first of these is the DAMAD Study, which was previously described [19]. This was a three year study of aspirin (325 mg tid) plus dipyridamole (75 mg tid) in 475 IDDM and NIDDM individuals. There was 1 myocardial infarction in the placebo group and 2 in the aspirin groups which caused therapy discontinuation. Thus, subgroup analyses in this study showed no effect of antiplatelet therapy on macrovascular endpoints. However, the number of such endpoints was very low, possibly because patients with apparent macrovascular disease were excluded. Further, no data were given on cerebrovascular endpoints or nonfatal myocardial infarctions in patients who stayed in the study.

A second study in which a subgroup of diabetic patients was analyzed was the Physician's Health Study [16]. There were 11 myocardial infarctions among the 275 diabetic individuals on aspirin therapy (4.0%), and 26 myocardial infarctions in those 258 men randomized to the placebo group (10.1%). This gave a relative risk of 0.39 for the aspirin-treated group. This was one of the lowest relative risk figures among a number of coronary risk factors analyzed. Data from this study generally supported the view that antiplatelet therapy may be most effective as a primary prevention strategy in high risk groups, including individuals with diabetes mellitus.

Present treatment modalities

Aspirin (+ dipyridamole): benefits

The results of primary and secondary prevention trials in which aspirin ± dipyridamole therapy has been used are summarized in Table 2. The meta-analysis of secondary prevention trials in nondiabetic individuals considered the issue of aspirin alone or in combination with dipyridamole therapy, and found that combination therapy gave no clear advantage [13]. In the one

Table 2 Results of primary and secondary prevention trials

Secondary prevention trials – antiplatelet agents								
					Results			
	D. M.	Entry group	ASA*	DIP.⁺	Vasc. mort.	Non-fatal vasc.	CVA/ TIA	Total mort.
Antiplatelet trialists	No	Post CVA or MI	+	±	$\downarrow$	$\downarrow$	0	0
ISIS-2	No	Recent MI	+	0	$\downarrow$	$\downarrow$	0	0
VACS • 43	Yes	Amputation	+	+	0	0	$\downarrow$	0
AICLA (Subgroup)	Yes	Post CVA or TIA	+	+	0	0	$\downarrow$	0
					Microan. prog.	High risk ret.		Vis. acuity
DAMAD	Yes	Background retinopathy	+	±	$\downarrow$	0		0
ETDRS	Yes	Early prolif. retinopathy	+	0	——— No data ———			
Mayo	Yes	Early nephropathy	+	+	25%: Stable renal function			
Primary prevention trials – antiplatelet agents								
					Results			
	D. M.	Entry group	ASA*	DIP.⁺	Vasc. mort.	Non-fatal vasc.	CVA/ TIA	Total mort.
UK Study (MDs)	No	Normal males	+	0	0	0	0	0
US Study (MDs)	No	Normal males	+	0	0	$\downarrow$	$\downarrow$	0
(Subgroup)	Yes	No vasc. dis.	+	0	0	0	$\downarrow$	0
ETDRS	Yes	Early PDR	+	0	——— No data ———			

D. M. = Diabetes mellitus * = Aspirin ⁺ = Dipyridamole + = Yes ± = Yes or No 0 = no drug or no effect study in diabetes in which a direct comparison was made (The DAMAD Study [19]), no difference was seen in microaneurysm progression between the aspirin and the aspirin plus placebo group. Finally, all of the primary prevention trials have used aspirin alone (Table 2). These considerations suggest that antiplatelet therapy with aspirin alone is a wise strategy in diabetic patients with established macrovascular disease. Further, the primary prevention trials suggest that aspirin is also a prudent choice in diabetic individuals without established vascular disease. As previously discussed, one 325 mg enteric coated aspirin preparation daily is the appropriate choice, in order to inhibit platelet release and production of thromboxane in the face of persistent, relatively low, plasma aspirin levels.

Aspirin (+ dipyridamole): risk

Adverse side effects, such as gastrointestinal tract bleeding, gastric irritation, skin rash, etc. are generally less in trials in which 325 mg or less of aspirin is used vs. those in which up to 1500 mg are used. Although one primary prevention trial had a suggestion of an increase in hemorrhagic stroke among physicians assigned to 325 mg aspirin therapy every other day, the difference was not statistically significant.

In diabetic subjects, there has been concern that bleeding into the retina or into the vitreous may be increased with aspirin therapy. This was not shown to be the case, either in the DAMAD Study of individuals with background retinopathy [19] or in the ETDRS, in patients with early proliferative diabetic retinopathy [22, 23]. In both of these trials, rather high doses of aspirin (650 to 975 mg) were shown to be safe in this regard.

There is one disquieting report which suggests that aspirin (975 mg) plus dipyridamole (225 mg) is associated with an increase in sudden death among NIDDM males with advanced peripheral vascular disease and recent amputation history [30]. While we were careful to interpret the findings with caution, further studies appear indicated. Some support for this potential side effect is offered by three other secondary prevention trials and by one primary prevention trial. One mechanism which deserves investigation, based upon studies in diabetic animals [31] is the possibility that leukotriene-induced coronary vasoconstriction may be operative in diabetes after aspirin-induced cyclo-oxygenase inhibition. However, since the net effects of aspirin therapy appear to be beneficial regarding vascular mortality, non-fatal vascular events, and myocardial infarction (Table 2) aspirin therapy's benefits would appear to outweigh the risks.

Other agents

The emphasis on this chapter has been on aspirin as an antiplatelet agent, because of the large number of collaborative trials in nondiabetic and diabetic subjects. While there has been interest in other antiplatelet drugs such as Vitamin E [32], ticlopidine [33], metformin [34, 35], sulfonylureas [35], and thromboxane synthetase inhibitors [27], there are limited numbers of large scale randomized trials which allow assessment of these agents. Further, in view of the low toxicity and rather high effectiveness of aspirin as a preventive agent, it is unlikely that any of these agents will prove to be superior as an adjunctive approach.

There have been many studies of insulin therapy on platelet aggregation and thromboxane release. Early studies indicated that epinephrine-induced platelet aggregation was influenced by glycemic regulation [36]. Subsequently, it was shown that intensive insulin management would suppress platelet thromboxane release [37, 38], and that platelet-derived growth factor release was lowered by long-term intensive insulin-therapy [39]. Insulin addition *in vitro* will reduce platelet sensitivity to aggregating agents [40] suggesting a direct action of the hormone on platelets. Euglycemic insulin clamp studies have shown a reduction of platelet aggregation in normals [41], and production of normoglycemia either by insulin or sulfonylureas in noninsulin-dependent diabetic patients may reduce enhanced platelet aggregation rates to normal [42]. All of these studies strongly suggest that the first goal of antiplatelet therapy in diabetes should be the production of normoglycemia.

Future perspectives

Prevention of macrovascular disease in diabetes mellitus requires a multifactorial approach. A recent consensus Development conference from the American Diabetes Association concluded that this was the case [43]. Thus, it is likely, though unproven, that vigorous attempts to produce normoglycemia, normal plasma lipid and lipoprotein levels, normal blood pressure, cessation of smoking, and weight reduction would have great benefits in diabetic subjects. Nevertheless, our present methods of achieving these theoretically beneficial therapeutic results are inadequate, and many diabetic individuals are destined to have accelerated macrovascular disease. It is for this reason that an effective and relatively safe form of antiplatelet therapy, aspirin in doses of once daily, has become attractive to many physicians and patients.

Future research will delineate other approaches which may make this recommendation outdated. In particular, the medical community is anxiously awaiting the results from the landmark Diabetic Control and Complications Trial, in order to determine if intensive insulin therapy is justified as a preventive strategy in IDDM patients. However, this study will not answer the issue of glycemic control and macrovascular disease, either in IDDM and NIDDM patients. Fortunately, the Veterans Administration has just embarked on a feasibility study of intensive glycemic control in NIDDM patients, using microvascular and macrovascular endpoints. If this study should show a beneficial effect of intensive diabetic therapy on macrovascular disease, a major influence on therapy for NIDDM would emerge. This approach will be aided by new research advances in our understanding of altered lipoprotein metabolism, protein glycation, macrophage, endothelial, and vascular smooth muscle function, and altered coagulation in the diabetic state. It is likely that many or all of these mechanisms, in addition to altered platelet function, interact to produce accelerated macrovascular disease in diabetes. Once this pathophysiology is better understood, other drugs, in addition to aspirin, will become available to prevent or retard the development of atherosclerosis in diabetes mellitus.

References

[1] Direct and Indirect Costs of Diabetes in the United States in 1987. Center for Economic Studies in Medicine (Pracon, Inc.). American Diabetes Association, Inc., Alexandria, VA, 1988.

[2] Harris MI, Entmacher P. Mortality from diabetes. In: Diabetes in America, U.S. Department of Health and Human Services, Public Health Service, National Institutes of Health, Nation Institutes of Arthritis, Diabetes, and Kidney Diseases, NIH Publication No. 85–1468, Chapter XXIX, 1–48, 1985.

[3] Colwell JA, Lopes-Virella MF, Winocour PD et al. New concepts about the pathogenesis of atherosclerosis in diabetes mellitus. In: Levin ME, O'Neal LW, eds. The Diabetic Foot. St. Louis: C.V. Mosby Co, 1988; 51–70.

[4] Ruderman NB, Haudenschild C. Diabetes as an atherogenic factor. Prog Cardiovasc Dis 1984; 26: 373–412.

[5] Colwell JA, Lopes-Virella MF, Halushka PV. Pathogenesis of atherosclerosis in diabetes mellitus. Diabetes Care 1981; 4: 121–133.

[6] Colwell JA. Macroangiopathy. In: Alberti KGMM, Krall LP, eds. Diabetes Annual 4. Amsterdam: Elsevier Science Publishers, 1988; 355–383.

[7] Colwell JA, Macroangiopathy. In: Alberti KGMM, Krall LP, eds. Diabetes Annual 5. Amsterdam: Elsevier Science Publishers, 1989, in press.

[8] Banga, JD, Sixma JJ. Diabetes mellitus, vascular disease and thrombosis. Clinics in Haematology 1986; 15: 465–492.

[9] Ross R, Glomset JA. The pathogenesis of atherosclerosis. N Engl J Med 1976; 295: 369–377, 420–425.

[10] Ross R. The pathogenesis of atherosclerosis: an update. N Engl J Med 1986; 488–500.

[11] Mustard JF, Packham MA, Kinlough-Rathbone RL. Platelets and atherosclerosis. In: Miller ME, ed. Atherosclerosis: Mechanisms and Approaches to Therapy. New York: Raven Press, 1983; 29–43.

[12] Hirsh J, Salzman EW, Harker L et al. Aspirin and other platelet active drugs. Chest 1989; 95: 12 S – 18 S.
[13] Antiplatelet Trialists' Collaboration. Secondary prevention of vascular disease by prolonged antiplatelet treatment. Br Med J 1988; 296: 310 – 331.
[14] ISIS-2 (Second International Study of Infarct Survival) Collaborative Group. Randomized trial of intravenous streptokinase, oral aspirin, both, or neither among 17,187 cases of suspected acute myocardial infarction: ISIS-2. Lancet 1988; 349 – 360.
[15] Peto R, Gray R, Collins R et al. Randomized trial of prophylactic daily aspirin in British male doctors. Br Med J 1988; 296: 313 – 316.
[16] Steering Committee of the Physicians' Health Study Research Group. Final report on the aspirin component of the ongoing physicians' health study. N Engl J Med 1989; 321: 129 – 135.
[17] Colwell JA, Bingham SF, Abraira C et al. Cooperative study on antiplatelet agents in diabetic patients after amputation for gangrene: II. Effects of aspirin and dipyridamole on atherosclerotic vascular disease rates. Diabetes Care 1986; 9: 140 – 148.
[18] Honour AJ, Hockaday TDR, Mann JI. The synergistic effect of aspirin and dipyridamole upon platelet thrombi in living blood vessels. Br J Exp Path 1977; 58: 268 – 272.
[19] The DAMAD Study Group. Effect of aspirin alone and aspirin plus dipyridamole in early diabetic retinopathy. A multicenter randomized controlled clinical trial. Diabetes 1989; 38: 491 – 498.
[20] Bousser MG, Eschwege E, Haguenau M et al. "AICLA" controlled trial of aspirin and dipyridamole in the secondary prevention of athero-thrombotic cerebral ischemia. Stroke 1983; 14: 5 – 14.
[21] Early Treatment Diabetic Retinopathy Study Reserach Group. Photocoagulation for diabetic macular edema. Early Treatment Diabetic Retinopathy Study Report Number 1. Arch Ophthalmol 1985; 103: 1796 – 1806.
[22] Scientific Reporting Section, National Institutes of Health. Conclusions of the Early Treatment Diabetic Retinopathy Study, October 1989.
[23] Fact Sheet. National Eye Institute, National Institutes of Health. November, 1989.
[24] Donadio JV Jr, Ilstrup DM, Holley KE et al. Platelet-inhibitor treatment of diabetic nephropathy: a 10-year prospective study. Mayo Clin Proc 1988; 63: 3 – 15.
[25] Nath, KA. Platelets, antiplatelet therapy, and diabetic nephropathy. Mayo Clin Proc 1988; 63: 80 – 85.
[26] Moel DI, Safirstein RL, McEvoy RC et al. Effect of aspirin on experimental diabetic nephropathy. J Lab Clin Med 1987; 10: 300 – 307.
[27] Barnett AH, Leatherdale BA, Polak A et al. Specific thromboxane synthetase inhibition and albumin excretion rate in insulin-dependent diabetes. Lancet 1984; 1322 – 1325.
[28] Baudoin C, Bousser M-G, Haguenau M et al. Secondary prevention of strokes: Role of platelet antiaggregant drugs in diabetic and non-diabetic patients. Diabetic Med 1985; 2: 145 – 146.
[29] DeMinno G, Silver MJ, Cerbone AM et al. Trial of repeated low-dose asprin in diabetic angiopathy. Blood 1986; 68: 886 – 889.
[30] Colwell JA, Bingham SF, Abraira C et al. V.A. cooperative study of antiplatelet agents in diabetic patients after amputation for gangrene: Unobserved, sudden, and unexpected deaths. J Diabetic Compl 1989; 3: 191 – 197.
[31] Takiguchi Y, Umemura K, Hashimoto H et al. Involvement of thromboxane and leukotriene in arachidonate induced coronary constriction in diabetic rats. Diabetologia 1989; 32: 337 – 341.
[32] Gisinger C, Jeremy J, Speiser P et al. Effect of vitamin E supplementation on platelet thromboxane A_2 production in type I diabetic patients. Diabetes 1988: 37: 1260 – 1264.
[33] Akazawa Y, Oishi M, Koide M et al. Antiplatelet effect of ticlopidine in diabetes (Part II) – The efficiency of the platelet antiaggregating agent, ticlopidine in preventing background diabetic retinopathy. Japanese A ch Intern Med 1985; 32: 313 – 325.

[34] Gin H, Freyburger G, Boisseau M et al. Study of the effect of metformin on platelet aggregation in insulin-dependent diabetics. Diabetes Res Clin Practice 1989; 6: 61–67.
[35] McAlpine LG, McAlpine CH, Waclawski ER et al. A comparison of treatment with metformin and gliclazide in patients with non-insulin-dependent diabetes. Eur J Clin Pharmacol 1988; 34: 129–132.
[36] Peterson CM, Jones RL, Koenig RJ et al. Reversible hematologic sequelae of diabetes mellitus. Ann Intern Med 1977; 86: 425–429.
[37] Mayfield, RK, Halushka PV, Wohltmann HJ et al. Platelet function during continuous insulin infusion treatment in insulin-dependent diabetic patient. Diabetes 1985; 34: 1127–1133.
[38] McDonald JWD, Dupre J, Rodger NW et al. Comparison of platelet thromboxane synthesis in diabetic patients on conventional insulin therapy and continuous insulin infusion. Thromb Res 1982; 28: 705–712.
[39] Hamet P, Sugimoto H, Umeda F et al. Abnormalities of platelet-derived growth factors in insulin-dependent diabetes. Diabetes 1987; 36: 667–672.
[40] Trovati M, Anfossi G, Cavalot F et al. Insulin directly reduces platelet sensitivity to aggregating agents. Diabetes 1988; 37: 780–786.
[41] Hiramatsu K, Nozaki H, Arimori S. Reduction of platelet aggregation induced by euglycaemic insulin clamp. Diabetologia 1987; 30: 310–313.
[42] Evans, RJ, Lane J, Holman RR et al. Induced basal normoglycemia and altered platelet aggregation in non-insulin-dependent diabetes. Diabetes Care 1982; 5: 433–437.
[43] Colwell JA et al. Consensus Statement: Role of cardiovascular risk factors in prevention and treatment of macrovascular disease in diabetes. Diabetes Care 1989; 12: 573–579.

Glycosylation inhibition

I. Giardino, M. Brownlee

Diabetic complications, altered metabolic pathways, and Advanced Glycosylation Endproducts (AGE)

The primary cause of most diabetic complications is the exposure of susceptible target tissues to abnormally high levels of glucose for many years. Increased intracellular levels of glucose and its derivatives are thought to contribute to diabetic tissue dysfunction by acutely altering polyol pathway activity [1], the redox state of pyridine nucleotides [2], myoinositol levels in selected sub-cellular pools [3], and the rate of *de novo* diacylglycerol synthesis and protein kinase C activation [4]. However, the development of diabetic microvascular disease in dogs *following* the long-term normalization of these metabolic abnormalities with insulin [5] suggests that additional, irreversible mechanisms must also be involved. The accumulation of irreversible, glucose-derived chemical modifications (Advanced Glycosylation Endproducts, AGE) on long-lived macromolecules such as matrix components and DNA is the irreversible mechanism most consonant with the observed experimental and clinical epidemiology.

AGE accumulation begins with the formation of chemically reversible early glycosylation products, resulting in the formation of Schiff base adducts at a rate proportional to glucose concentration and to duration of exposure to sugar (Fig. 1, ①) [6]. These Schiff base adducts then rearrange to form the more stable Amadori product (Fig. 1, ②). This type of early glycosylation product reaches equilibrium levels over a period of several weeks. Opposing this process is a newly described pathway for the oxidative degradation of Amadori products, involving oxidative cleavage into peptide bound carboxymethyllysine and erythronic acid [7].

On collagen, DNA, and other long lived macromolecules in the vessel walls, certain highly reactive early glycosylation products are not degraded. Instead, they undergo a slow complex series of chemical rearrangements to form AGEs. There are two general types of AGEs described in the literature [8, 9]. One type is formed by the condensation of two Amadori products (Fig. 1, ④), and it resembles the heterocyclic imidazole derivative, 2-furoyl-4[(5)]-

(2-furanyl)1-*H*-imidazole [8]. The second general type of AGE crosslink appears to form from the reaction of an Amadori product with the Amadori-derived compound 3-deoxyglucosone [9] to form a heterocyclic pyrrole structure (Fig. 1, ③). The formation of other AGEs appears to involve generation of glycolaldehyde from Schiff bases via a reverse aldol condensation reaction. This product is an even more reactive cross-linking agent than 3-deoxyglucosone.

Since AGEs are irreversibly bound to proteins they accumulate continuously on long-lived vessel proteins, where they may contribute to the development of diabetic complications by production of crosslinks on extracellular matrix proteins, by interaction with specific cellular receptors, and by modifications of nucleic acids (Table 1).

Pathologic consequences of AGE accumulation

Extracellular protein crosslinking

The characteristic increase in vascular permeability and the progressive narrowing of blood vessels lumina reflect in part qualitative and quantitative alterations in diabetic extracellular matrix components. These alterations arise in part as a consequence of AGE-derived protein crosslinking involving both matrix and plasma proteins [10]. In vitro experiments using collagen as a model matrix protein have shown that glucose-derived AGEs form covalent, heat-stable, intermolecular bonds between adjacent matrix components [11]. These bonds occur only on two peptides at the N- and C-terminal ends of the molecule. Similar changes were found in vivo, where aortic collagen from diabetic rats was 3 times more cross-linked than aortic collagen from non-diabetic animals [12].

Diabetic vessels with significant AGE accumulation have thicker walls in part because their susceptibility to proteolytic degradation is reduced. In vitro, nonenzymatically glycosylated glomerular basement membrane is considerably more resistant to digestion by pepsin, papain, trypsin, and endogenous glomerular proteases than is normal basement membrane [13]. Glomerular basement membranes with AGEs formed in vivo are also much less digestible [14].

In addition to reduced proteolytic degradation, the formation of AGEs on matrix proteins also interferes with the geometrically ordered self-assembly process of basement membrane structure involving site-specific end-to-end and lateral interactions of type IV collagen, laminin, heparin sulfate proteoglycan and entactin. These changes may contribute to distorted three-dimen-

Table 1 Biological effects of AGEs

Extracellular matrix	Cellular receptors	Nuclear proteins/DNA
↑ Resistance to proteolysis	↓ Integrin-mediated cell-adhesion	↑ Altered DNA/protein binding
↓ BM associative binding properties	↑ Growth-promoting cytokines	↑ DNA breaks/superhelicity
	↑ Procoagulatory endothelial cell surface	
	↑ Macrophage chemotaxis	↑ Genetic mutation

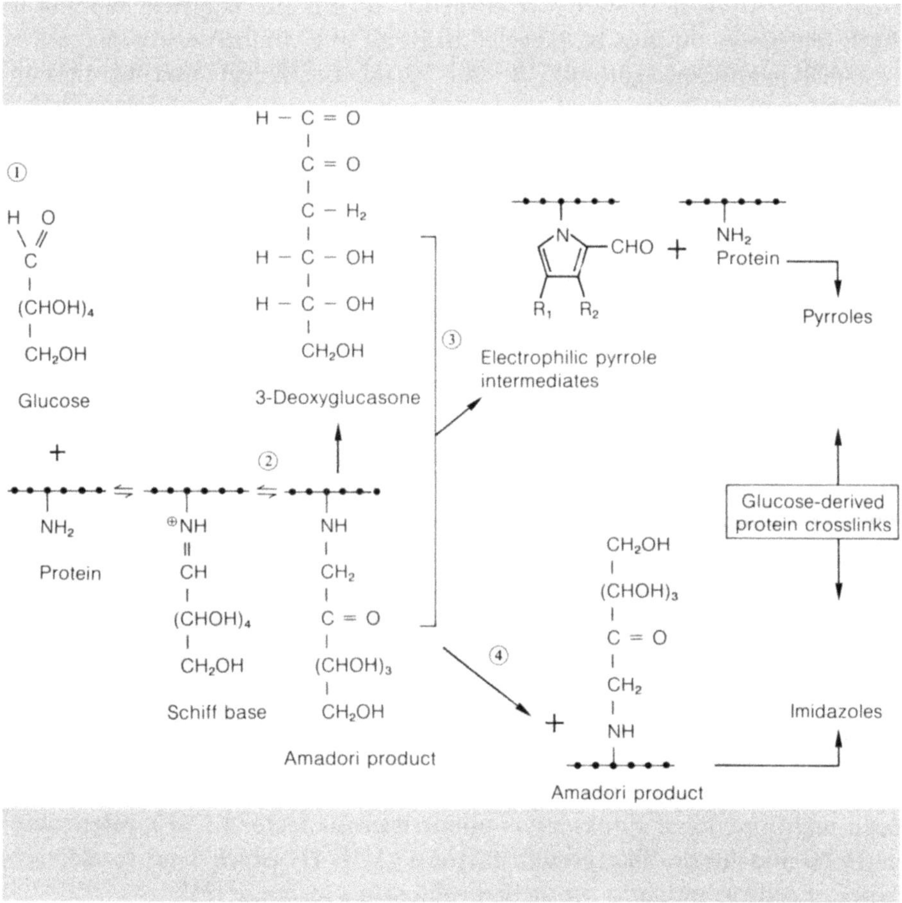

Fig. 1 Schematic representation of Early and Advanced Glycosylation Endproduct formation on extracellular matrix proteins (See text for details).

sional matrix structure, with increased effective intermolecular pore size [15] associated with permanent changes in vascular permeability and with permanently reduced associative properties of basement membrane components [16]. One particularly important consequence of reduced AGE-matrix component association appears to be a decrease in the amount of heparin sulfate proteoglycan in diabetic basement membranes.

Heparin sulfate proteoglycans are thought to down-modulate the proliferative activity of adherent cells [17], either through direct transmembrane inhibition of cellular activation via specific glycosaminoglycan (GAG) receptors, or indirectly via down-regulation of receptors for growth factors such as interleukin-1 (Il-1), insulin-like growth factor 1(IGF-1), and platelet-derived growth factor (PDGF). A reduction of this proteoglycan binding to AGE matrix would thus be expected to result in a compensatory increase of basement membrane synthesis [18 – 20]. Together with decreased degradation, this increased synthesis would produce the characteristic matrix accumulation of diabetic vasculopathy.

Accumulation of extravasated plasma proteins in the vascular basement membrane may also contribute to diabetic vascular occlusion. In vitro and in vivo experiments indicate that short-lived plasma proteins such as low density lipoprotein (LDL) and IgG, are bound specifically by reactive products generated by non enzymatic glycosylation of matrix proteins [21 – 25]. AGE-induced conformational changes in such matrix components as fibronectin, laminin, vitronectin, and collagen are likely to cause further abnormalities in diabetic blood vessels by altering matrix interactions with platelets and vascular wall cells [27, 28].

Interaction with cellular receptors

The progressive occlusion of diabetic blood vessels by matrix components is further accelerated by excessive cytokine stimulation of matrix synthesis. These growth-promoting cytokines are secreted by macrophages in response to AGE-protein binding to discrete cellular receptors. High affinity receptors for AGE proteins have been found in murine and human monocytes and macrophages and they may also exist in endothelial cells [29, 30]. The binding between AGE-matrix proteins and their receptors causes the production of such multifunctional cytokines as tumor necrosis factor (TNF), interleukin-1 (IL1), and insulin-like growth factor 1 (IGF-1), which bind to different types of cells to induce a synthetic/proliferative response [31].

The synthetic/proliferative cascade initiated by AGE-protein binding involves both direct growth-promoting effects of the cytokines produced, and indirect growth-promoting effects mediated by endothelial cells [32, 33]. The growth-promoting effects of TNF that are mediated by TNF-binding to specific endothelial cell receptors involve the induction of a precoagulatory state, which in turn results in the release of platelet-derived growth factor-like activity in response to thrombin and factor Xa stimulation [34]. Thrombus formation in diabetic vessels is also facilitated by a rapid reduction in thrombomodulin activity caused by direct interactions between endothelial cell AGE-receptors and AGE-matrix proteins [35].

Intracellular nucleic acid crosslinking

Some features of diabetic vascular complications such as the early loss of pericytes from retinal capillaries may reflect altered gene expression caused by irreversible AGE-induced damage to DNA [36]. Amadori products have been identified in the nucleus of cells from diabetic patients [37], and in vitro experiments have demonstrated that the glycosylating sugars can react with amino groups of both DNA nucleotides and all types of histones to form AGEs [38, 39].

Formation of AGEs on DNA has been associated with structural changes, mutations, and altered gene expression in prokaryotic and eukaryotic cells [40 – 42]. When human endothelial cells are cultured in 30mM glucose, there is an increase in single strand breaks and an increase in DNA repair synthesis. Increased single strand breaks in DNA also occur in lymphocytes from chronically hyperglycemic diabetic patients. In in vitro models, this AGE-damage appears to result in part from generation of specific purinic sites [42]. The nature of the endogenous repair systems for AGE-induced DNA damage are currently under investigation.

Glycosylation inhibition

Since AGE formation appears to play an essential role in the pathogenesis of diabetic complications, pharmacologic agents were sought that could inhibit this process by selectively blocking reactive carbonyls on early glycosylation products and on their derivatives such as 3-deoxyglucosone and glycolaldehyde. Aminoguanidine HCl, a small non-toxic nucleophilic hydrazine compound (LD50 = 1800 mg/kg in rodents) was found to prevent the chemical steps involved in AGE formation, while not interfering with normal lysyl oxidase dependent cross-links [12].

The site of aminoguanidine's pharmacological action could theoretically involve several steps in the AGEs formation process (Fig. 1). One possibility is that this compound is reacting with glucose, thereby lowering the ambient sugar concentration. However, since aminoguanidine effectively inhibits AGE formation when the glucose concentration is fifty times greater, this hypothesis cannot be correct [43]. Similarly, the possibilities that aminoguanidine is affecting either the rate of the Amadori rearrangement or the reaction of Amadori fragmentation products have both been shown to be inconsistent with the observed experimental data [44]. The data indicate that aminoguanidine acts primarily by binding covalently particular Amadori products, which are then rendered incapable to forming AGEs, although a small amount (<10%) may reflect reaction with 3-deoxyglucosone (Fig. 2) [41]).

In vitro experiments have demonstrated that aminoguanidine effectively inhibits AGE-crosslinking of soluble proteins to matrix. In addition, this compound inhibits AGE-induced crosslinking of collagen, and prevents crosslink-induced defects of heparin binding to collagen/fibronectin and crosslink-induced defects of heparin-sulfate proteoglycan binding to basement membrane ([12, 44], and Brownlee M., et al., unpublished data). Aminoguanidine also prevents AGE-induced defects in the normal growth properties of glomerular mesangial cells [45].

In vivo, the pharmacological effects of aminoguanidine have been investigated in a number of organs (Table 2). The presence of microaneurysms, PAS-positive intercapillary deposits of extravasated proteins, and acellular capillaries is dramatically reduced in the retinae of long-term diabetic rats treated with aminoguanidine [46]. Aminoguanidine also prevents diabetes induced increases in retinal vascular permeability and blood flow [47, 48].

In kidney, aminoguanidine treatment decreases GBM AGE content, and reduces the 400% increase in urinary albumin excretion induced by 10 weeks of diabetes to near-normal values [49]. Glomerular basement membrane from aminoguanidine-treated diabetic rats shows the same pattern of peptides after proteolytic digestion as non-diabetic controls, indicating that in vivo, the AGE-induced resistance to GBM degradation has been prevented [14].

Table 2 In vivo pharmacological effects of aminoguanidine

Retina	Kidney	Aorta
↓ Microaneurysms	↓ GBM AGE content	↓ AGE content
↓ Intercapillary deposits	↓ Urinary albumin excretion	↓ Lipoprotein deposits
↓ Acellular capillaries	↓ GBM thickness	
↓ Blood flow	Normal proteolytic degradation of GBM proteins	
↓ Vascular permeability		

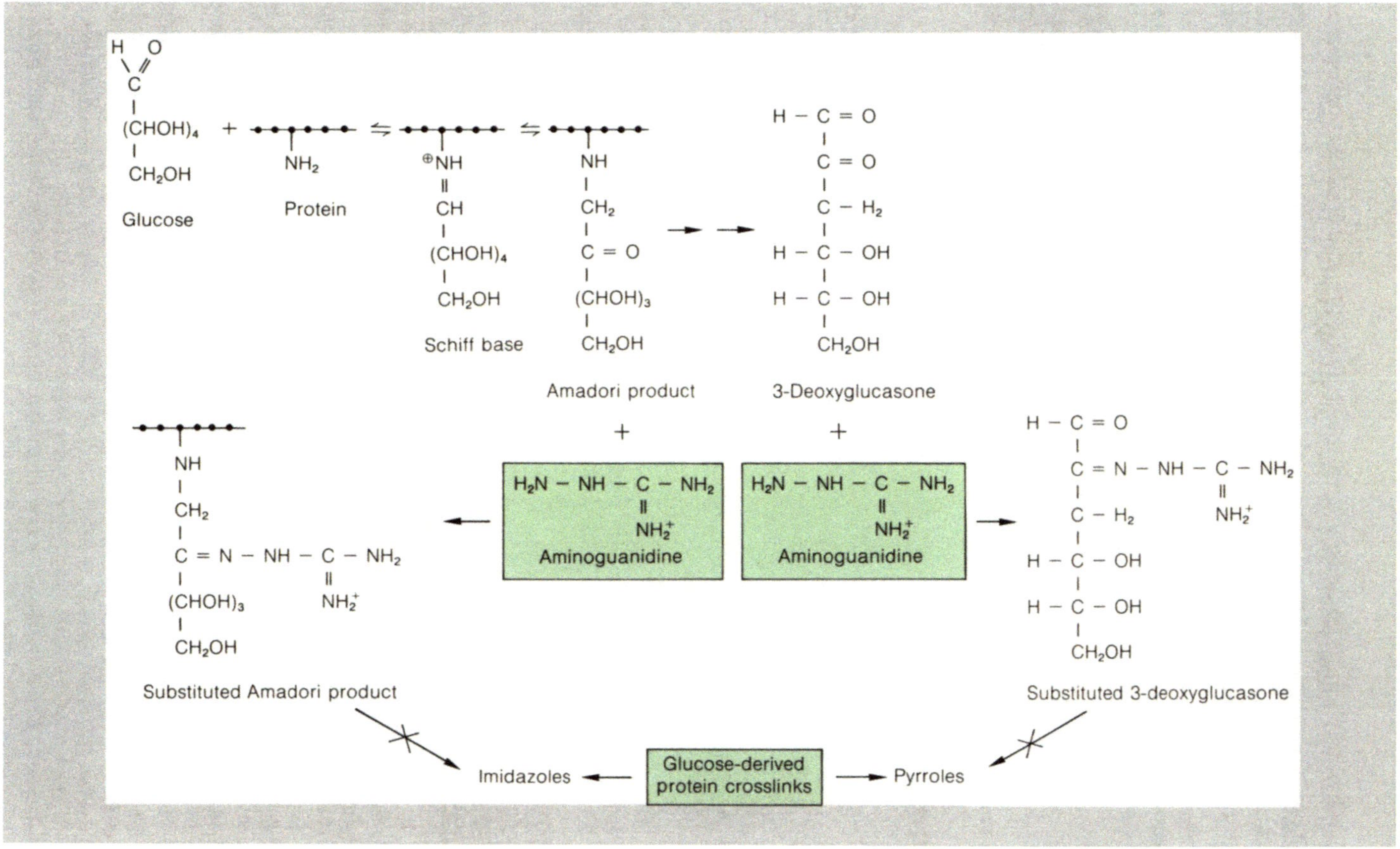

Fig. 2 Pharmacologic inhibition of AGE formation by aminoguanidine (See text for details).

Finally, the aminoguanidine treatment prevents the diabetes-associated increase in laminin B1 mRNA production, indicating that AGE-induced alterations in matrix-cell interactions are no longer stimulating excess matrix production [50]. In aortic wall of diabetic rats, aminoguanidine reduces AGE content while decreasing both the quantity of plasma proteins crosslinked to diabetic matrix, and the excess crosslinking of aortic matrix protein itself [14, 51, 52].

The therapeutic potential of aminoguanidine and its analogues is currently being more extensively evaluated in several animal and cell culture model systems, while the pharmacokinetics and potential toxicity of aminoguanidine are being determined in concurrent human studies [53].

References

[1] Greene, DA, Lattimer SA, Sima AAF. Sorbitol, phophoinositides, and sodium-potassium-ATPase in the pathogenesis of diabetic complications. N Engl J Med 1987; 316: 599–606.

[2] Williamson JR, Change K, Ostrow E et al. Sorbitol-induced increases in vascular albumin clearance are prevented by pyruvate but not by myoinositol. Diabetes 1989; 38 (suppl. 2): 94A.

[3] Winegrad AI. Does a common mechanism induce the diverse complications of diabetes? Diabetes 1987; 36: 396–406.

[4] Lee TS, Saltsman KA, Ohashi H et al. Activation of protein kinase C by elevation of glucose concentration: Proposal for a mechanism in the development of diabetic vascular complications. Proc Natl Acad Sci 1989; 86: 5141–5145.

[5] Engerman RL, Kern TS. Progression of incipient diabetic retinopathy during good glycemic control. Diabetes 1987; 36: 808–812.

[6] Brownlee M, Vlassara H, Cerami A. Nonenzymatic glycosylation and the pathogenesis of diabetic complications. Ann Intern Med 1984; 101: 527–537.

[7] Ahmed MU, Thorpe SR, Baynes JW. Identification of N-Carboxymethyllysine as a degradation product of fructosyllysine in glycated protein. J Biol Chem 1986; 261: 4889–4894.

[8] Chang JCF, Ulrich PC, Bucala R et al. Detection of an advanced glycosylation product bound to protein in situ. J Biol Chem 1985, 260: 7970–7974.

[9] The NIH Conference on the Maillard Reaction in Aging, Diabetes and Nutrition, Baines JW, Monnier VM, eds. Alan R. Liss, Inc. NY, 1989.

[10] Brownlee M, Spiro RG. Glomerular basement membrane metabolism in the diabetic rat. In vivo studies. Diabetes 1979; 28: 121–125.

[11] Kent MJC, Light ND, Bailey AJ. Evidence for glucose-mediated covalent cross-linking of collagen after glycosylation in vitro. Biochem J 1985; 225: 745–752.

[12] Brownlee M, Vlassara H, Kooney T et al. Aminoguanidine prevents diabetes-induced arterial wall protein cross-linking. Science 1986; 232: 1629–1632.

[13] Lubec G, Pollak A. Reduced susceptibility of nonenzymatically glucosylated glomerular basement membrane to proteases: is thickening of diabetic glomerular basement due to reduced proteolytic degradation? Renal Physiol 1980; 3: 4–8.

[14] Kempe HP, Engelmann K, Hasslacher Ch et al. Effect of aminoguanidine in degradation of glomerular basement membrane. Diabetologica 1989; 32: 502–503.

[15] Tanaka S, Avigad G, Brodsky B et al. Glycation induces expansion of the molecular packing of collagen J Med Biol 1988; 203: 495–505.

[16] Tsilibary EC, Charonis AS, Reger LA et al. The effect of nonenzymatic glucosylation on the binding of the main noncollgenous NC1 domain at to type IV collagen. J Biol Chem 1988; 263 (9): 4302–4308.
[17] Klahr S, Schreiner G, Ichikawa I. The progression of renal disease. N Eng J Med 1988; 318: 1657–1666.
[18] Klein DJ, Brown DM, Oegema TR. Glomerular proteoglycans: partial structural characterization and metabolism of de novo synthesized heparin-35SO4 proteoglycan in streptozotocin-induced diabetic rats. Diabetes 1986; 35: 1130–1142.
[19] Shimomura H, Spiro RG. Studies on macromolecular components of human glomerular basement membrane and alterations in diabetes: decreased levels of heparin sulfate proteoglycan and laminin. Diabetes 1987; 36: 374–381.
[20] Rohrbach DH, Hassel JR, Kleinman HK et al. Alterations in basement membrane (heparan sulfate) proteoglycan in diabetic mice. Diabetes 1982; 31: 185–188.
[21] Brownlee M, Vlassara H, Cerami A. Nonenzymatic glycosylation products on collagen covalently trap low -density lipoprotein. Diabetes 1985; 34: 938–941.
[22] Michael AF, Brown DM. Increased concentration of albumin in kidney basement membranes in diabetes mellitus. Diabetes 1981; 30: 843–846.
[23] Graham AR, Johnson PC. Direct immunofluorescence findings in peripheral nerve from patients with diabetic neuropathy. Ann Neurol 1985; 17: 450–454.
[24] Brownlee M, Pongor S, Cerami A. Covalent attachement of soluble proteins by nonenzymatically glycosylated collagen: Role in the in situ formation of immune complexes. J Exp Med 1983; 158: 1739–1744.
[25] Sensi M, Tanzi P, Bruno MR et al. Human glomerular basement membrane: altered binding characteristics following in vitro nonenzymatic glycosylation. Ann NY Acad Sci 1986; 488: 549–552.
[26] Smith EB, Massie IB, Alexander KM. The release of an immobilized lipoprotein fraction from atherosclerotic lesions by incubation with plasmin. Atherosclerosis 1976; 25: 71–84.
[27] Ruoslahti E, Pierschbacher MD. New perspectives in cell adhesion: RGD and integrins. Science 1987; 238: 491–497.
[28] Crowley S, Schlondorff D, Brownlee M. Effect of glycated matrix on mesangial cell function. (manuscript in preparation).
[29] Vlassara H, Brownlee M, Cerami A. High-affinity receptor-mediated uptake and degradation of glucose -modified proteins: A potential mechanism for the removal of senescent macromolecules. Proc Natl Acad Sci USA 1985; 82: 5588–5592.
[30] Williams SK, Devenny JJ, Bitensky MW. Micropinocytic ingestion of glyosylated albumin by isolated microvessels: possible role in pathogenesis of diabetic microangiopathy. Proc Natl Acad Sci USA 1981; 78: 2393–2397.
[31] Vlassara H, Brownlee M, Monogue K et al. Cachectin/TNF and IL-1 induced by glucose-modified proteins: role in normal tissue remodeling. Science 1988; 240: 1546–1548.
[32] Lovett DH, Ryan JL, Sterzel RB. Stimulation of rat mesangial cell proliferation by macrophage interleukin 1. J Immunol 1983; 136: 3700–05.
[33] Libby P, Warner SJC, Freidman GB. Interleukin 1: A mitogen for human vascular smooth muscle cells that induces the release of inhibitory prostanoids. J Clin Invest (in press).
[34] Bevilacqua MP, Pober JS, Majeau GR et al. Recombinant tumor necrosis factor induces procoagulant activity in cultured human vascular endothelium: Characterization and comparison with the actions of interleukin 1. Proc Natl Acad Sci USA 1986; 83: 4533–4537.
[35] Vlassara H, Esposito C, Gerlach H et al. Receptor-mediated binding of glycosytlated albumin to endothelium induces tissue factor and acts synergistically with TNF procoagulant activity. Diabetes 1989; 38 (Suppl. 2): 329.
[36] Penn A, Garte SJ, Warren L et al. Transforming gene in human atherosclerotic plaque DNA. Proc Natl Acad Sci USA 1986; 83: 7951.
[37] Kelly SB, Olerud JE, Witztum JL et al. A method for localizing the early products of nonenzymatic glycosylation in fixed tissue. J Invest Derm 1989; 93: 327–331.

[38] Bucala R, Model P, Cerami A. Modification of DNA by reducing sugars: a possible mechanism for nucleic acid aging and age-related dysfunction in gene expression. Proc Natl Acad Sci USA 1984; 81: 105–109.
[39] De Bellis D, Horowitz MI. In vitro studies of histone glycation. Biochem Biophys Acta 1987; 926: 365–368.
[40] Lee AT, Cerami A. Elevated glucose 6-phosphate levels are associated with plasmid mutations in vivo. Proc Natl Acad Sci USA 1987; 84: 8311–8314.
[41] Lornezi M, Montisano DF, Toledo S et al. High glucose and DNA damage in endothelial cells. J Clin Invest 1986; 77: 322–325.
[42] Carroll Z, Brownlee M, Yoacum G. Breakage of supercoiled DNA by stable products of Glucose-6-P or Glyceraldehyde-3-P with lysine. (Manuscript in preparation).
[43] Edelstein D, Brownlee M. Mechanistic studies of advanced glycation endoproduct inhibition by Aminoguanidine. (Submitted for publication.)
[44] Brownlee M, Vlassara H, Cerami A. Aminoguanidine prevents hyperglycemia-induced defect in binding of heparin by matrix molecules. Diabetes 1987; 36: 85A.
[45] Crowley S, Brownlee M, Singhal P et al. Effects of nonenzymatic glycosylation (NEG) of matrix on rat mesangial cell (MC) function. Am Soc Neph 1990; 32, 55: 30A.
[46] Hammes HP, Martin S, Federlin K et al. Aminoguanidine treatment inhibits the development of experimental diabetic retinopathy. Diabetes 1990; 39 (Suppl. 1), 248: 62A.
[47] Tilton RG, Chang K, Ostrow E et al. Aminoguanidine redices increased 131I-Albumin permeation of retinal and uveal vessels in streptozoticin -diabetic rats. Invest Ophthal VIS. SCI. 1990; 31 (Suppl. 4): 43.
[48] Ido Y, Chang K, Ostrow E et al. Aminoguanidine prevents regional blood flow increases in Streptozotocin- diabetic Rats. Diabetes 1990; 39 (Suppl. 1), 372: 93A.
[49] Yamashita H, Yoshikawa C, Bannai D et al. Glycation of basement membrane collagen and proteinuria. Diabetes 1989; 38 (Suppl. 2): 25A.
[50] Ellis EN, Bowen W. Aminoguanidine ameliorates glomerular basement membrane (GBM) thickening in experimental diabetes. Diabetes 1990; 30 (Suppl. 1), 282: 71A.
[51] Brownlee M, Vlassara H, Kooney T, Ulrich P, Cerami A. Aminoguanidien prevents diabetes-induced arterial wall protein cross-linking. Science 1986; 232: 1629–1632.
[52] Nicholls K, Mandel TE. Advanced glyosylation end-products in experimental murine diabetic nephropathy: effect of islet isografting and aminoguanidine. Lab Invest 1989; 60: 486–493.
[53] Makita Z, Radoff S, Rayfield E et al. Radioreceptor Assay (RRA) for human serum and arterial tissue advanced glycosylation endproducts (AGE). Diabetes 1990; 39 (Suppl. 1), 113: 29A.

Pharmacologic prevention and treatment of diabetic foot problems

E. Standl, H. Stiegler, R. Mathies, R. Standl, B. Weichenhain

Introduction

Foot disorders are the most common complications requiring hospitalisation of diabetic patients [1–9). In addition to being a devastating situation for the individual, treatment of diabetic foot ulcers and gangrene is a huge economic burden for the health care system [10]. In a recent survey, diabetic patients accounted for 50% of all amputations performed in the United States [11], and one out of ten diabetic patients is faced with this problem at some time during his life. A larger proportion of these complications, however, can be prevented when appropriate education of the patients and proper foot care are provided [8, 12] and early lesions are managed effectively and by avoiding further hazards. The present chapter, therefore, deals with the adequate pharmacology of both the preventive foot care and the treatment of foot lesions in diabetic patients with special reference to problems associated with peripheral vascular disease and to potentially harmful or useless measures.

Pathogenetic background

The etiology and pathogenesis of diabetic foot problems – leading to a 20 to 50 times greater risk for gangrene as compared to nondiabetics – are rather complex (for review see [13]). Fig. 1 outlines the most important factors. In addition to the at least fivefold increase of peripheral arterial disease [1, 2, 4, 6, 9], peripheral polyneuropathy is another major contributor to serious foot complications in diabetics [4, 7, 29]. The disordered nerve function may not only lead to trophical tissue changes, but also cause a significant loss in the pain and temperature perception, both of which render the foot vulnerable to injuries which go unnoticed for days. Absent or low grade symptomatology must never be mistaken as a favorable prognostic sign, but rather as a typical feature of foot lesions in a diabetic. This phenomenon, an insensitive yet

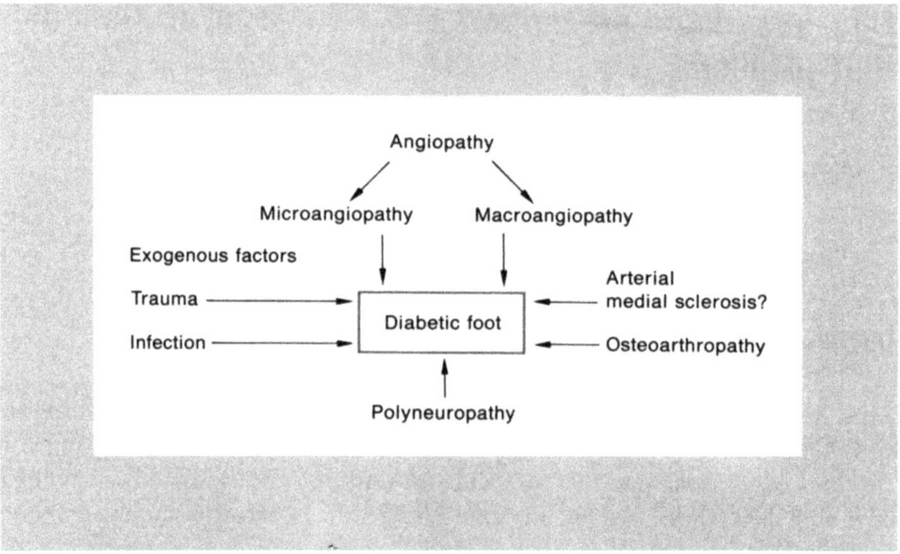

Fig. 1 Etiology and pathogenesis of the diabetic foot

vulnerable foot, must also be kept particularly in mind in the context of any pharmacologic treatment attempts or any other manipulations at the foot of a diabetic patient.

Arterial mediasclerosis of the Mönckeberg type, complex microvascular abnormalities and osteoarthropathy may be other distinct manifestations in the foot of a diabetic [7, 8, 14] and should be looked for when planning the therapeutical approach to a given foot lesion. The diagnostic work up of diabetic foot problems is shown in Table 1. Systolic ankle blood pressure below 40 to 50 mmHg is usually incompatible with primary healing of significant foot lesions, unless macrocirculation can be improved by angioplasty or vascular surgery, whereas a systolic toe presure of > 45 mmHg (in cases without mediasclerosis) seems to offer an 85% chance of primary wound healing [28]. In addition to arterial blood supply, the severity of the lesion also determines the possible outcome of any pharmacotherapy applied. Initial classification of the lesion, e.g. according to Wagner [14], is strongly recommended. In short, the type of lesion is characterized as superficial (grade 1) up to a necrosis through the full thickness of the dermis; deep (grade 2), if subcutaneous tissue is also involved; abscess and/or osteomyelitis (grade 3); minor gangrene (grade 4) as defined by continuous necrosis of the skin and underlying structures (muscle, tendon, joint, or bone) mainly located on the forefoot; or major gangrene (grade 5), if continuous necrosis as described above involves most of the foot. A significant proportion of grade 3 lesions and most grade 4 and 5 lesions will need at least some local amputation, especially in case of progressive gangrene, intolerable pain despite analgesic treatment, and toxic or septic conditions not responding to medical treatment [28]. Of course, all lesions must undergo surgical debridement when necessary and pharmacotherapy without this prerequisite is a major mistake!

The risk profile associated with the excessive morbidity of macrovascular, microvascular and neurological disease contributing to diabetic foot problems has been more clearly defined in recent years. Table 2 (for review see [1, 2, 3,

Table 1 Diagnostic measures for peripheral vascular disease and diabetic foot problems

- History of the duration and control of diabetes; identification of cardiovascular risk factors, previous or existing claudication, rest pain, foot ulcers, neuropathy, infection or trauma
- Examination for trophic changes, deformities, local inflammation, pressure points of the feet
- Palpation of pulses, temperature differences
- Auscultation of arteries in typical sites, eventually immediately following exercise
- Angiologic investigations (electronic oscillometry, Doppler ultrasound measurements, CW-Doppler tracings, duplex sonography)
- Neurological investigations (electrophysiological measurements)
- Bacteriologic analysis in case of foot infections
- Pedographic tracing for identification of pressure points or changes in foot mechanics
- Identification of microangiography (fundus examination, microalbuminuria, capillary microscopy)
- Radiological investigations (x-rays of the feet for identification of osteomyelitis, osteo-arthropathy, angiographic examination if necessary)

Table 2 Risk factors or indicators of micro- and macroangiopathy in diabetic patients

Microangiopathy	Macroangiopathy
Hyperglycemia	Age
(duration of diabetes, quality of control)	Hypertension (incl. syst. hypertension)
Hypertension	Nephropathy (incl. microalbuminuria)
Smoking	Dyslipoproteinemia (incl. hypertriglyceridemia)
	Hyperglycemia
	Insulin resistance/hyperinsulinemia
	Smoking
Hemostasiological and hemorheological abnormalities	

5, 6, 9, 13]) lists the most pertinent items in terms of microangiopathy and macroangiopathy. Peripheral neuropathy shows many similarities with microangiopathy. Correction of dehydration and improvement of hemorheology by rather aggressive compensation of metabolic control is an indispensable requirement and short-term goal for any pharmacotherapy of foot complications. For the appropriate long-term therapy, the eliminiation – as far as possible – of the other risk ingredients comes into focus and good metabolic control and weight reduction will also favorably influence hypertension, lipids, and the insulin resistance/hyperinsulinemia syndrome.

Pathophysiologically, macrovascular disease and, in particular, peripheral vascular disease in diabetics seem to be characterized by multiple imbalances in the blood clotting and fibrinolytic systems, including in the prostaglandine pathways, and by an abnormal hemorheology [15, 16, 56, 57]. Induced by an increase of acute phase proteins (e. g. a_2-macroglobulin or fibrinogen) in serum, especially in the context of foot infections, and decreased red cell fluidity, both whole blood and plasma viscosity may be markedly increased [31, 40, 57]. This seems to be especially important in the microcirculation of patients with advanced arterial insufficiency, in whom large areas of non perfused capillaries are found. At the same time, even physiologically, erythrocyte fluidity is strongly decreased in the more acid milieu of underperfused tissues [54]. Acidosis and infection induced activation of granulocytes and macrophages with free radical formation, lipid peroxidation and lysosomal enzyme release also contribute to profound tissue damage [8].

A 5-year prospective study on a large group of non-insulin dependent diabetics has shown the significant predictive power of increased platelet aggregation and fibrinogen concentration in the occurrence of severe macrovascular complications in male patients [17]. In view of these observations, it is not surprising that practically all pharmacological attempts to treat large vessel disease in diabetic patients, beyond good glycemic and lipid control, have been directed towards a normalization of the disordered hemostasis and hemorheology.

Survey of clinical trials

"Vasoactive" drugs

Drugs targeted against arteriosclerotic disease have been in use since as early as the 1930s [32, 33]. Although numerous new agents have since then been developed for "vasoactive" therapy and countless studies have been performed, it is only a few years ago that it was stated how unsatisfactory our notions were [42]. In fact it had been argued that "vasodilator" drugs in pheripheral vascular disease might be useless or even harmful in that they might hamper ischemic tissues by "borrowing – lending mechanisms" [32, 33, 42, 54]. In addition, complaints have been made about the poor comparability of the many studies. The following points were of particular concern:

1) The aims of the studies had often not been clearly defined.
2) Patients studied were somewhat inhomogeneous with respect to severity, duration, localisation, and etiology of vascular disease.
3) The severity of large vessel disease was somewhat ill defined and Doppler examinations or grading according to Fontaine were often missing.
4) Inclusion and exclusion criteria for patients were not disclosed.
5) No information was given about accompanying diseases.
6) Claudication was not assessed in a standardized manner.
7) Studies were organized as open trials without randomisation for comparison and placebo control.

On the other hand, the quantification of peripheral occlusive arterial disease is especially complex. Any newly occurring process obliterating the lumen of a main artery will induce collateral circulation, which will in turn improve for example the ability to walk spontaneously, for up to one year [32]. Furthermore, another confounding factor may be the fact that regular physical exercise has been shown to improve the walking capacity of patients with intermittent claudication as much as 200 – 300 per cent, depending on the localisation of the occlusion [32, 43, 44, 45, 53]. Physical exercise has been established as a treatment of choice for patients with claudication, and beneficial effects attributed to drug intervention have often not been better than the potential exercise effect.

In recent years however, several scientific angiologic committees or associations have issued guidelines for the evaluation of "vasoactive" agents [47, 48, 61]. In the meantime, a few longer-term double blind, placebo-controlled trials with well defined protocols and agents without "steel-effects" have been completed and will be reported here in brief [26, 27, 30, 34, 35, 38 – 40, 45, 46, 48, 50 – 52, 59, 61]. How far the results really apply to diabetic patients is yet another problem, since nondiabetics and diabetics have been usually incorporated into the same study groups or diabetic patients have even been excluded. Concomitant microvascular and neuropathic complications in a diabetic may significantly alter the outcome of any given intervention [13].

These limitations admitted, Table 3 indicates a few widely used "vasocative" compounds which have been tested in a well controlled, double blind manner, their suggested mechanisms of action, and the stage of peripheral vascular

Table 3 Evaluation of "vasoactive" compounds in relation to severity of peripheral vascular disease (Fontaine grades II–IV)

"Vasoactive" compound	Suggested action	Efficacy tested in Fontaine stage		
		II	III	IV
(1) Buflomedil	Improved hemorheology. Effect on metabolic and cellular factors	+	+	
(2) Naftidrofuryl	As for (1) + aggregation inhibition	+	+	+
(3) Pentoxifylline	Improved hemorheology Aggregation inhibition	+		+
(4) Prostaglandine E_1	As for (1) and (2) + vasodilatation and activation of fibrinolysis	+	+	+

disease according to Fontaine in which efficacy has been evaluated [26, 27, 30, 34, 35, 38–40, 45, 46, 50–52, 59, 61]. Table 4 depicts in more detail the "state of art" as to Fontaine stage II b, the stage of seriously limiting intermittent claudication. Walking capacity has usually been assessed on treadmills, which give the most reliable results. As may be seen, an increase of 50 to 100% of the pain-free walking distance can be expected subsequently to the blinded, standardized application of "vasoactive" drugs. It is of particular note that in some of the more recent studies, patients were assigned to the active drug trial only after a 6 month period of regular physical exercise during which a considerable gain in the walking capacity was achieved [45, 52, 59, 61]. Nevertheless, the studies indicated the drugs to be beneficial on top of the exercise effect.

These statistically established differences are most likely of clinical relevance in patients with a severely decreased walking tolerance (Fontaine grade II b) who are not suited to angioplastic or local thrombolytic procedures or have only very peripheral occlusive disease below the knee and who can reach an almost unlimited walking capacity with a regular physical exercise program in combination with the use of an approved "vasoactive" agent. Furthermore, adjuvant "vasoactive" pharmacotherapy in patients with rest pain (Fontaine grade III) has been shown to significantly reduce the acute ischemic pain in placebo-controlled, double blind studies with the compounds listed in Table 3 [40, 48, 50, 60]. Similarly, the amputation rate could be significantly decreased and primary healing of arterial ulcerations or necrosis of the foot significantly

Table 4 "Vasoactive" agents: Double blind, placebo controlled, prospective studies with significant improvement of intermittent claudication

First author	Agent	Year	Length of treatment	Total patients (on "vasoactive" compound)	Per cent gain of pain-free walking distance
Becker	Naftidrofuryl	1979	i. v. 14 days	210 (106)	183
Trübestein	Buflomedil	1982	12 weeks	93 (47)	97
Porter	Pentoxifylline	1982	24 weeks	128 (61)	56
Maas	Naftidrofuryl	1984	12 weeks	104 (54)	68
Adhoute	Naftidrofuryl	1986	24 weeks	118 (54)	94
Kiesewetter	Pentoxifylline*	1987	4 weeks	30 (15)	23
Rudofsky	Pentoxifylline	1988	i. v. 14 days	154 (75)	70
Kriessmann	Naftidrofuryl*	1988	12 weeks	136 (71)	77
Rudofsky	Prostaglandine E_1*	1988	i. v. 28 days	50 (25)	73
Diehm +	Prostaglandine E_1*	1989	i. v. 21 days	(24)	99
	Naftidrofuryl*			(24)	97
Lindgärde	Pentoxifylline	1989	24 weeks	150 (75)	80

* Trial following long-term exercise program;
\+ Randomized prospective trail

improved (Fontaine grade IV, Table 3, [48, 50, 51, 60]. In the latter context, prostaglandine E_1 seems to yield superior results in comparison to other compounds [51, 56].

Continuing controversies, however, can not be denied [26, 32, 33, 56]. Negative results have been obtained even with the compounds listed in Table 3, although it must be realized that these studies were performed in the early days of the respective compounds and the dosages were too small [36, 37]. With regard to the intravenous administration of prostaglandine E_1 it should be pointed out that 80–90% of the active compound is eliminated in the first lung passage and the recently applied 60 ug/d or 2 × 40 ug/d during a 2 h saline infusion period need to be titrated against side effects like venous discomfort, headache, flush etc. [56]. Lower dose intraarterial administration of PGE_1 into the extremity at risk is preferable and probably superior in this context, but may introduce other problems during long-term application and is not everywhere available [49, 56, 60]. More disturbingly, diabetic patients have been found to be less responsive to PGE_1 in some studies [55] and eliminated in others [59], so that information is still scarce with respect to the particular topic discussed in this chapter.

Many more substances have been tested and even found beneficial in some studies, but results could not be confirmed by others (for review see [32, 54]). Obviously, these should not be used. In contrast, isovolemic and hypervolemic hemodilution have been universally assessed as effective in controlled randomized trials concerning patients with hemoconcentration (PVC > 45%) or increased plasma viscosity (> 1.4 mPas) and grade II b–IV of peripheral occlusive arterial disease [18, 19, 54, 57, 58]. The volume replacement with 6 or 10% hydroxyethyl starch in correspondence to venesection seems to be preferable compared to dextrane infusion for several reasons, including efficacy [18, 58]. The combination of hemodilution and "vasoactive" pharmacotherapy has been observed to yield additive effects in patients with intermittent claudication [57]. In theory, the combination of hemodilution with defibrinogenisation (e. g. by means of ancrod) would also appear reasonable in patients with high fibrinogen levels and plasma viscosity, but this could not be validated so far in larger scale, controlled trials [31, 54]. Diabetic patients in particular often show markedly increased plasma fibrinogen concentrations [17], and perhaps the most efficient way to lower these excessive concentrations is by means of bag plasmapheresis [57].

Local thrombolysis

One of the rare major breakthroughs in clinical pharmacotherapy in recent years has been the introduction of local thrombolysis through a catheter to occlusive arterial disease, subsequently to the development of catheter angioplasty in the 1960s [7, 20, 21, 22]. As far as the lower limbs are concerned, obliterated segments from the pelvic arteries down to the crural arteries beyond the trifurcation are accessible to the local thrombolytic action of low dose streptokinase, urokinase, and – more recently – tissue plasminogen activator. This therapeutic option of choice in patients with grade II to IV peripheral artery disease – frequently used in conjunction with balloon catheter angioplasty – has also been evaluated in diabetic patients compared to nondiabetics [23]. The primary success rate of this procedure seems to be almost the same in diabetics as in nondiabetics (75% vs 91%), and the long-term outcome is indeed equally good in both groups (approx. 79% patency after 30 months). Thus, there is no reason why diabetics should not undergo local thrombolysis, even though many of them show signs of accelerated blood clotting or hyperaggregation.

Secondary prevention

Long-term secondary preventive pharmacotherapy appears to be warranted after arterial lumen reconstructive measures, e. g. endarterectomy, bypass, angioplasty, or local thrombolysis. Generally, antiplatelet therapy with acetyl salicylic acid provides the best results, whereas coumadines and anticoagulation are superior following bypass surgery [32]. For details including dosage and ordinary secondary prevention of arterial disease with antiplatelet drugs, the separate chapter on the topic in this book should be consulted.

Local care

As far as diabetic foot infections, including ulcers and gangrene are concerned, several prospective studies have indicated that bacteriologic results obtained are not dissimilar compared to nondiabetics [7, 24]. Usually, a mixed bacterial flora is involved, including aerobic, facultatively anaerobic, and anaerobic microorganisms. Staphylococcus species, Enterococcus species, Corynebacterium species are most commonly isolated along with various species of Enterobacteriaceae, Peptostreptococcus magnus or prevotil, and Bacteroides species. Specimens should be obtained from infected tissue that does not communicate directly with the foot ulcer if possible.

Local treatment of foot lesions – except total contact casting for neuropathic plantar ulcers [29] – has not been specifically evaluated for diabetic patients and the same applies to pharmacological measures of ordinary preventive foot care. It has been shown, however, that more than half of all amputations in diabetic patients can be prevented by appropriate education of the patient and that proper foot care is of the utmost importance [12]!

Present treatment modalities

Fig. 2 outlines the complex prophylactic and therapeutical approach to diabetic foot problems in relation to the clinical situation and severity.

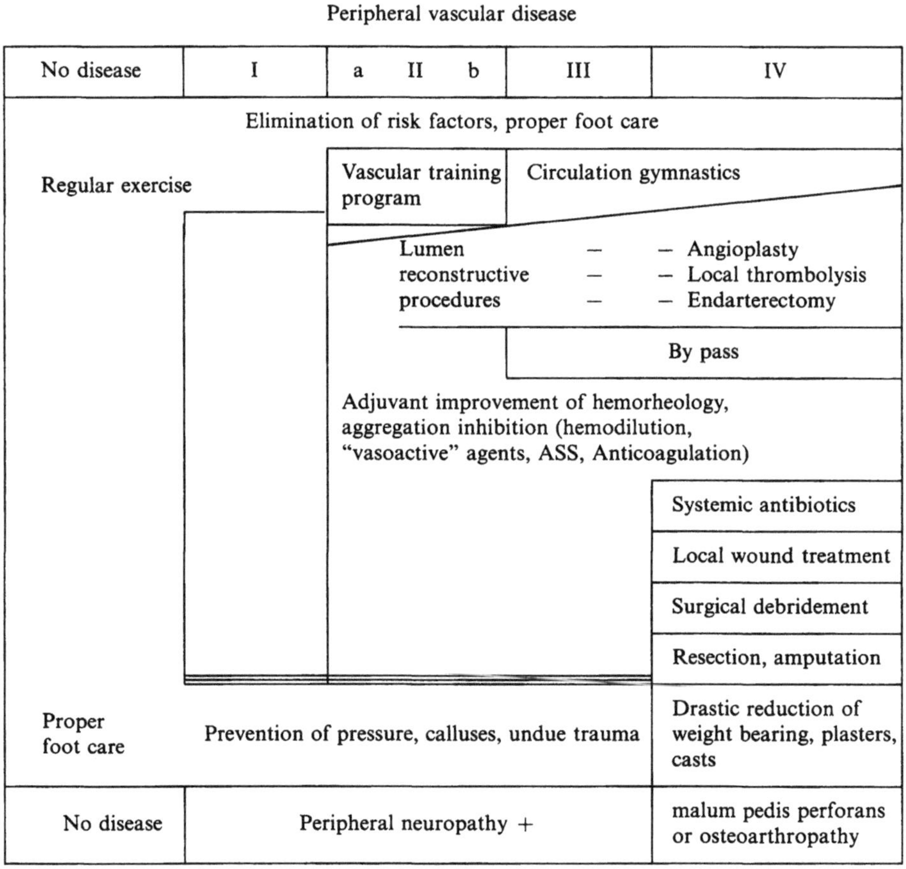

Fig. 2 Prevention and treatment of diabetic foot problems

Preventive foot care

Proper foot care is essential in all diabetic patients, even in those without any other detectable complications. It can, however, literally determine the fate of the individual diabetic, once the specific risk factors for foot problems have emerged. The principles of good foot care, therefore, are reiterated here, although this book deals mainly with pharmacologic aspects:

1. Give your feet good preventive care
2. Look at your feet regularly or have someone else do so
3. Avoid injury to your feet
4. Wear well-fitting shoes and socks
5. Provide good circulation through regular exercise

For appropriate skin care, feet should be washed daily, but not soaked (!), in lukewarm (to be tested), soapy water. Soaking the feet softens the skin and makes it more susceptible to infection. Patients with dry skin should apply a moisturizing lotion containing lanolin or pH5-Eucerin cream nightly to the feet. The web spaces, however, should be spared. Lotions containing alcohol dry the skin further and must be avoided. When the skin of the foot is too moist, talcum or baby powder should be used daily to absorb the moisture. The skin must never be nicked with scissors or sharp instruments. Calluses can be trimmed or removed by the use of limestone or a (mechanical) "quick-lime" device. Concentrated salicylic acid ointments may be harmful. For small bruises, a mild uncoloured antiseptic should be used, e. g. uncoloured merfen (phenyl-mercuryl(11)-acetate). Coloured fluids applied may mask significant inflammation. In case of athlete's foot, an antifungal ointment must be used on the affected skin for an extended period of time, but without macerating the epidermis. At the same time an antifungal powder should be applied to the shoes.

Local treatment of foot lesions

Lesions on the foot of a diabetic must be subjected to the differential diagnosis as to macrovascular disease, microangiopathy or neuropathy as the predominant underlying pathogenic factor. In addition, the severity of the lesion should be classified according to Wagner and the presence of an abscess, necrotizing cellulitis, fasciitis, osteomyelitis or osteoarthropathy be considered. If possible, a reliable specimen avoiding contamination with the ulcer or the open lesion should be obtained for bacteriological testing prior to antibacterial testing. It is best if specimens are taken by aspiration of bullae or abscesses, or by surgical biopsy of soft tissues or bone. Other specimens may be unreliable and cultures not adequately reflect the infecting microorganisms, but can still give useful information on which to base decisions about antibiotic therapy. Bacteriology should be repeated weekly since both the resident and the pathogenic organisms may change. Specimens must promptly be transferred to the laboratory and processed aerobically and anerobically [24].

Dry ischemic lesions should be kept dry and – except protective dry dressings – no other local manipulations applied. Wet lesions often need surgical debridement which may have to be repeated every other day. In case of neuropathic plantar ulcers the removal of the surrounding callus is essential. Strict avoidance of weight bearing on the diseased area is a must for successful therapy of this type of lesions and in the absence of gross infection, osteomyelitis, or gangrene, total contact casting is a favourable option of treatment. This reduces pressure at the ulcer site while allowing the patient to remain ambulatory and protects the lesion from further contamination [29]. In contrast, severely infected or wet ischemic lesions need an initial period of bed rest up to 3 weeks. In addition to surgical care, three strategies of local pharmacotherapy may be pursued: local antisepsis, fibrinolysis, and induction of granulation. But, before starting any local therapy the supreme goal of "nil nocere (avoid injury)" must be remembered. This includes the testing for contact allergies, since many people exhibit this problem in one way or another. Antibiotic ointments or powders may have only deleterious and no beneficial effects on ischemic lesions and should be strictly avoided.

Antiseptics should be gentle (potassium permanganate, ethacridin lactate, 8-chinolinol sulfate plus potassium sulfate, H_2O_2, poly (1-vinyl-pyrrolidon) iodine complex) and their effects should be reexamined at least every other day. The tissue surrounding the lesion must not be macerated and if antiseptic foot baths are used, they should be no longer than 3 – 5 minutes and the skin thoroughly dried afterwards (without rubbing). As far as torpid areas are concerned (covered with excessive amounts of fibrous tissue) the cautious application of fibrinolytic substances (streptokinase plus streptodornase, collagenase, plasmin plus desoxiribonuclease) may be recommended. Again, a close follow up on the effects is warranted. With regard to clean wounds, induction of granulation can be helpful, using dressing with saline, chlor (IV)-oxid-O_2-complex or actovegin or by exposure to hyperbaric oxygen, CO_2 etc.

Systemic antibiotic therapy of foot lesions

Diabetic foot infections require an appropriate systemic antibiotic treatment. Antibiotic therapy should be selected, based on reliable bacteriologic analysis.

Broad-spectrum β-lactam antibiotics or a combination of antibiotics active against facultatively anaerobic cocci and bacilli as well as anaerobes usually provide the best empirical antimicrobial coverage. Combinations of cefotaxim, piperacillin, and gentamicin or of moxalactam and ampicillin or third generation cephalosporin may be used. Other approved antibiotics include flucloxacyllin and gyrase inhibitors. In patients with severe ischemic problems, the additional intraarterial administration of certain antibiotics (tetracycline, cefotaxim, ceftriaxon) may be helpful to achieve higher tissue levels in the extremity at risk.

Local thrombolysis

Reconstructive procedures of the arterial lumen are of predominant importance in patients with grade II b – IV peripheral vascular disease (Fig. 2). Among these, local thrombolysis using small amounts of streptokinase, urokinase, or tissue plasminogen activator is the treatment of choice for longer occluded arterial segments. On the average, 40,000 – 60,000 U streptokinase, 150,000 – 200,000 U urokinase, and 5 – 10 mg tissue plasminogen activator applied locally through a catheter into the thrombotic obliterate are needed. Although some systemic fibrinolytic action of these rather small dosages of fibrinolytic substances must be accepted, diabetic retinopathy in general is no contraindication for this type of treatment, except fresh major hemorrhages into the vitreous or intraretinally. Usual contraindications are uncontrolled hypertension, recent cerebrovascular events and fresh gastrointestinal ulcers.

Adjuvant systemic pharmacotherapy of peripheral occlusive arterial disease

Beginning with the stage of intermittent claudication, there are several alternatives for adjuvant pharmacotherapy in patients with grade II – IV peripheral vascular disease. As outlined in Fig. 2, improvement of hemorheology and reduction of the increased aggregation tendeny can be principally achieved by hemodilution, "vasoactive" agents, acetyl salicylic acid and anticoagulation. Correction of hemoconcentration by adequate blood glucose control however, should always be considered as the therapeutical option of choice. Patients experiencing hemoconcentration (hematocrit > 45%) or increased plasma viscosity [> 1.39 mPas) beyond hyperglycemia induced hemoconcentration, and despite proper hydration should have a venesection of 250 – 400 cc blood and a parallel infusion of 500 cc HAES. If plasma viscosity is < 1.39 mPas, HAES 200/0.5 10% is recommended for volume substitution, whereas HAES 200/0.5 6% or HAES 40/05 6% is suggested for patients with higher plasma viscosity. For patients with exclusively increased plasma viscosity and fibrinogen concentrations, the same rules for volume substitution may be applied, but instead of removal of blood, plasmapheresis may be performed. In patients with rest pain or acral lesions Wagner grade 1 and 2, additional, but temporary effect on increased fibrinogen levels may be obtained by the use of ancrod in conjunction with low dose heparin.

In addition to isovolemic and hypervolemic hemodilution, "vasoactive" compounds like bufledil, naftidrofuryl or pentoxifylline can also improve hemorheology and reduce the aggregation tendency in patients without hemoconcentration or increased plasma viscosity. Although usually applied orally, intravenous infusion seems to be superior to grade IV arterial disease [27, 48, 51, 52]. Pentoxifylline has been described as equally effective both in diabetics and nondiabetics [25], whereas i.v. prostaglandine E_1 infusions apparently exhibit lesser efficacy in diabetic patients [55, 56].

Although the situation seems to have become more complex as outlined in details in chapter 12, acetyl salicylic acid is also widely used in grade II arterial disease or for secondary prevention [32]. Following angioplasty, local thrombolysis and endarterectomy, however, long-term treatment with acetyl salicylic acid in particular has been established as an effective means for the prevention of vessel reocclusion [32] and is probably effective in a daily dose of 300 mg [32]. Anticoagulation is the principal preventive treatment after bypass surgery of the lower limbs (especially after a femero-popliteal or -crural bypass) or in patients with morbus embolicus into peripheral arteries or with dilatative angiopathy [32].

No place in the rational adjuvant pharmacotherapy of peripheral vascular disease should be given to the many insufficiently evaluated "miraculous drugs" [32]. They may even have detrimental effects. This applies especially to "cures" like "fresh cell therapy", calcium-chelating treatment or oxygen insufflation into peripheral arteries.

Future perspectives

Due to the still not fully understood nature of arteriosclerosis, or macrovascular disease in diabetes in particular, and the complex etiopathogenesis of diabetic foot lesions, real progress in the pharmacologic prevention and treatment of diabetic foot problems is rather slow. Perhaps the early reduction of the hyperinsulinemia/insulin resistance syndrome, e.g. by the use of alphaglucosidase inhibitors will be able to slow down the accelerated atherogenesis in diabetes. More specific and efficient fibrinolytic substances could increase the success rate of local catheter thrombolysis and may make even small arteries accessible to this approach. It is also conceivable that stable prostacycline analogues would be the most effective "vasoactive" agents. Furthermore, the combination of an antithrombotic substance like acetyl salicylic acid with other proven "vasoactive" compounds might display a greater effectivity. Finally, the availability and applicability of powerful growth factors, like PDGF, TNF, and others for local therapy could improve primary wound healing considerably. For the time being however, proper education of all diabetic patients, good metabolic control, elimination of risk factors, and regular physical activity are the best measures for preventing diabetic foot problems.

References

[1] Kannel WB, McGee DL. Diabetes and glucose tolerance as risk factors for cardiovascular disease: The Framingham Study. Diabetes Care 1979; 2: 120–126.

[2] Krolewski AS, Warram JH, Christlieb AR. Onset, course, complications, and prognosis of diabetes mellitus. In: Marble A, Krall LP, Bradley RF et al, eds. Joslin's Diabetes mellitus, 12th ed., Philadelphia: Lea & Febiger 1985; 251–277.

[3] Prevalence of small and large vessel disease in diabetic patients from 14 centres. The WHO Multinational Study of Vascular Disease in Diabetics. Diabetologia 1985; 28 (Suppl): 615–640.

[4] Panzram G, Zabel-Langhenning R. Diabetes mellitus: Bedingte Gesundheit oder schicksalhafte Erkrankung. Med Klin 1984; 70: 282–289.

[5] Janka HU. Five year incidence of major macrovascular complications in diabetes mellitus. Horm Metabol Res 1985: (Suppl 15): 15–19.

[6] Standl E. Die Angiopathien des Typ II-Diabetes. Verh Dtsch Ges Inn Med 1986; 92: 579–586.

[7] Stiegler H, Frey S, Standl E. Diagnostische und therapeutische Überlegungen beim „diabetischen Fuß". Med Klin 1988; 83: 263–269.

[8] Levine ME, O'Neal IW. The diabetic foot. 3rd ed. St. Louis–Toronto–London: Mosby, 1983.

[9] Standl E, Stiegler H, Janka HU et al. Risk profile of macrovascular disease in diabetes mellitus. Diabete Metabolisme 1988; 14: 505–511.

[10] Jönsson B, Persson U. Diabetes – eine gesundheitsökonomische Studie. Swedish Institute for Health Economics, Copenhagen; 1981.

[11] National Health Interview Survey. Harris MI, Hamman RF, eds. Diabetes in America. US Government Printing Office, NIH Publication 1985; No 85–1468.

[12] Davidson JK, Alogna MT, Goldsmith MP et al. Assessment of program effectiveness at Grady Memorial Hospital. In: Lawrence P, Steiner G, eds. Educating of the diabetic patient. New York: Springer Publishing Co, 1981; 329–348.

[13] Standl E, Stiegler H, Janka HU et al. Cerebral and peripheral vascular disease. In: Mogensen CE, Standl E, eds. Prevention and treatment of diabetic late complications. Berlin, New York: de Gruyter, 1989; 169–198.

[14] Wagner FW. The dysvascular foot: a system for diagnosis and treatment. Foot Ankle 1981; 2: 64–122.

[15] Standl E. Intravascular clotting factors. Diab Res Clin Pract 1988; 4 (Suppl I): 11–14.

[16] Janka HU, Standl E, Schramm W et al. Platelet enzyme activities in diabetes mellitus in relation to endothelial damage. Diabetes 1983; 32 (Suppl 2): 47–51.

[17] Breddin HK, Krzywanek HJ, Althoff P et al. PARD Platelet aggregation as a risk factor in diabetics: Results of a prospective study. Horm Metabol Res 1985; (Suppl 15): 63–68.
[18] Haaß A, Kroemer H, Jäger H et al. Dextran 40 or HAES 200/05? Dtsch Med Wschr 1986; 111: 1681–1686.
[19] Rudofsky G, Meyer P, Strohmeyer HG. Effect of hemodilution on resting flow and reactive hyperemia in lower limbs. Bibl Haemat 1982; 47: 157–161.
[20] Stiegler H, Lander Th, Standl E. Angioplastie einschließlich lokaler Thrombolyse beim diabetischen Patienten. Akt Endokrin Stoffw 1987; 8: 40–43.
[21] Roth FJ, Krings W, Cappius G et al. Die lokale, niedrig dosierte fibrinolytische Therapie. Indikation, Technik und Resultat. Vasa 1984; 12: 52–56.
[22] Bollinger A, Schlumpf M, Grüntzig A et al. Perkutane transluminale Angioplastie (PTA) bei Diabetikern mit peripherer arterieller Verschlußkrankheit. Akt Endokr Stoffw 1983; 2: 62–65.
[23] Stiegler H, Hufen V, Weichenhain B et al. Ergebnisse der lokalen Thrombolyse unter besonderer Berücksichtigung einer diabetischen Stoffwechsellage. Med Klinik 1990; 171–175.
[24] Wheat JJ, Allen SD, Henry M et al. Diabetic foot infections. Bacteriologic analysis. Arch Intern Med 1986; 146: 1935–1940.
[25] Rössner M, Müller R. On the assessment of the efficacy of pentoxifylline. J Med 1987; 18: 1–15.
[26] Kjellström T, Palmquist I, Stavenow L. Conservative drug-treatment in patients with moderately severe chronic occlusive peripheral arterial disease. Circulation 1989; 80: 1549–1556.
[27] Rudofsky G, Hanssler KF, Künkel HP et al. Zur intravenösen Pentoxifyllin-Behandlung der chronischen arteriellen Verschlußkrankheit. Med Welt 1988; 39: 1136–1140.
[28] Apelqvist J, Castenfors J, Larsson J et al. Prognostic value of systolic ankle and toe blood pressure levels in outcome of diabetic foot ulcer. Diab Care 1989; 12: 373–378.
[29] Blair VP, Drury DA, Rose SJ. Total contact casting in treatment of diabetic plantar ulcers. Controlled clinical trial. Diab Care 1989; 12: 384–388.
[30] Reich T, Cutler BC, Lee BY et al. Pentoxifylline in the treatment of intermittent claudication of the lower limbs. Angiology 1984; 35: 389–295.
[31] Ehrly AM. Verbesserung der nutritiven Durchblutung bei peripheren ischämischen Erkrankungen. Vasa 1983; (Suppl 11): 1–21.
[32] Bollinger A. Medikamentöse Therapie bei peripherer arterieller Verschlußkrankheit. Schweiz med Wschr 1988; 118: 1283–89.
[33] Heidrich H. Vasoaktive Pharmaka bei peripheren arteriellen Durchblutungsstörungen. Dtsch med Wschr 1985; 110: 1219–1224.
[34] Porter JM, Cutler BS, Lee BY et al. Pentoxifylline efficacy in the treatment of intermittent claudication: Multicenter controlled double-blind trial with objective assessment of chronic occlusive arterial disease patients. Amer Heart J 1982; 104: 66–72.
[35] Becker MH, Ehlert O, Häring R et al. Wirksamkeitsnachweise von Dusodril-PI bei arterieller Verschlußkrankheit in einer multizentrisch angelegten Doppelblindstudie. Med Welt 1979; 30: 1062–1606.
[36] Boobis LH, Bell PRF. Can drugs help patients with lower limb ischemia? Brit J Surg 1982; 69 (Suppl): 17–23.
[37] Clyne CAC, Galland RB, Fox MJ et al. A controlled trial of naftidrofuryl in the treatment of intermittent claudication. Brit J Surg 1980; 67: 347–348.
[38] Maass U, Amberger HG, Böhme H et al. Naftidrofuryl bei arterieller Verschlußkrankheit: Kontrollierte multizentrische Doppelblindstudie mit oraler Applikation. Dtsch med Wschr 1984; 109: 745–750.
[39] Trübestein G, Balzer K, Bisler H et al. Buflomedil bei arterieller Verschlußkrankheit. Dtsch med Wschr 1982; 107: 1957–1961.

[40] Meßmer K, ed. Makro- und Mikrozirkulation bei ischämischer Verschlußkrankheit, 2. Internationales Bufedil-Sysmposium. München, Bern, Wien, San Franzisco: Zuckschwerdt, 1987.
[41] Bonnameaux H, Holditch T, Hellemans H et al. Placebo-controlled, double-blind, two-center trial of Ketanserin in intermittent claudication. Lancet 1985; II: 1268–71.
[42] Coffman JD. Vasodilator drugs in peripheral vascular disease? New Engl J Med 1979; 300: 713–17.
[43] Clifford PC, Davies PW, Hayne JA et al. Intermittent claudication. Is a supervised exercise class worthwhile? Brit med J 1980; 280: 1503–1505.
[44] Maass U. Ergebnisse der physikalischen Therapie bei arterieller Verschlußkrankheit. In: Trübestein, ed. Therapie der arteriellen Verschlußkrankheit. München, Bern, Wien, San Franzisco: Zuckschwerdt, 1987.
[45] Kiesewetter H, Blume J, Jung F et al. Gehtraining und medikamentöse Therapie bei der peripheren arteriellen Verschlußkrankheit. Dtsch med Wschr 1987; 112: 873–878.
[46] Adhoute G, Bacourt F, Barral M et al. Naftidrofuryl bei chronischer arterieller Verschlußkrankheit. Angiology 1986; 37: 160–166.
[47] Widmer LK. Provisorische Richtlinien zur Prüfung der therapeutischen Wirksamkeit peripher vasoaktiver Medikamente bei arterieller Durchblutungsstörung. Vasa 1981; 4: 337–341.
[48] Böhme H, Heidrich H. Naftidrofuryl. Vasa 1988; (Suppl 24): 1–75.
[49] Böhme H, Brülisamer M, Härtel U et al. Kontrollierte Zweizentren-Studie zur Wirksamkeit von intraarteriellen Prostaglandin E_1-Infusionen bei peripherer arterieller Verschlußkrankheit im Stadium III und IV. In: Heidrich H, Böhme H, Rogatti W, eds. Prostaglandin E_1-Wirkungen und therapeutische Wirksamkeit. Berlin, Heidelberg, New York: Springer, 1988; 118–126.
[50] Trübestein G, Ludwig M, Diehm C et al. Prostaglandin E_1 bei arterieller Verschlußkrankheit im Stadium III und IV. Dtsch med Wschr 1987; 112: 955–959.
[51] Trübestein G, von Bary S, Breddin K et al. Intravenous prostaglandin E_1 versus pentoxifylline therapy in chronic arterial occlusive disease – a controlled randomised multicenter study. Vasa 1989; (Suppl 28): 44–49.
[52] Diehm C, Kühn A, Strauss R et al. Effects of regular physical training in a supervised class and additional intravenous prostaglandin E_1 and naftidrofuryl infusion therapy in patients with intermittent claudication – a controlled study. Vasa 1989; (Suppl 28): 26–30.
[53] Ernst E. Physical exercise for peripheral vascular disease. A review. Vasa 1987; 16: 227–231.
[54] Trübestein G, ed. Conservative therapy of arterial occlusive disease. Stuttgart, New York: Thieme, 1986.
[55] Gruß JD, Fietze-Fischer B. Die advante PGE_1-Therapie bei femero-distalen Rekonstruktionen. In: Heidrich H, Böhme H, Rogatti W, eds. Prostaglandin E_1-Wirkungen und therapeutische Wirksamkeit. Berlin, Heidelberg, New York: Springer, 1988: 151–159.
[56] Alexander K. Prostaglandine einschließlich Prostacyclin in der Therapie peripherer arterieller Durchblutungsstörungen. Internist 1989; 30: 429–439.
[57] Kiesewetter H, Jung F, Spitzer S et al. Die Fließeigenschaften des Blutes und ihre klinische Bedeutung beim arteriellen Gefäßpatienten. Internist 1989; 30: 420–428.
[58] Kiesewetter H, Jung F, Blume J et al. Hemodilution in peripheral arterial occlusion disease stage II b. A prospective, randomized double blind comparison of middle molecular hydroxyethyl starch and low molecular dextrane solution. Klin Wochenschr 1987; 65: 324–330.
[59] Rudofsky G. Intravenöse PGE_1-Infusionsbehandlung bei Patienten mit arterieller Verschlußkrankheit im Stadium II b. In: Heidrich H, Böhme H, Rogatti W, eds. Prostaglandin E_1: Wirkungen und therapeutische Wirksamkeit. Berlin, Heidelberg, New York, London, Paris, Tokyo: Springer, 1988: 103–111.

[60] Heidrich H, Böhme H, Rogatti W, eds. Prostaglandin E_1: Wirkungen und therapeutische Wirksamkeit. Berlin, Heidelberg, New York, London, Paris, Tokyo: Springer, 1988; 1–184.

[61] Kriessmann A, Neiss A. Klinischer Wirksamkeitsnachweis von Naftidrofuryl bei Claudicatio intermittens. In: Böhme H, Heidrich H, eds. Naftidrofuryl. Vasa 1988; (Suppl 24): 27–32.

Pharmacologic treatment of erectile dysfunction by intracavernous injection

A. W. Zorgniotti

Introduction

That vascular disease might be the principal cause of all erectile failure is gradually being accepted by psychiatrists who have long taught that most impotence is psychogenic. Similarly, the vascular "explanation" has begun to make inroads into the view by diabetologists that erectile failure in diabetes is of neurogenic origin. This view has been engendered by the frequent observation by peripheral neurologic deficit and the presence of neurogenic bladder in diabetes. Since erection and bladder function share the same sacral nerve pathways, a neurological explanation becomes a logical assumption.

The conventional wisdom is that penile erection is a complex neurovascular event requiring autonomic and somatic nerve, vascular and endocrine contributions. In addition to these physiologic factors, there are psychologic ones. With arousal a large increase in blood flow into the corpus cavernosum with concomitant occlusion of outflow occurs as the result of neurotransmitter mediated smooth muscle relaxation. Arterial caliber increases and as the smooth muscle walls of the sinuses of the corpus cavernosum relax the outflow veins within the tunica albuginea are restricted. Aided by contraction of the striated perineal muscles, intracavernous pressure reaches near systolic levels giving erection the necessary stiffness for penetration. Thus blood dynamics are a common denominator in erectile function. In impotence, non-erection is a manifestation of altered blood flow, regardless of etiology. It has been my experience that, in the diabetic, impotence can be shown to have both vascular and neurogenic elements with the vascular predominating. In all instances, pharmacologic erection produces satisfactory results.

At this writing the Pharmacologic Erection Program (PEP) has emerged as a highly effective method for producing transitory erectile capability in the diabetic who is dysfunctional. In general, oral medications (yohimbine, vitamins); hormones (testosterone); diets; acupuncture; psychiatry and prayer produce only transitory, possibly placebo induced, improvement in well being and erection, but no real restoration of potency. The method of auto-injection of the penis is painless and not difficult for patients to master. Although there have been concerns expressed, the side effects and complications have not been proven to be serious, provided the patient has been correctly taught and supervised. What some men find unacceptable is the need to self inject each time coitus is desired. PEP is, in my opinion, safer for the diabetic than penile implant where infection is not uncommon. Since February of 1983 when I first began teaching intracavernous injections, I have never encountered the complication of infection at the puncture site or corpus cavernosum in any patient, diabetic or otherwise [1].

Penile microsurgical arterial bypass for arterial insufficiency does not yield good results in diabetics and is considered contraindicated in such patients. The fact that the surgery can take as long as ten hours also makes the risk to the diabetic unacceptable. When the corpora are not able to retain blood, owing to insufficiency of the venous occlusion mechanism, and erection is lost rapidly on intromisssion, diabetics will benefit from much less lengthy surgery to correct this entity with either return of erection or reversal of previously unsuccessful injection therapy. Before this is undertaken, it must be demonstrated that arterial inflow is unimpaired.

There is no doubt that the quality of life of diabetics, young and older, can be greatly enhanced by PEP. Clinical experience has been accumulating for less than eight years so that the useful duration of PEP for any one patient cannot be predicted at this time.

Diabetes: a major risk factor for impotence

The complaint of impotence requires that the clinician routinely investigate for diabetes mellitus. Except for differences in age at onset, there do not appear to be any demonstrable differences between insulin dependent and non-insulin dependent diabetes mellitus. It has been observed that ischemic heart disease and impotence share the same risk factors: age, smoking, diabetes, hypertension and hyperlipidemia [2]. Hypogonadism may also be a risk factor [3]. Vascular disease has long been considered a major contributor to morbidity and mortality in diabetes and there may be parallels between the arteries of the heart and those of the penis.

Vascular disease in diabetes can be demonstrated at the gross and microscopic levels. Biopsies of the corpus cavernosum in impotent diabetic patients show evidence of sclerosis of arterioles, capillaries and venules of varying degrees, apparently sufficient to interfere with erectile function. More recently, Saenz de Tejada has shown a decrease in Endothelium Derived Relaxing

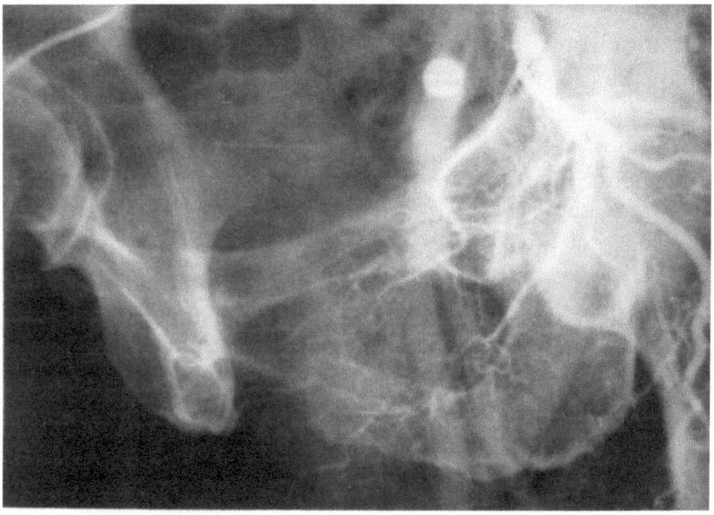

Fig. 1 Selective pudendal arteriogram shows severe vascular disease with non-filling of the cavernous arteries responsible for erection.

Factor (EDRF) in the corporal tissues of impotent diabetics [4]. The degree of alteration from normal is comparable to aging changes seen in non-diabetics who are 10 – 15 years older. Biopsies also demonstrate changes in the nerve structures of the corpus.

At the level of the penile arteries, autopsy specimens and selective pudendal arteriograms frequently demonstrate obstructive vascular abnormalities which can be assumed to alter blood flow to the penile structures (Fig. 1). This suggests that vascular disease is a major factor in men with secondary impotence.

Non-invasive testing for vascular insufficiency in the diabetic

Non-invasive studies of penile blood pressure often demonstrate a decrease in penile brachial mean presure. In general, penile systolic pressure is higher than brachial mean pressure. However, it can be shown that patients with severe Cavernous artery disease demonstrated on selective arteriography, can have normal penile blood pressures. It is now generally accepted that penile/brachial pressure determinations are diagnostic of vascular insufficiency only when these are abnormal.

A simple non-invasive test is the penile plethysmogram. While this is qualitative, it gives important information. Diminution in pulse wave size and disappearance of the dicrotic notch on the descending limb of the curve are considered evidence of vascular disease and are very frequent in diabetes regardless of type.

Recently, improvements in ultrasound have made possible study of the penis so that penile arteries < 0.1 cm can be demonstrated and their diameters measured before and after intracorporal injection of the smooth muscle relaxant, papaverine HCl. The instrument software permits estimation of normal and pathologic flow rates in these vessels. In the instance of diabetes, this examination can be bypassed unless there is a suspicion that the impotence is not of diabetic causation.

A simple office examination which has been gaining in popularity is the Papaverine Test. This consists of the intracavernous injection of papaverine HCl followed by observation of the penis over a period of an hour. If a rigid erection is obtained, without sexual stimulation, the arterial inflow and venous outflow restriction can be considered intact. If erection is partial, it is probable that there is either vascular insufficiency or corporol venous insufficiency. A far better approach is to arrange for the patient to rejoin his sex partner immediately after the injection in order to attempt coitus which, if successful, leads to the decision to go ahead with PEP.

Pharmacologic erection programs (PEP) address vascular insufficiency

Until the advent of PEP, the only way to assure that a patient could have vaginal penetration when desired was penile implantation. PEP provides an alternative for diabetic patients who may be reluctant to undergo surgery. Questions have arisen concerning its use in young men, including diabetics, as long term effects are still under study. If these patients accept the possibility that PEP may have to be abandoned and that implantation remains the only alternative treatment, then PEP becomes the preferred alternative.

Success lies in careful selection and rigorous supervision of the patient. Unreliable patients should be encouraged to have an implant. The urologist is well qualified to manage any problems which can arise, but must be temperamentally able to provide uncompromising supervision, necessary during the evaluative and maintenance phases of intracavernous self-injection.

After intracavernous injection of 30 mg of papeverine HCl to which 0.5 mg of phentolamine has been added, 78% of impotent men, regardless of age or etiology, are able, over a 2–3 hour span, to achieve ridigity with arousal. The initial injection is given by the physician and the patient is asked to rejoin his sex partner within 30–40 minutes. In order to assure that the injection works, to determine proper selection and dose of the agent and to treat possible prolonged erection, such a trial must take place before self-injection can be taught.

Scheme for self-injection program

1. Thorough evaluation and selection of patient including: history, physical examination, serum testosterone and prolactin, penile blood pressure determinations and/or plethysmography.
2. Trial injection with coitus must precede teaching. About 6% of patients develop an erection which does not subside and the practitioner will need to be available to treat this within four hours. The prolonged erection is high flow in nature and should not be called a priapism. This, more commonly, occurs with the initial injection and not subsequently. The practitioner adjusts the dose for optimum results.
3. It the trial is successful, it may be repeated with an increased dose or change of agent.
4. Alternative treatments are explained and he signs an informed consent.
5. The patient is instructed in the technic of self-injection at the base of the penis avoiding the urethra and the neurovascular bundle (Fig. 2).

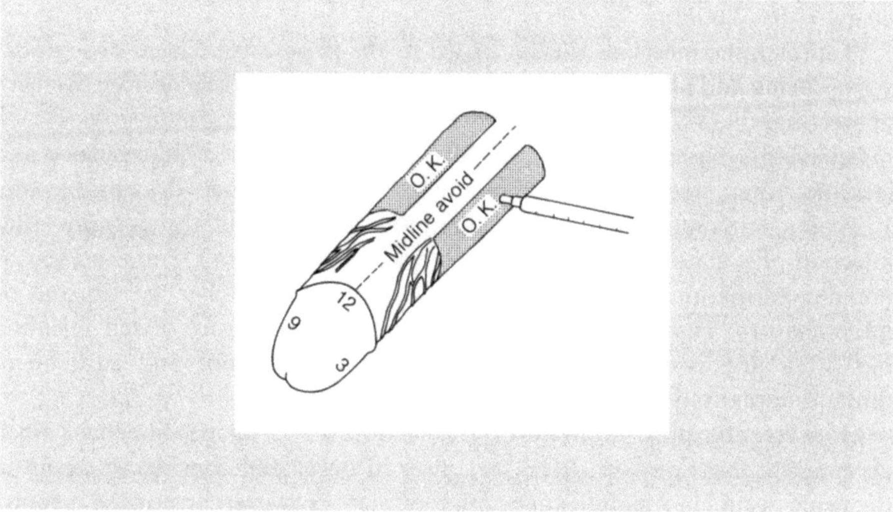

Fig. 2 Illustration used in patient teaching.

6. The patient receives a multiple dose vial with the pharmacologic agent, disposable syringes and alcohol pledgets, sufficient for ten doses/month.
7. The patient reports monthly to obtain new supplies and be examined. Once or twice during the year, a blood sample for liver function is suggested.

Results are generally satisfactory with coitus up to ten times a month. It is rare to encounter a prolonged erection after the initiation of treatment since this problem is eliminated at the time of the initial trial. Complications are rare and usually consist of transitory pains in the penis and ecchymosis due to perforation of superficial skin vein. After several months, 4% of patients will be found to have areas of induration of the penis which can be nodular and non-tender. These indurations do not always correspond to the site of injection and usually do not interfere with continuation of the injections. Most subside spontaneously with discontinuation of injection. This has been identified as fibrosis and could interfere with eventual penile prosthesis insertion. This problem may be due to the pH of the papaverine, but also may depend on injection technic, since it is important to avoid extravasation into the corporal tissues during the injection which is intended to be diffused within the sinuses.

Pharmacology

The original drug employed was papaverine HCL and this can produce erection with as little as 6.0 mg injected although the more usual dose is 30 – 60 mg (1.0 – 2.0 ml).

Phentolamine mesylate can be added to the papeverine (usual dose papaverine 30 mg and phentolamine 0.5 mg) resulting in considerable improvement in erection.

Papaverine based injections produce rapid induction of tumescence and erection often requires sexual foreplay. The principal drawbacks are: 1. Prolonged erection which might require aspiration of the corpora after injection or a suitable vasoconstrictor (e. g. phenylephrine). 2. Induration or nodular formations within the corpora which may either be fibrotic or inflammatory. These tend to disappear with discontinuance of self injection but often are associated with development of tolerance and subsequent difficult implantation.

More recently alprostadil (PGE_1) (Usual dose 5 – 15 μg in saline) has gained acceptance. Erection with PGE_1 is slower in onset and considerable pain in the penis occurs in a significant number of men. However, prolonged erection is less likely to occur and can be reversed with an oral dose of pseudoephedrine. The tissue changes seen with papaverine apparently do not occur with this agent which is most costly.

Mixtures of all three agents cited above have been shown to be effective in men who have not been able to obtain sufficient stiffness for erection with any single agent. The most commonly used dose will contain: papaverine HCL 60 mg, phentolamine 2.0 mg and PGE_1 40 μg.

In the United States, practitioners dispense owing to the fact that these drugs are approved by the U.S. Food and Drug Administration for uses other than impotence. As long as the practitioner assumes responsibility for the outcome of treatment, dispensing drugs for unapproved uses is permitted. The agents used for PEP have unusual uses. Papaverine HCl is for intra-arterial injection in the presence of impending gangrene of an extremity. Phentolamine is used for the diagnosis of a rare edrenal tumor, pheochromocytoma. Alprostadil is employed in neonates with severe cardiac malformation to maintain patency of the ductus arteriosus while cardiac surgery is being planned. Certainly not items to be found at the apothecary down the street!

Conclusion

Impotence is due to blood flow disturbance regardless of etiology. In diabetes there is strong evidence that the vascular component is critical. At present, the only reliable methods to permit coital penetration are Pharmacologic Erection Programs which address the problem of vascular insufficiency and penile implant which does not produce erection per se. In the future, treatment of impotence may be preventive, addressing the known risk factors for impotence, with special attention to smoking. Improved methods of insulin control and the use of enzyme blocking agents such as aldose reductase inhibitor may have a role in decreasing the incidence of impotence in diabetic men.

References

[1] Zorgniotti A. Self Administered Intracavernous Injection of a Vasoactive Substance for Impotence in Diabetics. J Urol 1984; 133: 210 A.

[2] Virag R et al. Is impotence an Arterial Disease? A study of arterial risk factors in 440 impotent men. Lancet 1985; I: 181.

[3] Swartz CM. Low Serum Testosterone: A Cardiovascular Risk in Elderly Men. Geriatric Med Today 1988; 7: 39.

[4] Saenz de Tejada I et al. Impaired Neurogenic and Endothelium Mediated Relaxation of Penile Smooth Muscle in Diabetic Patients with Impotence. New Eng J Med 1989; 320: 1025.

Suggested reading

Ellenberg M. Sexual function in diabetic patients. Ann Int Med 1980; 92: 331.
Goldstein I et al. Impotence in diabetes mellitus. In: Krane R, Siroky M, Goldstein I, eds. Male Sexual Dysfunction. Boston: Little Brown, 1983.
McMillan D. Deterioration of the microcirculation in diabetes. Diabetes 1975; 24: 944.
Zorgniotti A. Etiology of vascular impotence. In: Resnick M, Kursch E, eds. Current Therapy in Genitourinary Surgery. Toronto: Decker, 1987; 468.
Zorgniotti A, Lizza E. Diagnosis and treatment of impotence. Toronto: Decker, 1990 (In press).

Antihypertensive treatment in non-insulin-dependent diabetes mellitus (NIDDM)

A. Kribben, U. Heemann, Th. Philipp

Introduction

Arterial hypertension is confirmed when a diastolic blood pressure of above 90 mmHg is recorded in at least 2 of 3 measurements on two different occasions. The measurements should be performed in a sitting or supine position after at least 5 minutes of rest. The term mild hypertension is used for a diastolic blood pressure between 90 and 104 mmHg. Moderate hypertension is defined as diastolic blood pressure between 105 and 114 mmHg, whereas in severe hypertension diastolic blood pressure is at least 115 mmHg [50]. Isolated systolic hypertension is defined as a systolic blood pressure above 160 mmHg in the presence of a diastolic blood pressure below 90 mmHg.

Hypertension appears to be more frequent in patients with non-insulin-dependent diabetes mellitus (NIDDM), although there are not many controlled data concerning the prevalence of hypertension in NIDDM. Comparison of persons of equal age, sex and genetic predisposition is necessary for critical examination of the prevalence of hypertension in a population with NIDDM. In one such comparison of a prevalence of 58% hypertensive patients was reported for NIDDM compared to 21% in age and sex matched non-diabetics [47].

Apart from cardiovascular morbidity and mortality, the prognosis of NIDDM is mainly influenced by the degree of hypertension and the incidence of chronic renal failure [21, 47]. Antihypertensive therapy is therefore mandatory in the treatment of diabetes [11, 51, 53]. While in patients with type I diabetes diastolic blood pressure should be lowered to below 90 mmHg, in patients with NIDDM, who are on the average older, enforced normalization of blood pressure does not appear to be necessary [53].

Pathophysiology

Hypertension in diabetes mellitus has multiple causes. In NIDDM the onset of hypertension may be associated with diabetic nephropathy, arteriolosclerotic alterations of the kidney, obesity or the coexistence of essential hypertension. The mechanisms behind hypertension in diabetes are poorly understood. Osmotic effects, increased sodium retention, alteration of the renin-angiotensin-aldosterone-system and alterations of the sympathetic nervous system have been discussed [4, 25].

The secondary forms of hypertension such as pheochromocytoma, Cushing's disease or primary aldosteronism are no more common in diabetics than in non-diabetic patients and are in general uncommon. Despite accelerated atherosclerosis in diabetes mellitus, the incidence of renovascular hypertension was not found to be more frequent in diabetics than in the non-diabetic population [9], althouth this is still under debate [45].

Postural hypertension remains a special problem. Supine hypertension with orthostatic hypotension sometimes occurs in patients with autonomic neuropathy and is the most difficult blood pressure problem to treat in diabetic patients.

Sodium retention and insulin hypothesis

Hyperglycemia in patients with NIDDM is often followed by renal hyperfiltration of glucose prior to the appearance of glucosuria. The increased reabsorption of glucose stimulates sodium reabsorption due to proximal-tubular sodium-glucose-cotransport resulting in elevated body sodium [57]. Elevated body sodium may result in raised blood pressure.

Some epidemiologic studies have reported a correlation between insulin level and blood pressure [33]. This correlation was independent of body weight and glucose tolerance.

Reaven [42] postulated the following link between hyperinsulinemia and hypertension: in vitro insulin stimulates Na/K-ATPase [36] and, at least in acute studies, tubular sodium reabsorption [10]. This again would be followed by elevation of body sodium and volume load and could raise blood pressure. The higher blood pressure results in an increased excretion of sodium so that whole body sodium is only slightly above normal [57].

Increased activity of Na^+/H^+ exchange transport could also be the connecting link between hyperinsulinemia and hypertension [12]. Chronic hyperinsulinemia overstimulates Na^+/H^+-exchange resulting in intracellular accumulation of sodium and in turn in an increase in intracellular calcium which may increase reactivity to pressor stimuli such as norepinephrine and angiotensin II [6]. Increased activity of Na^+/H^+ exchange transport also leads to intracellular alkalosis. Chronic alkalosis may result in increased protein synthesis and cell proliferation [48], which might explain the hypertrophy of resistance vessels characteristic of hypersensitive patients.

Although the release of norepinephrine is stimulated by insulin, in healthy men the norepinephrine-mediated pressor effect is prevented by a simultaneous norepinephrine-antagonistic action of insulin. The latter is the reason for the fall in blood pressure seen after i. v. infusion of insulin in patients with autonomic dysfunction in whom there is no stimulation of norepinephrine release [32]. Exogenous insulin does not modify the pressor effect of angiotensin II in either healthy or diabetic men although it does impair the secretion of aldosterone during stimulation by a supraphysiological dose of angiotensin II [56].

Figure 1 summarizes the relations between insulin, hyperglycemia and the regulation of blood pressure and body sodium.

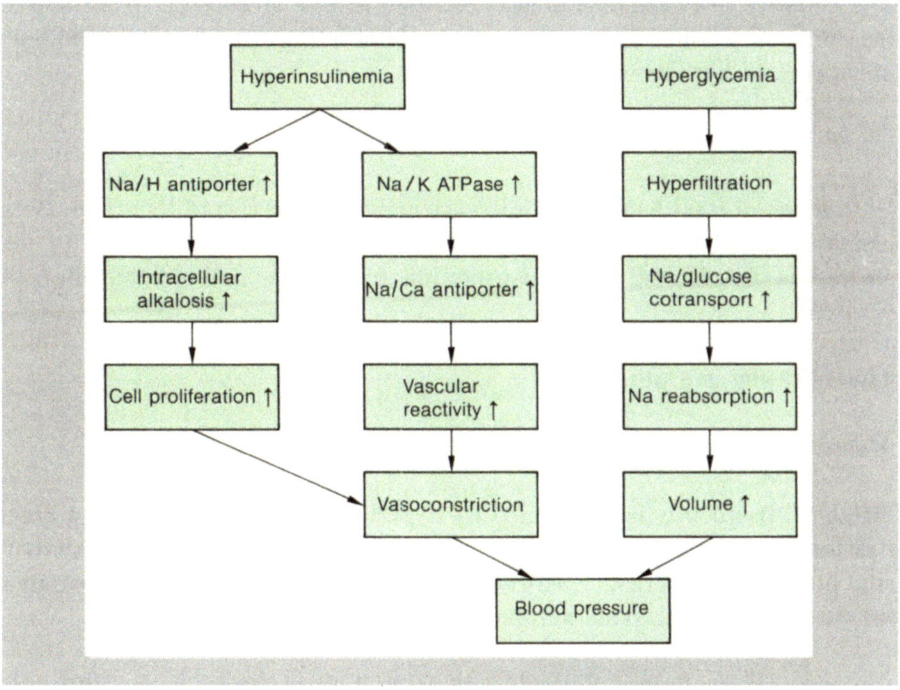

Fig. 1 Relation between insulin, hyperglycemia and the regulation of blood pressure.

Endocrine disorders

The renin-angiotensin-aldosterone system is involved in blood pressure regulation by means of vasoconstriction, renal blood flow regulation, and by regulation of sodium reabsorption in the kidney, which also leads to reabsorption of water. In small samples of diabetic patients the overall activity of the renin-angiotensin-system was found to be normal or slightly increased [4]. O'Hare, however, reported decreased renin activity in 18 patients with type II diabetes [37].

There is no consistent evidence that sympathetic nervous activity is changed in uncomplicated diabetes. Diminished sympathetic nervous activity in patients with secondary complications is so far not confirmed. A slight increase in circulatory reactivity to norepinephrine independent of the level of blood pressure has been described, however, data on diabetic patients with moderate and accelerated hypertension are not available [25].

Obesity

The majority of obese people have elevated insulin levels [10]. According to the above mentioned insulin hypothesis this finding would explain the high prevalence of hypertension in the obese.

Chronic renal failure

Chronic renal failure can induce hypertension irrespective of its origin. Both increased activity of the renin-angiotensin-aldosterone system due to decreased perfusion and reduced excretion of sodium and volume may be involved.

Morbidity and mortality

Macrovascular disease

NIDDM, frequently accompanied by hyperlipidemia and obesity, is a great risk for development of atherosclerosis and its secondary diseases. Hypertension potentiates this risk. Macrovascular disease is of remarkable importance for cardiac, cerebral, renal and peripheral blood flow.

Coronary artery disease: Patients with arterial hypertension have a threefold risk of developing coronary heart disease compared to normotensives [22].

Like hypertension, diabetes mellitus is a risk factor for development of cardiovascular disease. Even in patients with hyperinsulinemia and normal glucose tolerance an increased risk for the development of coronary heart disease has been confirmed [59]. However, whether hypertension in patients with diabetes mellitus further increases this risk is not proved at the present time, also there is strong evidence that this is the case [43].

Cerebrovascular disease: Hypertension is a major risk factor for cerebrovascular disease. The risk of hypertensive patients for the development of cerebrovascular disease is up to 10 times higher than that of normotensives [22]. Stroke occurs up to six times more frequently in diabetics compared to non diabetics. The incidence of development of cerebral vascular disease in hypertensive diabetics is double than in normotensive diabetics [26].

Renovascular disease: Atherosclerotic plaques can cause narrowing of one or both renal arteries resulting in renovascular hypertension. The occurrence of atherosclerotic renal artery stenosis with the pathophysiological consequence of renovascular hypertension has not been found to be significantly different in hypertensive diabetics compared to hypertensive non-diabetics [45].

Peripheral vascular disease: Hypertensive patients have a 2.5 times greater risk of developing intermittent claudication compared to normotensives [22], the risk for diabetics, however, is 30 times as high as that for non-diabetics. There is a strong correlation between systolic blood pressure and peripheral artery disease [19].

Microvascular disease

Microvascular disease is of major importance for the mortality and morbidity of diabetic patients. It is involved in the development of retinopathy, chronic renal failure and diabetic nephropathy.

Retinopathy: A positive correlation has been described between the prevalence of hypertension and of retinopathy in patients with diabetes. It has been suggested that at least systolic elevation of blood pressure plays a role in the development of diabetic retinopathy in NIDDM [19, 24].

Nephropathy (chronic renal failure): The development of chronic renal failure in NIDDM is common and due to different factors.

Only 20% of renal insufficiency in this population is due to diabetic nephropathy. More frequently renal insufficiency is a consequence of atherosclerotic complications, both micro- and macroangiopathy.
Chronic infection of the upper urinary tract is more frequent in diabetic patients, especially in those with a poorly controlled metabolism.
In the end-stage of type II diabetics with autonomic neuropathy, sclerosis of the bladder sphincter is often the cause of obstructive uropathy.

Diabetic nephropathy: As mentioned above, diabetic nephropathy has to be distinguished from microangiopathic nephropathy. The risk for the development of diabetic nephropathy in patients with type II diabetes is equal to that in type I diabetics [15]. State I nephropathy with glomerular hypertrophy and hyperfiltration is only seen in type I diabetics [46]. Further progression seems to be equal in type II and type I [15]. The average extent of hyperglycemia is positively correlated to the onset of proteinuria. The prognosis of renal insufficiency in patients with type II diabetes and proteinuria is related to the level of blood pressure [14, 34]. There is also a negative correlation between diastolic blood pressure and the beginning of proteinuria in type II diabetics [14].

Survey of clinical intervention trials

Various intervention trials have demonstrated a reduction in cardiovascular morbidity and mortality in patients with severe hypertension [55] and moderate hypertension as well as in patients with mild hypertension (Table 1). All the above mentioned trials were carried out in patients with essential hypertension. Comparable studies performed in patients with arterial hypertension and diabetes mellitus do not exist. However, a few of the studies mentioned in Table 1 included some patients with diabetes mellitus.

In a secondary prevention study in 99 hypertensive diabetics treated with the beta-blocker timolol after myocardial infarction the cardiovascular mortality was reduced by 66% compared to a placebo treated control group [13]. Some smaller studies indicate that a significant reduction in blood pressure has a positive influence on the progression of renal failure in patients with NIDDM (Table 2). In NIDDM at least the effect does not appear to be specific for the particular drug used (diuretic, CE-inhibitor, calcium antagonist, beta-blocker).

In recent studies diuretics and beta-blockers were used besides reserpine, hydralazine, methyldopa and clonidine, most of which are not in use as step 1 drugs today. In the medical research council trial [32a] and in the heart attack

Table 1 Effect of antihypertensive treatment on cardiovascular events in intervention trials on mild hypertension

Trial	n	diuretic	β-blocker	reserpine	hydralazine	methyldopa	clonidine	cardiovascular mortality	cerebrovascular insult	myocardial infarction
		Drugs used						Reduction (%)		
VA II	380	•		•	•			56*	74*	16
USPH	389	•		•				49*	83*	15
HDFP	10940	•		+	+	+		19	36*	48*
Australian	3427	•	+		+	+	+	56	46*	11
Oslo	785	•	+			+		7	100*	−30
MRC	17354	•	•			+		4	45*	6

• = basic drug + = additional drug * = significant reduction

VA II: Veterans administration study II [54]
USPH: U.S. public health service study [41]
HDFP: Hypertension detection and follow-up program [18]
Australian: The Australian therapeutic trial in mild hypertension [44]
Oslo: The Oslo study [16]
MRC: Medical research council trial (Medical research council working party 1985) [32a]

Table 2 Reduction of progression of diabetic nephropathy in diabetics

Author		Drug	(n)	Patients Characteristics		
Mogensen	1982	Furosemide	6	NIDDM + IDDM	proteinuria	hypertensive
Carrasco	1987	Captopril	21	NIDDM + IDDM	proteinuria	hypertensive
Marre	1987	Enalapril	10	NIDDM + IDDM	micro-proteinuria	normotensive
Baba	1989	Nicardipine	7	NIDDM	micro-proteinuria	hypertensive
Baba	1989	Enalapril	7	NIDDM	micro-proteinuria	hypertensive

primary prevention in hypertension trial (HAPPHY trial, 6569 patients) [58] diuretics and beta-blocker had similar effects on cardiovascular mortality. Diuretics and beta-blockers are thus accepted as substances which reduce cardiovascular complications in hypertensive patients. However, pharmacological lowering of blood pressure was not able to lower the incidence of stroke and coronary heart disease to estimated levels. The effect of blood pressure lowering on stroke reduction was about 80% and the effect on reduction of coronary heart disease about 36% of the figures estimated on the basis of prospective observational studies such as the Framingham study and the follow-up study of the Multiple risk factor intervention trial screenees [29]. On the one hand these differenes may reflect structural alterations, on the other hand diuretics and beta-blockers influence glycemic control. This may imply other cardiovascular risks.

Until now no influences on metabolism have been reported for calcium antagonists, CE-inhibitors and postsynaptic alpha receptor blockers. It is therefore possible that these substances cause a greater reduction in cardiovascular morbidity and mortality than diuretics or beta-blockers. However, there is a lack of studies testing the influence of these recent substances on cardiovascular morbidity and mortality. It is likewise not clear whether 90 mmHg or below is a suitable goal for the – mostly elderly – patients with NIDDM.

Treatment

Nonpharmacologic therapy

Nonpharmacologic therapy is to be preferred especially in patients with NIDDM. Reduction of weight in these mostly obese patients is the most important intervention at the beginning of therapy [11, 51, 53]. Weight reduction can result in a remarkable improvement of glucose metabolism and blood pressure. A mixed hypocaloric diet coupled with physical activity is the best measure to reach this goal. A reduction of alcohol intake to less than 30 g/day can reduce the level of blood pressure. Salt intake should be reduced to 6 g/day [11].

Pharmacologic treatment of hypertension

The different drugs commonly used will be discussed with special regard to their interference with glucose metabolism.

Beta-blockers: The exact antihypertensive mechanism of beta-blockers is very complex. A distinction is made between cardioselective (preponderantly β_1-activity) and non-selective beta-blockers.

It is mainly the β_1-component which is responsible for the reduction of blood pressure. β_1-blockade reduces cardiac output (and heart rate). Peripheral resistance often increases initially and then decreases after long term beta blockade. The mechanism underlying the reduction of peripheral resistance is not clear. An additional factor in the reduction of blood pressure is the β_1 suppression of the renin angiotensin system. The blood pressure lowering effect of beta-blockers is therefore more pronounced in patients with high renin levels than in those with low renin [7].

The β_2-component is of special interest because of the interference with the carbohydrate metabolism. β_2-receptors influence insulin- and glucose release as well as relaxation of peripheral vessels. β_2-blockade inhibits glucose release, leading to a longer persistence of hypoglycemia [8]. In hypoglycemia β_2-blockade additionally induces an increase in blood pressure, because the alpha-mediated vasoconstrictory activity of catecholamines cannot be antagonized [8]. Moreover, β_2-blockade influences the cellular potassium homeostasis, inhibits muscle-glycogenolyses and suppresses catecholamine induced lipolysis.

For the above mentioned reasons cardioselective beta-blockers seem to be preferable to nonselective ones in treating diabetic patients. However, even β_1-blockers are not without problems: in hypoglycemic events the release of catecholamines leads to β_1-mediated symptoms such as tachycardia, palpitations or anxiety. Consequently, β_1-receptor blockade may veil warnings of hypoglycemia. However, this is apparently of little clinical significance [3].

Diuretics: Diuretics are divided into 3 different types: thiazides, loop diuretics and potassium sparing diuretics.

For antihypertensive treatment, thiazides are the group most frequently evaluated (Table 1). They diminish vessel reactivity to pressor substances resulting in a decrease in peripheral resistance [39]. Moreover they counteract sodium- and water retention. Their efficacy diminishes at creatinine levels above 2 mg/dl. The most important side effect is potassium deficiency. Hypokalemia results in decreasing insulin release, possibly in addition to a direct effect of the thiazides itself. This leads to a disturbance of glucose metabolism. Furthermore thiazides inhibit glycolytic enzymes of glucose transport resulting in hyperglycemia [20]. The changes in glucose tolerance seem to be fully reversible: Lewis performed a long term study in 51 hypertensive patients treated with four different diuretic agents (chlorthalidone, chlorexolon, chlorothiazide, furosemide) over a period of 6 years. He noticed elevated fasting glucose levels and a diminished glucose tolerance. However, one year after discontinuation of the diuretics all parameters mentioned had returned to normal levels [27].

Loop diuretics inhibit $Na^+/Bl^{2-}K^+$-Cotransport in the ascending limb of Henle followed by substantial diuresis. In long term treatment this leads to dehydration with counteracting mechanisms of compensation, so the long term diuretic effect is no more impressive than in thiazides. The extrarenal antihypertensive effect of loop diuretics seems to be equal to that of thiazides. Loop diuretics may also induce hypokalemia. In contrast to the other kinds of diuretics, loop diuretics are still effective in renal insufficiency.

Potassium sparing diuretics have minor diuretic effects. The mechanism of their antihypertensive action is based on diminishing vessel reactivity to pressor substances. In renal insufficiency these agents can induce dangerous hyperkalemia. Therefore they should not be used if the creatinine level is above 1.5 mg/dl. In elderly patients with diabetes mellitus hyperkalemia can occur even if renal function is normal. This can be explained by diminished aldosterone secretion (hypoaldosteronism; Schambelan's syndrome). Potassium sparing diuretics should be used in combination with thiacides.

Calcium antagonists: These substances inhibit calcium influx from the extracellular space resulting in relaxation of smooth muscle. This leads to vasodilation and decreases peripheral resistance. In renal insufficiency calcium antagonists are able to reduce hyperfiltration. This is, however, only of importance for patients with IDDM, since hyperfiltration was not found in NIDDM (see above). Calcium antagonists do not alter glucose homeostasis [52]. Whether they are of advantage for diabetic patients is still not clear.

Converting enzyme inhibitors: Inhibition of angiotensin converting enzyme reduces the synthesis of angiotensin II, which has vasoconstrictory, aldosterone stimulating and thirst regulating properties. Converting enzyme inhibitors (CE-inhibitors) induce vasodilation, reduce peripheral resistance and induce a minor diuresis. CE-inhibitors also block kininase II and thus lead to an increase in endogeneous vasodilatory kinins.

CE-inhibitors do not interfere with carbohydrate metabolism [53]. However, there is some preliminary evidence of a positive effect of CE-inhibitors on glucose tolerance [40]. After short term treatment of hypertensive patients with CE-inhibitors Pollare noticed increased insulin sensitivity. Whether CE-inhibitors can inhibit or decrease progression of diabetic nephropathy in patients with NIDDM is not entirely clear.

There is evidence that CE-inhibitors decrease progression of renal insufficiency in type I diabetes. This effect might be due to the effect of angiotensin II on hyperfiltration mentioned above. On the other hand the benefit of CE-inhibitors might be due only to their unspecific antihypertensive action. However, treatment with CE-inhibitors especially in old patients with NIDDM is not without risk. In patients with bilateral renal artery stenosis acute renal failure was observed following treatment with CE-inhibitors [17]; this renal damage appears to be totally reversible after discontinuation of the CE-inhibitor.

In patients with renal insufficiency the dosage has to be adapted to renal function, since CE-inhibitors are excreted via the kidneys and can accumulate. Combination with diuretics or vasodilatators can result in severe hypotension. The use of CE-inhibitors must thus be monitored closely especially at the beginning.

Postsynaptic alpha$_1$-antagonists: Postsynaptic alpha$_1$-antagonists do not interfere with carbohydrate metabolism, but frequently result in orthostatic complications especially in patients with peripheral neuropathy [49]. Besides, a moderate degree of sodium- and water retention is often seen during treatment with postsynaptic alpha$_1$-antagonists. These substances should therefore be used primarily in combination with diuretics.

Other antihypertensive substances: If hypertension can not be treated sufficiently with the above mentioned substances, antihypertensive drugs with more important side effects have to be employed.

Hydralazine or dihydralazine is often used in combination with beta-blockers and diuretics. Interference with carbohydrate metabolism is not known.

Minoxidil, the most potent oral vasodilator, causes tachycardia and edema, and must therefore be given in combination with loop diuretics and beta-blockers. The diuretic dosage has to be adjusted to the degree of water retention; in some patients dosages up to 250 mg furosemide/day are required for compensation of water retention. These large doses of diuretics can interfere with carbohydrate metabolism, although minoxidil itself causes no interference.

Central alpha$_2$-agonists may worsen existing mental problems (loss of mental power, tiredness), which can easily be overlooked in long term treatment of elderly diabetics, but they do not influence carbohydrate metabolism.

Stepped-care approach to drug treatment: Superiority of any one of the above mentioned basic substances in hypertensive treatment has not yet been demonstrated, especially not in patients with NIDDM. Lowering of blood pressure independently of the substance employed is of major importance. The antihypertensive drug should be individually adapted to the patients' situation with respect to age, concomitant diseases and treatment of further metabolic disorders.

Beta-blockers seem to have a higher efficacy in younger patients, whereas in elderly patients cardiopulmonar side effects and contraindications are more frequent. In contrast diuretics seem to be more effective in older patients. This may result from the inverse relation between antihypertensive action and plasma renin activity, because in elderly patients lower plasma renin levels are more frequently observed [7].

Calcium antagonists more often cause hemodynamic side effects (headache, palpitations) in younger patients than in elderly ones, due to the intact baroreflexes in the former. They also appear to be more effective in elderly patients [7]. CE-inhibitors seem to have a higher degree of efficacy if plasma renin activity is increased. The number of patients with low plasma renin levels increases with age; CE-inhibitors thus reduce blood pressure more effectively in younger patients than in older ones.

In patients with coronary artery disease beta-blockers and calcium antagonists are to be preferred whereas in patients with cardiac failure preference should be given to diuretics and CE-inhibitors.

Table 3 Stepped care treatment in diabetics

	FRG	Switzerland	US
mono-therapy	β_1-blocker or diuretic or (calcium antagonist) or (CE inhibitor)	calcium antagonist or CE inhibitor or (a_1-blocker) or (β_1-blocker) or (diuretic)	diuretic or β_1-blocker or a_1-blocker or CE inhibitor or calcium antagonist
combi-nation	diuretic + β_1-blocker or calcium antagonist or CE inhibitor or a_1-blocker or calcium antagonist + β_1-blocker or CE inhibitor	any combination of the above mentioned drugs	diuretic + β_1-blocker or central adrenergic inhibitor or a_1-blocker or CE inhibitor or calcium antagonist

FRG [11], Switzerland [53], and USA [51]

The interference of beta-blockers and diuretics in carbohydrate metabolism should be considered in each patient. It should not, however, be overinterpreted nor should this interaction be grounds for dogmatic recommendations. Up to now equivocal evidence for a reduction in cerebrovascular mortality exists only for beta-blockers and diuretics, but not for the newer antihypertensive drugs such as CE-inhibitors and calcium antagonists. Patients who report repeated episodes of hypoglycemia, have problems in noticing warning symptoms of hypoglycemia or have severe visceral polyneuropathy should perhaps not be treated with a beta-blocker in the first place.

In patients with NIDDM, treatment with diuretics should be discontinued if metabolic control deteriorates during such treatment. In coexisting hyperlipemia the frequently observed beta-blocker or diuretic induced elevation of serum lipids should be taken into consideration [1, 28].

In conclusion, in younger patients low dosages of β_1-receptor blockers are preferable, in older ones diuretics. CE-inhibitors or calcium antagonists seem to be possible alternatives.

This is not sufficient for management of all hypertensive patients. For example, beta-blockers as well as diuretics result in normalisation in only 40 – 50% of all hypertensive patients. If monotherapy is not sufficient blood pressure treatment should be modified by using a combination of drugs according to the stepped care approach. The stepped care approaches of different organisations are shown in Table 3.

A combination of 2 drugs increases the possibility of lowering blood pressure sufficiently compared to monotherapy. For example: the primary combination of diuretics and β-receptor blockers lowers blood pressure sufficiently in more than 70%. The greater efficacy of combining two drugs of different classes can result in diminishing side effects as well due to lower dosages.

However, side effects in monotherapy are easier to handle and there is more experience of long term treatment, especially with diuretics and β-receptor blockers. Thus, all stepped care approaches shown in Table 2 begin with monotherapy. However, in stable or severe hypertension it might be reasonable to begin with a combination of drugs. There is still discussion as to whether an alternative monotherapy is superior to a combination of drugs if one drug fails to lower blood pressure sufficiently.

Future perspectives

At the present time more studies are necessary to test the new promising drugs used for antihypertensive therapy such as calcium antagonists and CE-inhibitors in order to decide whether these substances are preferable to the established diuretics and beta-blockers.

References

[1] Ames RP, Hill P. Increase in serum lipids during treatment of hypertension with chlorthalidone. Lancet 1976; I: 721.
[2] Baba T, Murabayashi S, Takebe K. Comparison of the renal effects of angiotensin converting enzyme inhibitor and calcium antagonist in hypertension type 2 (non-insulin-dependent) diabetic patients with microalbuminuria: a randomised controlled trial. Diabetologia 1989; 32: 40–44.
[3] Barnett, AH, Leslie D, Watkins PJ. Can insulin-treated diabetics be given beta-adrenergic blocking drugs. British Medical Journal 1980; 280: 976–978.
[4] Beretta-Piccoli C, Weidmann P. Body sodium and renin activity in diabetes mellitus. Diabete et Metabolisme 1989; 15: 296–300.
[5] Berglund G, Andersson O, Widgren B. Low-dose antihypertensive treatment with a thiazide diuretic is not diabetogenic. A 10-year controlled trial with bendroflumethiazide. Acta Med Scand 1986; 220: 419–424.
[6] Blaustein MP. Sodium ions, calcium ions, blood pressure regulation and hypertension: a reassessment and a hypothesis. Am J Physiol 1977; 232: C165–C173.
[7] Bühler FR. Age and cardiovascular response adaptation: determinants of an antihypertensive treatment concept primarily based on betablockers and calcium entry blockers. Hypertension 1983; 5 (Suppl. III): 94–100.
[8] Christlieb AR, Maki PC. The effect of beta-blocker therapy on glucose and lipid metabolism. Primary Cardiology 1980: (Suppl.): 47–54.
[9] Christlieb AR. Treating hypertension in the patient with diabetes mellitus. Med Clin North Am 1982; 66: 1373–1388.
[10] DeFronzo RA. The effect of insulin on renal sodium metabolism. Diabetologia 1981; 21: 165–171.
[11] Deutsche Liga zur Bekämpfung des hohen Blutdrucks: Empfehlungen für die Behandlung des Hochdrucks bei Diabetes. Heidelberg, 1989.
[12] Ferrannini E, Hommel E, Mauer SM et al. Hypertension: A metabolic disorder? Diabete et Metabolisme 1989; 15: 284–291.
[13] Gundersen T, Kjekshus J. Timolol treatment after myocardial infarction in diabetic patients. Diabetes Care 1983; 6: 285–290.
[14] Hasslacher CH, Wolfrum M, Stech G et al. Diabetische Nephropathie bei Type-II-Diabetes. Einfluß von Stoffwechselkontrolle und Blutdruck auf Entwicklung und Verlauf. Dtsch med Wschr 1987; 112: 1445–1449.
[15] Hasslacher CH. Nephropathie bei Typ-II-Diabetes. GIT Labor-Medizin 1988; 5: 278–280.
[16] Helgeland A. Treatment of mild hypertension: A five year controlled drug trial. The Oslo study. Am J Med 1980; 69: 725–732.
[17] Hricik DE, Browning PJ, Kozelman R et al. Captopril-induced functional renal insufficiency in patients with bilateral renal-artery stenoses or renal-artery stenosis in a solitary kidney. N Eng J Med 1983; 308: 373–376.
[18] Hypertension detection and follow-up program cooperative group. The effect of treatment on mortality in mild hypertension. Results of the hypertension detection and follow-up program. N Engl J Med 1982; 307: 976–980.
[19] Janka HU, Dirschedl P. Systolic blood pressure as a predictor for cardiovascular disease in diabetes. Hypertension 1985; 7 (Suppl. II): 90–94.
[20] Jung CY, Mookerjee BK. Inhibitory effect of furosemide on glucose transport. J Lab Clin Med 1976; 87: 960.

[21] Kannel WB, McGee DL. Diabetes and cardiovascular risk factors. The Framingham Study. Circulation 1979; 59: 8–13.
[22] Kannel WB. Status of risk factors and their consideration in antihypertensive therapy. Am J Cardiol 1987; 59: 80 A–90 A.
[23] Kirkendall WM: Treatment of hypertension in the elderly. Am J Cardiol 1983; 57: 63 C–68 C.
[24] Klein R, Klein BEK, Moss SE et al. The Wisconsin epidemiologic study of diabetic retinopathy. III. Prevalence and risk of diabetic retinopathy when age at diagnosis is 30 or more years. Arch Ophthalmol 1984; 12: 527–532.
[25] Kribben A, Philipp Th. The contribution of the sympathetic nervous system to hypertension in diabetes mellitus. Diabete et Metabolisme 1989; 15: 313–317.
[26] Kuller LH, Dorman JS, Wolf PA. Chapter XVII: Cerebrovascular disease and diabetes, in: Diabetes in America. U.S. Department of Health and Human Services, NIH Publication 1985; No. 85–1468, XVIII-1–XVIII-18.
[27] Lewis PJ, Kohner EM, Petrie A et al. Deterioration of glucose tolerance in hypertensive patients on prolonged diuretic treatment. Lancet 1976; I: 564–566.
[28] Lohmann FW. Die Beeinflussung des Stoffwechsels durch β-Rezeptorenblocker. Klin Wschr 1981; 59: 49.
[29] MacMahon SW, Cutler JA, Neaton JD et al. For the Multiple Factor Intervention Trial Research Group: Relationship of blood pressure to coronary and stroke morbidity and mortality in clinical trials and epidemiological studies. J Hypertension 1986; 4 (Suppl. 6): 14–17.
[30] Management Committee of the Australian national blood pressure study. Prognostic factors in the treatment of mild hypertension. Circulation 1984; 69: 668–676.
[31] Marre M, Leblanc H, Suarez L et al. Converting enzyme inhibition and kidney function in normotensive diabetic patients with persistent microalbuminuria. Br Med J 1987; 294: 1448–1452.
[32] Mathias CJ, Frankel LH, Turner RC et al. Physiological response to insulin hypoglycemic in spinal man. Paraplegia 1980; 17: 319–326.
[32a] Medical research council working party: MRC trial of treatment of mild hypertension: principal results. Br Med J 1985; 291: 97–104.
[33] Modan M, Halkin H, Almog S et al. Hyperinsulinemia. A link between hypertension obesity and glucose intolerance. J Clin Invest 1985; 75: 809–817.
[34] Mogensen CE. A complete screening of urinary albumin concentration in an unselected diabetes out-patient clinic population. Diabetic Nephropathy 1983; 11–18.
[35] Mogensen CE. Long-term antihypertensive treatment inhibiting progression of diabetic nephropathy. Br Med J 1982; 285: 685–688.
[36] Moore RD. Effects of insulin upon ion transport. Biochem Biophys Acta 1983; 737: 1–49.
[37] O'Hare JA, Ferris JB, Brady D et al. Exchangable sodium and renin in hypertensive diabetic patients with and without nephropathy. Hypertension 1985; 7 (Suppl. II): 43–48.
[38] Parving HH, Anderson AR, Hommel E et al. Effects of long-term antihypertensive treatment on kidney function in diabetic nephropathy. Hypertension 1985; 7 (Suppl. II): 114–117.
[39] Philipp Th. Diuretika und Gefäßreagibilität. In: Bock KD, Schrey A, eds. Natrium und Hypertonie. München: Wolf, 1981; 71–77.
[40] Pollare T, Lithell H, Berne C. A comparison of the effects of hydrochlorothiazide and captopril on glucose and lipid metabolism in patients with hypertension. N Engl J Med 1989; 321: 868–873.
[41] Public health service hospitals cooperative group; W McFate Smith: Treatment of mild hypertension: results of a ten year intervention trial. Hypertension 1977; 15 (suppl. I) Circ Res 40: 108–105.
[42] Reaven GM, Hoffman BB. A role for insulin in the aetiology and course of hypertension? Lancet 1987; II: 435–437.

[43] Reid DD, Brett GZ, Hamilton PJS et al. Cardiorespiratory disease and diabetes among middle-aged male civil servants: a study of screening and intervention. Lancet 1974; I: 469–473.
[44] Report by the management committee: The Australian therapeutic trial in mild hypertension. Lancet 1980; II: 1261–1267.
[45] Ritchie CM, McIlrath E, Hadden DR et al. Renal artery stenosis in hypertensive diabetic patients. Diabetic Med 1988; 5: 265–267.
[46] Schmitz A, Jorgen H, Gundersen G et al. Glomerular morphology by light microscopy in non-insulin dependent diabetes mellitus. Lack of glomerular hypertrophy. Diabetes 1988; 37: 38–43.
[47] Standl E, Stiegler H, Roth R et al. On the impact of hypertension on prognosis of NIDDM. Results of the Schwabing G.P.-program. Diabete et Metabolisme 1989; 15: 352–358.
[48] Stout RW, Biermann EL, Ross R. The effect of insulin on the proliferation of cultured primate arterial smooth muscle cells. Circ Res 1975; 36: 319–327.
[49] Takabataka T et al. Effects of long-term prazosin therapy on lipoprotein metabolism in hypertensive patients. Am J Med 1985; 79: 113–116.
[50] The 1984 report of the Joint National Committee on Detection, Evaluation and Treatment of High Blood Pressure. Arch Intern Med 1984; 140: 1280–1285.
[51] The working group on hypertension in diabetes: Statement on hypertension in diabetes mellitus. Final report. The working Group on Hypertension in Diabetes. Arch Intern Med 1987; 147: 830–842.
[52] Trost BN, Weidmann P. Effects of calcium antagonists on glucose hemostasis and serum lipids in non diabetic and diabetic subjects. J Hypertension 1987; 5: 81–104.
[53] Trost BN. Hypertension in the diabetic patient. Selection and optimum use of antihypertensive drugs. Drugs 1989; 38: 621–633.
[54] Veterans administration cooperative study group on antihypertensive agents. Effects of treatment on morbidity in hypertension. II. Results in patients with diastolic blood pressures averaging 90 through 114 mm Hg. JAMA 1970; 213: 1143–1152.
[55] Veterans administration cooperative study group on antihypertensive agents. Effects of treatment on morbidity in hypertension. Results in patients with diastolic blood pressures averaging 115 through 129 mm Hg. JAMA 1967; 202: 116–122.
[56] Vierhapper H. Effect of exogeneous insulin on blood pressure regulation in healthy and diabetic subjects. Hypertension 1985; 7 (Suppl. II): 49–53.
[57] Weidmann P. Pathogenesis of hypertension accompanying diabetes mellitus. Contrib Nephrol 1989; 73: 73–90.
[58] Wilhelmsen I, Berglund G, Elmfeldt D et al. Betablockers versus diuretics in hypertensive men. Main results from the HAPPHY trial. Hypertension 1987; 5: 561–572.
[59] Zavorini I, Bonora E, Pagliara M et al. Risk factors for coronary artery disease in healthy persons with hyperinsulinemia and normal glucose tolerance. N Engl J Med 1989; 320: 702–706.

Pharmacology of the kidney in IDDM patients

C. E. Mogensen

Introduction

End-stage renal failure in IDDM patients remains a major medical problem [1], although we have witnessed some progress within this area in the last few years [2–4]. End-stage renal failure in these patients is the final result of a long-term complicated process involving not only metabolic, but also hormonal and metabolic factors possibly modulated by genetic features in the diabetic patient [5–9]. In most cases end-stage diabetic nephropathy takes about three decades or more to develop and marked renal changes are present right from the diagnosis of diabetes.

Initially a very characteristic feature is seen in these patients, namely hyperfiltration and renal hypertrophy, which is found at clinical diagnosis, and as a major abnormality in these patients during the first decade of the disease when uncontrolled. Over the following decade many of the poorly controlled patients may develop microalbuminuria, which, without intervention, is progressive, and eventuates in clinical proteinuria. Microalbuminuria is defined as elevated urinary albumin excretion rate (UAER) in the absence of overt proteinuria. The stage with proteinuria is associated with increasing blood pressure and a fairly constant and linear rate of decline of GFR.

It is understood that this complicated process may require different pharmacological approaches according to the stage of disease. Fig. 1 outlines the natural history of the renal changes in diabetes and the sequence of markers and characteristics for diabetic nephropathy is shown in Table 1, referring to changes shown in Fig. 1. It is, however, important to know that with more and more widespread knowledge of the nature of disease and more and more effective intervention, the natural history of the disease may change. The disease process is likely to be retarded, but in principle the same stages may be described.

It has been clear that early intervention in diabetic nephropathy mainly deals with optimized insulin treatment along with proper diet and life-style. The diabetic diet has changed considerably during the last few decades and may change further [10–11]. Maybe the most important and effective inter-

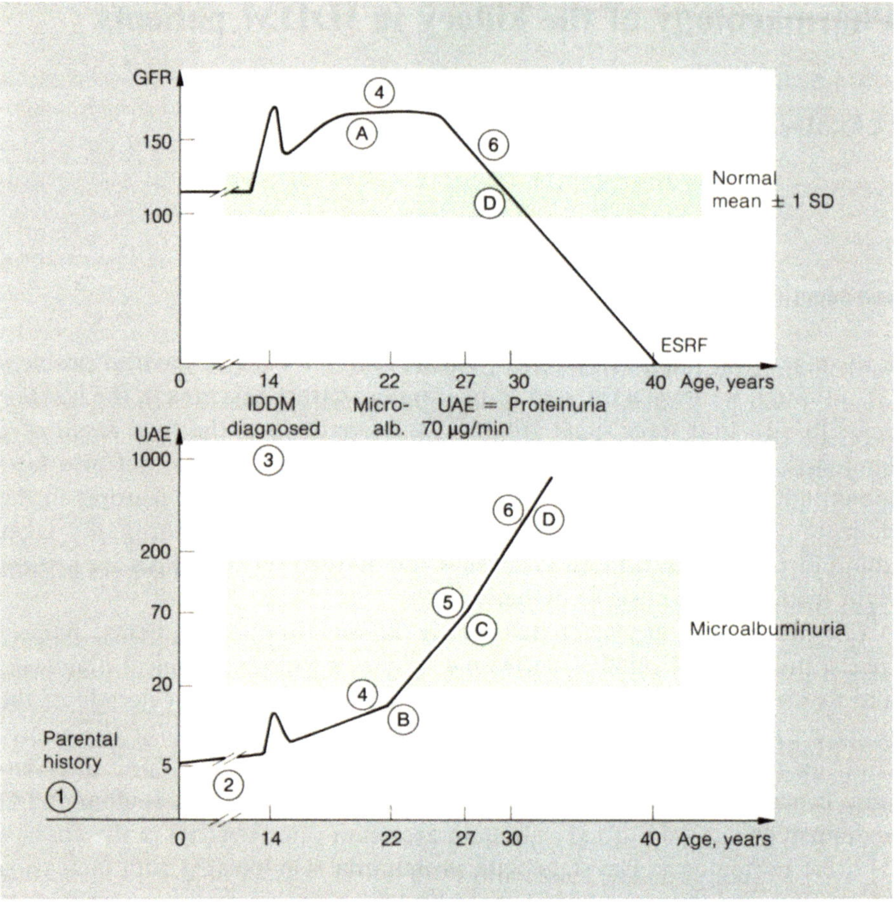

Fig. 1 The figure provides a summary of the natural history of diabetic nephropathy in IDDM patients. The figure also includes the possibilities of intervention in the various stages of diabetic nephropathy. GFR values in normals are shown by the hatched area in the upper part of the figure. The lower part shows development of albuminuria. The level 20—200 µg/min is the microalbuminuric range. Parental history of hypertension (1) or prediabetic hypertension (2) is difficult to use in the prediction of nephropathy. Also, nephropathy cannot be predicted at the clinical diagnosis (3), but extreme hyperfiltration (4) and more convincingly microalbuminuria (5) is related to subsequent nephropathy. Proteinuria (6) usually predicts progression of nephropathy to end-stage renal failure (ESRF).

The figure shows a typical course in a patient developing diabetes at the age of 14 years. The patient showed poor metabolic control as indicated by the high level of GFR (> 150 ml/min) and the increasing albumin excretion rate. At the age of 22 years the patient developed microalbuminuria and later clinical nephropathy at age 30 years, typically after 16 years of diabetes. Blood pressure rises, and GFR starts to decline during incipient diabetic nephropathy with increasing microalbuminuria (> 70 µg/min) and end-stage renal failure reached at the age of 40 years — if intervention is not undertaken.

Intervention (A → D) is possible as discussed in the section on present treatment modalities.

Table 1 *Sequence of markers/end-points in diabetic nephropathy*

Hyperfiltration (+ increased renal size)	Early extreme hyperfiltration associated to late DN in some studies
Microalbuminuria	Probable laboratory sign of early glomerulopathy
Proteinuria	Degree well-established marker of severity
Fall-rate of GFR (+ clar BP-elevation)	Important parameter (if carefully measured)
ESRF	Important and-point
Death	Final end-point

Table 2 *Pathogenesis of diabetic nephropathy*

Are risk factors related to pathogenesis?	
Possible risk factor	Reversal by intervention
1) Genetic factors	
a) Predisposition to hypertension?	Genetically related hypertension treatable
b) Family clustering of nephropathy?	?
2) Poor metabolic control	Optimized treatment
a) Glycemic changes	$HbA_{1C}\downarrow$
b) Non-glycemic changes	metabolic/hormonal
(e. g. hyperfiltration)	haemodynamic inhibition
3) Dietary factors	
High protein intake	Normalizing protein intake
High lipid intake	Diet
High sodium	Sodium-reduction in diet
Tobacco smoking	Anti-smoking campaigns?
4) Blood pressure elevation	Reducing BP by a) Diuretics b) β_1-blocker c) ACE-inhibitors d) Ca-antagonists
5) Increased vascular permeability	e. g. BP reduction
6) Charge defects in BM	Not possible today

vention modality, somewhat later in the course, is antihypertensive treatment. These modalities of intervention are also linked to the pathophysiology or pathogenesis of diabetic nephropathy as outlined in Table 2.

Pathophysiology and pathogenesis of renal function in IDDM patients

The pathophysiology of renal changes in diabetes varies considerably according to the stage of the disease. During the first decades increased renal function or hyperfiltration is a characteristic feature associated with poor metabolic control. The pathophysiology behind the increase in renal size and hyperfiltration is not clearly understood, but a number of abnormalities have been proposed as outlined in Table 3 [12–13].

Other factors may be involved in pathogenesis, especially in the late stages of the disease as outlined in Table 2. Identification of risk factors is important, but obviously it cannot be taken for granted that a particular risk factor is in fact involved in the pathogenetic process. However, if intervention appears to be successful, evidence then suggests that the risk factor is actually involved in the disease process, – unless intervention is given too late or in too small amounts, possibly for too short a period of time.

The pharmacologic approach [14] will be dealt with in accordance with risk factors as related to pathogenesis as outlined in Table 2. Monitoring of treatment effect is clearly important, and the parameters shown in Table 1 may be used as effect parameters or end-points. Obviously, the most critical approach would require increased longevity as a result of treatment. However, such criteria would require extremely long-term follow-up, and some substitutes or surrogates for a firm end-point must therefore be considered. For instance if fall rate of GFR can be reduced it may be likely that end-stage renal failure can also be postponed. Also, reduction in microalbuminuria may

Table 3 Possible causes for high GFR in IDDM*

Candidate	Acute effect	Long-term effect	Comments
Glucose	≈ 5% increase or less	Unknown	Correlation between GFR/HbA_{1c}
Glucagon	≈ 6% increase	Unknown	Requires rather high levels of plasma glucagon
Growth hormone	None	≈ 6% increase	Requires 4–7 days of administration
Ketone bodies	Increase?	Unknown	Controversial
Dietary protein content	Enhancement of GFR	Enhancement of GFR	As judged from dietary intervention studies

*Best correlated to renal size

be considered beneficial, because microalbuminuria is probably the earliest laboratory sign of the main disease process in the kidney. An even earlier abnormality is, as mentioned, hyperfiltration, but the significance of the amelioration of this early physiological process may for a long period remain unproven. So far, quantitative evaluation of renal biopsies has not been used in documenting effect of treatment, but form the theoretical point of view, structural analysis might be considered as an extremely important parameter [4].

Classification of patients

Table 4 outlines a schematic illustration of the natural history of diabetic nephropathy including concomitant changes in renal and systemic hemodynamics [3]. The scheme also suggests some basic pathophysiological changes and structural counterparts. This outline of changes will be a guideline for intervention as discussed in the following [14]. Even without any clinical trials, suggestions for intervention are clearly possible. Diabetic nephropathy only develops after many years of diabetes and its metabolic aberrations. Therefore, it is conceivable that the disease is in some way produced by the diabetic state. Usually there is an association between high blood pressure and rate of progression of renal disease, irrespective of the nature of the original renal injury. Based on these observations, the clinical approach would a priori be to obtain the best possible metabolic control within practical limits, simply because the lesions of diabetic nephropathy do not develop without these metabolic aberrations. Along this line, a close to normal blood pressure level would also seem a priori justified, knowing that high blood pressure is associated with progressive renal disorders. Also, no radical changes should be proposed in the diet as compared with the background population. This would be the arm-chair approach. Indeed, considerable evidence from clinical trials now supports the view that good metabolic control and satisfactory blood pressure control ameliorate the initiation and progression of diabetic renal disease, as well as does a protein-reduced diet [11, 15].

Survey of clinical trials

Table 5 outlines recent results regarding clinical trials in diabetic renal involvement in IDDM patients. Antihypertensive treatment in NIDDM patients will be discussed in this book by Kribben et al. and modalities of insulin-treatment in chapter 2.

Table 4 Schematic natural history outline of diabetic nephropathy (IDDM)

Stage	I At diagnosis, acute changes	II FIRST DECADE (or first ≈ 7–13 y)	III SECOND DECADE (≈ 7–25 years duration)	IV THIRD DECADE (or last ≈ 8–12 y)	V ESRF (after ≈ 30 y)
GFR	High*	Hyperfiltration (HF) (total and single nephron)	Still HF, but declining GFR	Fall rate 12 ml/y. Single-nephron-HF likely	Close to zero
UAER	High* or normal	Normal, but slightly increasing	Increasing microalbuminuria	Increasing proteinuria (P)	Still P
BP or hyperten-sion (HT)	BP usually normal	BP comparable to background popula-tion (HT seen in ≈ 2–10%)	Increasing blood pressure, 3% per year	HT increasing, 7% per year	High BP
Suggested basic changes	Metabol. and hemodynam. changes, plus hyperphagia	*Metabol.*: ↑ Glycemia, ↑ AR**, ↑ Hormones *Hemodynam.*: Normal BP but intra-renal HT likely *Diet*: Usually high in protein	*Metabol.*: ↑ Glycemia, ↑ AR**, ↑ Hormones *Hemodynam.*: Systemic + intrarenal HT *Diet*: Usually high in protein	*Metabol.*: ↑ Glycemia, ↑ AR**, ↑ Hormones *Hemodynam.*: Systemic + intrarenal HT *Diet*: Usually high in protein	Nephron closure
Progressing to next stage	100%	30–40%	> 80%	Close to 100%	
Other con-comitant abnormality	HbA_{1c}↑ and many meta-bolic changes	Possible hyperperfusion	Retinopathy + Neuropathy Lipid changes and vascular disease in general	As III, but increasing in severity	Uremia
Main structural counterparts	Hypertrophy of nephrons	Hypertrophy of nephrons, BM-thickening after ≈ 2 years Mesang. expansion after ≈ 5 years	Microalb. associated with more ad-vanced hist. and ultrastruct. lesions	Advancing structural lesion especially mesangial expansion and glom. closure	Nephron closure

* = Reversible
** = Aldose reductase activity

Table 5 Recent results regarding clinical trials in diabetic renal involvement in IDDM patients

	Hyperfiltration	Microalbuminuria	Proteinuria, fall in GFR
Optimized insulin treatment	Hyperfiltration reduced, but reduction difficult to sustain in some patients	Stabilized or reduced if BP does not rise	Effect not documented
Dietary modification: Protein reduced diet	Hyperfiltration reduced by normalizing dietary proteins	Microalbuminuria reduced in short-term studies	Fall rate of GFR and proteinuria reduced
Hormonal inhibition (by somatostatin: growth hormone and glucagon reduced)	Hyperfiltration reduced in acute studies	No data	No data
Metabolic-pathway-inhibition (Aldose reductase inhibition)	Hyperfiltration reduced	Microalbuminuria possibly reduced in short-term studies	No data
Hemodynamic modification by ACE-inhibition	Filtration fraction reduced, UAER reduced, no change in GFR	Microalbuminuria reduced, GFR may be preserved No proteinuria seen	Proteinuria reduced, fall rate of GFR reduced
Long-term treatment with β_1-blockers (+ diuretics)	No data	Microlabuminruria reduced, GFR may be preserved	Proteinuria reduced, fall rate of GFR reduced

Optimized insulin treatment

The test parameters to be monitored early in the course of renal involvement, besides known risk factors, are hyperfiltration and UAER, which may be in the upper normal range. Later, microalbuminuria/proteinuria, as well as fall rate in GFR, are the main parameters.

Hyperfiltration: It is now clear that optimized insulin treatment can reduce hyperfiltration, at least in short-term studies over a few years [12]. A number of patients develop severe hyperfiltration, exceeding 150 ml/min, which is usually associated with very poor metabolic control [13], but standard intensified treatment with insulin pens is often able to reduce such degrees of hyperfiltration in compliant patients.

Upper normal range of UAER: The longest insulin-pump study published to date is the Oslo study, where patients were monitored for 4 years [16]. Upper-normal-range-UAER was reduced significantly by long-term intensified treatment as compared with conventional treatment. Such patients with upper normal range values may of course be those who later develop microalbuminuria [17].

Microalbuminuria: It is probably very important to intervene effectively in patients with microalbuminuria. Regarding optimized insulin treatment, the Steno Study II and its extension certainly suggest that good metabolic control can ameliorate the progression of microalbuminuria as discussed in volume 2 of this series [19]. This concept will be further established, if the DCCT study is able to confirm the Danish results. Part of the Steno study was continued for more than two years [20], but some patients had to be treated with antihypertensive agents which are likely to decrease UAER more than optimised insulin treatment.

The proteinuric phase: In patients with clinical proteinuria no dramatic effect of optimised insulin treatment has been noted, but it should be kept in mind that it is likely that very large groups of patients are required to document such an effect [21]. An association between progression in nephropathy and metabolic control has been noted by Nyberg et al. [22] and glycemic control may therefore still play an important role in the progression of renal disease in these patients.

Low protein diet

Although this is not strictly a pharmacological approach, a low protein diet will be discussed briefly in this chapter.

Hyperfiltration: It has been shown that protein restriction generally lowers GFR [10]. In a recent study [15] diabetic patients were randomized to follow four weeks of their usual protein intake (19% of energy) alternating with four weeks of a limited protein intake (12% of energy). Kidney function was investigated after the two dietary periods. It was found that the limited protein diet reduced GFR by about 10%. S-urea was significantly reduced on limited protein intake suggesting that patients were compliant to the diet, which was accepted very well by the patients. Thus, limitation of the often high protein intake in diabetics might be valuable and realistic, and there is no obvious reason to prescribe a diet with as much as 20% of the calories derived from proteins [10].

Microalbuminuria: A single study suggests that microalbuminuria can be reduced on a short-term basis by a low protein diet [23], but so far, no long-term results are available.

Overt nephropathy: In diabetic nephropathy new data have recently been published indicating that the rate of decline of GFR can be considerably reduced by a low protein diet [11]. Patients were monitored on their usual dietary intake of proteins and thereafter patients were put on a low protein diet. A remarkable reduction in the fall rate of GFR was observed, although the response varied considerably. The mean fall rate of GFR was reduced from 0.61 to 0.14 ml/min/month. Patients served as their own controls without a parallel non-treated group and it cannot be excluded that late or long-term action of antihypertensive treatment may explain at least part of observed beneficial effect. As discussed earlier, dietary advice over the last years has resulted in a rather high protein intake, and it cannot be excluded that such a dietary program may contribute to the development of renal disease. There has been considerable debate regarding a protein-reduced diet in non-diabetic nephropathy, but protein-restriction now seems generally to be effective in some of these patients [24].

Antihypertensive treatment, including ACE-inhibition

Much attention has been paid to antihypetensive treatment in IDDM patients, mostly in patients with incipient or overt nephropathy, but also in patients with hyperfiltration.

Hyperfiltration: In a recent study the possible beneficial effect of ACE-inhibition in normo-albuminuric patients was investigated [25]. After 3 months of enalapril treatment, FF and UAER were significantly decreased but no significant changes in GFR, RPF, mean arterial pressure were observed. Thus, long-term and acute [25] ACE-inhibition in normotensive, normoalbuminuric insulin-dependent diabetic patients may be associated with some beneficial changes in renal hemodynamics and albumin excretion rate, possibly as a result of a reduction in glomerular capillary hydrostatic pressure. These observations are interesting, but cannot at present be applied to ordinary treatment, since long-term effets are unknown. In a similar study a reduction in FF and UAER was not observed [26].

Microalbuminuria or incipient nephropathy: From a theoretical point of view ACE-inhibitors may offer advantages in the treatment of early and late hypertension of diabetic nephropathy [27]. As an example, Marre et al. [28] in a one-year study examined the effect of chronic ACE-inhibition in microalbuminuric normotensive patients and documented a long-term beneficial effect (Table 5 and 6). In the ACE-treated group, UAER was reduced and GFR remained stable. β-blockers combined with diuretics also appear to be effective in long-term studies [29].

New studies have confirmed the effect by ACE-inhibitors on microalbuminuria [30]. In a randomized, but non-blind study, captopril treatment combined with a thiazide diuretic, was evaluated in 21 patients during a three year follow-up period. Patients treated with ACE-inhibition plus diuretics exhibited a fall in albumin excretion rate as shown in Table 6. Fractional albumin clearance fell with 16 per cent per year during captopril treatment, rose with 6 per cent per year during placebo. These results confirm earlier long-term studies with β-blockers also combined with diuretics [29]. In a short-term study similar results were obtained [31]. This overall beneficial pattern (also to some extent in the controls) may partly be due to closer follow-up of patients in this study. It is a general impression that patients with low grade microalbuminuria, from 20 to 70 microgram/min, may stay rather stable if blood pressure does not increase, and if glycemic control is fairly satisfactory.

Table 6 ACE-inhibition in young IDDM patients with incipient and overt nephropathy

Group of patients	Treatment/ plecebo/ control	N	Years of treat- ment	Blood pressure (mmHg)			UAER (µg/min)			GFR (ml/min)		Remarks
				Before		During	Before		During	Initial value	Change per year	
Incipient nephropathy (micro- albuminuric) (Marre, 1988)	Enalapril	10	1	≈ 100 (MAP)	*	85□	18.6+	*	3.6+	131	−7	Rapid progression in the placebo group
	Placebo	10		≈ 99 (MAP)	*	102□	11.4+	*	41.9+	129	−20*	
(Mathiesen, 1990)	Captopril (+ Diuretics)	21	3	129/79	(n. s.)	127/76	57	*	33	unchanged	unchanged	0/21 developed DN x
	No treatment	23		125/77	(n. s.)	124/74	73	*	94	unchanged	unchanged	7/23 developed DN
Early nephropathy (Christensen, 1990)	Enalapril added to Metropolol and Thiazide	8	½	129/84	(n. s.)	123/79	175	*	70	121	no change	UAE and BP rose after dis- continuation of enalapril
Proteinuria without hypertension (Parving, 1989)	Captopril	15	1	128/78		122/77	378		Fall by 11%	111	−3.1	Fall rate of GFR not significant different
	Placebo	17		127/79	*	134/84	471		Increase by 55%*	115	−6.4	
Overt nephropathy (Parving, 1988)	Captopril	18	2.5	146/93	*	136/85	982	*	390	98	−5.8 *	Historical controls
	Historical controls	13		137/95	*	145/98	936	*	1367	96	−10.0	

+ = Fractional albumin clearance ($x10^6$)
* = Significant change
□ At end of one year

Conventional antihypertensive agents or ACE-inhibitors given as monotherapy may not always reduce UAER in diabetes. The aim of a recent study [32, 33] was to investigate the renal effect of the addition of an ACE-inhibitor to conventional antihypertensive treatment comprising β_1-blockers plus diuretics in diabetics with early nephropathy. Thus, the patients would be on triple treatment (β_1-blockers, thiazide-diuretics and ACE-inhibitors, all in moderate doses). Importantly, UAER was reduced from 175 to 70 μg/min ($2p < 1\%$). The combination therapy was well tolerated. Thus, ACE-inhibition plus conventional AHT produces a marked reduction of UAER in spite of minor or no changes in hemodynamic parameters [33].

Overt nephropathy with proteinuria: The first studies suggesting a beneficial effect on renal function of antihypertensive treatment in overt diabetic nephropathy were published as long as 15 years ago [34, 35]. In these studies it was documented that antihypertensive treatment with β-blockers and diuretics not only reduced albumin excretion [35], but also seemed to reduce the rate of decline of GFR [34], as now confirmed in long-term studies [36, 37].

Recently, a series of important clinical trials has been conducted by Parving et al., with ACE-inhibitors as the proposed major reno-protective agent [38–40]. In an interesting study [39], patients were monitored for 2.5 years with captopril and furosemide, and compared with a historical control group. The most important parameter, namely the rate of decline of GFR, was lower with captopril, 5.8 ml/min/year versus 10.0 ml/year in the historical controls (Table 5). The rate of decline of GFR in patients on captopril and furosemide is quite comparable to β-blockers and diuretics given in combination [33]. Earlier Björck et al. also observed a beneficial effect by adding ACE-inhibitors to conventional antihypertensive treatment [41]. In a new study, a special group of patients was studied, namely patients with proteinuria, but without clear hypertension [40]. These patients were randomized to treatment for 12 months with ACE-inhibitors or placebo (Table 6). In these patients without overt hypertension BP was reduced by captopril, but rose as expected in the control group. In addition, albumin excretion declined in the captopril treated group. The fall rate of GFR was 3.1 ml/min/year in the captopril group versus 6.4 ml/min/year in the control group, a difference which failed to reach statistical significance. Thus, ACE-inhibition appears to arrest the progressive rise in albuminuria in normotensive insulin dependent patients, but the effect on the fall rate of GFR was not clearly established.

The same effect on GFR-fall-rate and proteinuria seems to be obtained by most antihypertensive agents and one main issue is therefore side-effects during antihypertensive treatment. Some evidence suggests that fewer side effects are seen when using ACE-inhibitors as discussed in volume II in this series, although long-term follow-up is not yet available [19, 33]. There is little experience with calcium-antagonists in IDDM patients.

Hormonal intervention

As hyperfiltration in IDDM is associated with the development of late diabetic nephropathy, new methods of lowering this hyperfunction are being researched, e. g. reduction of growth hormone and glucagon hypersecretion [42]. To elucidate the acute effect of the somatostatin analogue SMS 201 – 995 (Sandostatin®) renal function was measured in normoalbuminuric IDDM patients. GFR and RPF were reduced by 5% and 9% respectively (Table 7). The elevated serum GH-level was reduced to normal values and a significant drop was also seen in serum glucagon. Thus, SMS 201 – 995 acutely lowers hyperperfusion and hyperfiltration in IDDM, and this effect on kidney function is most likely a direct one, possibly mediated via a reduction in serum glucagon.

Metabolic intervention, ameliorating the sorbitol pathway by aldose reductase inhibition

In tissues not requiring insulin for glucose absorption, hyperglycemia causes enhanced glucose metabolism via the polyol pathway. It has been suggested that the high level of aldose reductase activity may cause functional and structural abnormalities in diabetes and may be involved in the development of late complications [43]. In order to elucidate the effect of an aldose reductase inhibitor (Statil, ICI 128436), normoalbuminuric diabetic patients were randomized to follow either 6 months of treatment with Statil or placebo (Table 7). GFR was significantly reduced by 8% in the Statil treated patients.

Table 7 Changes in renal hemodynamics in normoalbuminuric IDDM

ACE-I (3 months)	SMS (acute)	Preotein limitation (1 month)	AR-I (6 months)
GFR –	GFR ↓	GFR ↓	GFR ↓
RPF –	RPF ↓	RPF (↓)	RPF –
FF ↓	FF ↑	FF –	FF –
UAER ↓	UAE –	UAE –	UAE –

The RPF, UAER, fractional albumin clearance, and renal vascular resistance were unchanged in both groups. Thus, inhibition of aldose reductase reduces the characteristic hyperfiltration in uncomplicated Type 1 diabetes, but here too the long-term effect is unknown [43].

Present treatment modalities

Early in the course of diabetes, metabolic aberrations seem to determine renal changes as well as renal prognosis and great emphasis should therefore be put on relative near-normalization of glycemic control without side-effects as related to hypoglycemic attacks and too rigid a life-style (A + B in Fig. 1). This is also important later in the course of diabetes, especially in patients with microalbuminuria (C). In patients with overt nephropathy, good metabolic control becomes increasingly difficult. In general, the main goal should be to reduce glycated hemoglobin to less than 7.5–8% (mean reference-value 5.5% ± 0.5 (SD)), although this goal should be less rigid in overt nephropathy. Regarding the dietary approach, a reduction in protein intake should be attempted (A), down to the background population level of around 12% of calories, but 14% would be more practical to achieve, although not at all easy [10]. With advancing renal disease a further reduction should be attempted (D). Antihypertensive treatment has an important place in the management of diabetic nephropathy (C + D). With advancing renal changes, which start with microalbuminuria, the blood pressure begins to increase. The apropriate level of blood pressure is likely to be around 135/85 in the average younger patient. Pharmacological antihypertensive treatment should probably be given in patients where blood pressure continuously equals or exceeds 140/90. Care should be taken to avoid overtreatment by careful monitoring of blood pressure, possibly by 24-hour recording [44]. So far there are no clinical indications for treatment with aldose reductase inhibitors, or somatostatin analogues, and these agents still remain under investigation. ACE-inhibition in normoalbuminuric, normotensive patients is also not indicated.

Recently, several papers have reported that survival is considerably improved in diabetic patients with proteinuria, apparently owing to the introduction of antihypertensive treatment in the seventies [45–47]. Certainly prognosis may have improved even more in recent years. It is now likely that patients with microalbuminuria carry a better prognosis with early antihypertensive treatment and improved metabolic control, as outlined above. Therefore, we may expect that clinical proteinuria can be considerably postponed with these treatment modalities. However, we are still awaiting the long-term results from the DCCT study [48].

Future perspectives

Obviously, rational treatment must rely on detailed knowledge of pathogenesis of the disease, but unfortunately there are many unknown elements within the field of diabetic nephropathy. A main feature, expansion of the mesangial area, seems rather closely related to the disease process. Factors that determine rate of expansion in the mesangial area have not yet been clarified. However, patients may be divided into those with a slow rate of expansion and those with a rapid rate of expansion of the mesangium. It is clear that blood pressure elevation is associated with mesangial expansion, but this is probably not the sole explanation. The relation to glycemic control is not so clear. Thus, we have to await for the studies clarifying the mechanism of mesangial expansion, before further therapeutic manoeuvres can be proposed. Also, important new achievements [49] have been made within the field of biochemical changes regarding molecular constituents in glomeruli, but so far treatment on the basis of these ideas is hardly possible.

Another related pathogenetic mechanism that has attracted much attention in recent years is the possible loss of negative charges in the glomerular filter. Although loss of an ionic barrier for plasma proteins is not clearly established, this is certainly an interesting hypothesis [50]. There may be genetic polymorphism and the anionic loss may be related to low N-deacetylase activity in glomeruli and subsequent low density of heparan sulphate units and thereafter development of albuminuria and loss of renal function. Thus far, this hypotheses has not been confirmed, and there are no possibilities of intervention.

The disease process seems clearly related to glomerular hypertension [51], and as discussed in this chapter there are many ways of reducing hyperfiltration. However, we still lack knowledge of the clear mechanisms behind the elevated GFR and renal hypertrophy in diabetes, and intervention modalities must therefore rely largely on symptomatic treatment. Another interesting treatment modality also related to poor metabolic control is inhibition of non-enzymatic glycosylation, which is discussed in chapter 12.

As discussed in the present chapter, inhibition of glucagon and growth hormone hypersecretion may be an interesting avenue for intervention. Short-term studies show a reduction in hyperfiltration, but long-term studies are clearly needed in patients not only with hyperfiltration, but also with microalbuminuria. New stimulatory data have revealed that increased plasma prorenin [52] and increased sodium lithium counter-transport activity [53], seem to be associated with increased risk of nephropathy. Further clarification of the pathogenetic mechanisms involved may well result in new treatment proposals. Importantly, microalbuminuria continues to be a key parameter [54].

Finally, a key question regarding the management of early diabetic renal disease remains to be clarified, but studies are in progress to solve this issue. When should antihypertensive treatment, e. g. ACE-inhibitors, be given to patients with persistent microalbuminuria? There is good evidence to suggest that microalbuminuria by such treatment is reduced, irrespective of blood pressure level, but it is not yet clearly settled whether treatment will prevent development of overt diabetic nephropathy. Additional treatment programs (at which blood-pressure level?) also remain to be worked out, e. g. if ACE-inhibitors are not effective (mainly in reducing microalbuminuria but also BP), should diuretics and β-blockers be added or should a low sodium diet be proposed? Some preliminary evidence suggests that such treatment programs could be worthwhile. Until final results are available we have adapted the policy to start antihypertensive treatment in microalbuminuric diabetics without BP-elevation only if microalbuminuria is convincingly increasing. Usually such patients show rises in blood pressure with time, if left untreated. New studies show that microalbuminuria also can be reduced by an ACE-inhibitor in diabetic children with this abnormality [55].

References

[1] Editorial. Rocher L. Diabetic Nephropathy. The Internist's Role. Arch Intern Med 1990; 150: 26–28.

[2] Reddi AS, Camerini-Davalos RA. Diabetic Nephropathy. An Update. Arch Inter Med 1990; 150: 31–43.

[3] Mogensen CE. Natural history of renal functional abnormalities in human diabetes mellitus, from normoalbuminuria to incipient and overt nephropathy. In: Brenner BM, Stein JH, eds. The Kidney in Diabetes Mellitus. New York, Edinburgh, London, Melbourne: Churchill Livingstone, 1989; 19–49.

[4] Mogensen CE. Prediction of clinical diabetic nephropathy in IDDM patients: are there alternatives to microalbuminuria? Diabetes 1990; 39: 761–767.

[5] Seaquist ER, Goetz FC, Rich S et al. Familial clustering of diabetic kidney disease. N Engl J Med 1989; 320: 1161–1165.

[6] Viberti GC, Keen H, Wiseman MJ. Raised arterial presure in parents of proteinuric insulin dependent diabetics. Br Med J 1987; 295: 515–517.

[7] Krolewski AS, Canessa M, Warram JH et al. Predisposition to hypertension and susceptibility to renal disease in insulin-dependent diabetes mellitus. N Engl J Med 1988; 318: 140–145.

[8] Mangili R, Bending JJ, Scott G et al. Increased sodium-lithium countertransport activity in red cells of patients with insulin-dependent diabetes and nephropathy. N Engl J Med 1988; 31: 146–150.
[9] Nørgaard K, Jensen JS, Mathiesen ER et al. Increased blood pressure and red cell sodium/lithium countertransport activity are not inherited in diabetic nephropathy. Diabetes 1989; 38 (suppl.) 2: 15 A.
[10] Pedersen MM, Winther E, Mogensen CE. Reducing the protein in the diabetic diet. Diabete Metab (Paris) 1990 (in press).
[11] Walker JD, Dodds RA, Murrells TJ et al. Restriction of dietary protein and progression of renal failure in diabetic nephropathy. Lancet 1989; II: 1411–1415.
[12] Christensen CK, Christiansen JS, Schmitz A et al. Effect of continuous subcutaneous insulin infusion on kidney function and size in IDDM patients a two years controlled study. J Diabetic Compl 1987; 1: 91–95.
[13] Mogensen CE, Christensen CK, Christiansen JS et al. Early hyperfiltration and late renal damage in insulin-dependent diabetes. Proceedings of an International Workshop of Diabetic Angiopathy in Children, Berlin, September 25–26, 1986. In: Weber B, ed. Early Vascular Complications in Children with Diabetes Mellitus. Basel: Karger, Pediat Adolesc Endocr 1988; vol 7: 197–205.
[14] Mogensen CE. Management of diabetic renal involvement and disease. Lancet 1988; I: 867–870.
[15] Pedersen MM, Mogensen CE Jørgensen FS et al. Renal effects from limitation of high dietary protein in normoalbuminuric insulin-dependent diabetic patients. Kidney Int suppl. 1989; 27: S 115–S 121.
[16] Dahl-Jørgensen K, Hanssen KF, Kierulf P et al. Reduction of urinary albumin excretion after 4 years of continuous subcutaneous insulin infusion in insulin-dependent diabetes mellitus. Acta Endocrinol (Copenh) 1988; 117: 19–25.
[17] Mathiesen ER, Rønn B, Jensen T et al. Relationship between blood pressure and urinary albumin excretion in development of microalbuminuria. Diabetes 1990; 39: 245–249.
[18] Feldt-Rasmussen B, Mathiesen E, Deckert T. Effect of two years of strict metabolic control on the progression of incipient nephropathy in insulin-dependent diabetes. Lancet 1986; II: 1300–1304.
[19] Mogensen CE. Microalbuminuria and diabetic renal disease. In: Mogensen CE, Standl E, eds. Prevention and Treatment of Diabetic Late Complications. Berlin, New York: de Gruyter, 1989; 41–77.
[20] Feldt-Rasmussen B. Association of poor metabolic control for five to eight years and progression of diabetic renal disease. Diabetologia 1989; 32: 486 A.
[21] Drury PL, Watkins PJ, Viberti GC et al. Diabetic nephropathy. Br Med Bull 1989; 45: 127–147.
[22] Nyberg G, Blohmé G, Nordén G. Impact of metabolic control on progression of clinical diabetic nephropathy. Diabetologia 1987; 30: 82–86.
[23] Cohen DL, Dodds R, Viberti GC. Effect of protein restriction in insulin dependent diabetics at risk of nephropathy. Br Med J 1987; 294: 795–798.
[24] Ihle BU, Becker GJ, Whitworth JA et al. The effect of protein restriction on the progression of renal insufficiency. N Engl J Med 1989; 321: 1773–1777.
[25] Pedersen MM, Schmitz A, Pedersen EB et al. Acute and long-term renal effects of angiotensin converting enzyme-inhibition in normotensive, normoalbuminuric insulin-dependent diabetic patients. Diabetic Med 1988; 5: 562–569.
[26] Drummond K, Levy-Marchal C, Laborde K et al. Enalapril does not alter renal function in normotensive, normoalbuminuric, hyperfiltering Type 1 (insulin-dependent) diabetic children. Diabetologia 1989; 32: 255–260.
[27] Keane WF, Anderson S, Aurell M et al. Angiotensin converting enzyme inhibitors and progressive renal insufficiency. Current experience and future directions. Ann Intern Med 1989; 111: 503–516.

[28] Marre M, Chatellier G, Leblanc H et al. Prevention of diabetic nephropathy with enalapril in normotensive diabetics with microalbuminuria. Br Med J 1988; 297: 1092–1095.
[29] Christensen CK, Mogensen CE. Antihypertensive treatment: long-term reversal of progression of albuminuria in incipient diabetic nephropathy. A longitudinal study of renal function. J Diabetic Compl 1987; 1: 45–52.
[30] Mathiesen ER, Hommel E, Giese J et al. Captopril postpones and may even prevent development of diabetic nephropathy. European Diabetic Nephropathy Study Group, May 1990.
[31] Rudbergs, Aperia A, Freyschuss et al. Enalapril reduces microalbuminuria in young normotensive Type 1 (insulin-dependent) diabetic patients irrespective of its hypotensive effect. Diabetologia 1990; 33: 470–476.
[32] Christensen CK, Pedersen MM, Mogensen CE. Combining antihypertensive agents in early diabetic nephropathy. J Diabetic Compl 1990; 4: 88–90.
[33] Mogensen CE, Pedersen MM, Christiansen JS et al. Potential renal protective effect of ACE inhibitors in early and overt diabetic nephropathy as compared with other antihypertensive agents. In: Dollery CT, Sherwood LM, eds. Cardiac and Renal Failure: An Expanding Role for ACE Inhibitors. Philadelphia: Hanley & Belfus, Inc., 1989; 287–331.
[34] Mogensen CE. Renal function changes in diabetes. Diabetes 1976; 25: 872–879.
[35] Mogensen CE. Progression of nephropathy in long-term diabetics with proteinuria and effect of initial anti-hypertensive treatment. Scand J Clin Lab Invest 1976; 36: 383–388.
[36] Mogensen CE. Long-term antihypertensive treatment inhibiting progression of diabetic nephropathy. Br Med J 1982; 285: 685–689.
[37] Parving H-H, Andersen AR, Smidt UM et al. Effect of antihypertensive treatment on kidney function in diabetic nephropathy. Br Med J 1987; 294: 1443–1447.
[38] Hommel E, Parving H-H, Mathiesen E et al. Effect of captopril on kidney function in insulin-dependent diabetic patients with nephropathy. Br Med J 1986; 293: 467–470.
[39] Parving H-H, Hommel E, Smidt UM. Protection of kidney function and decrease in albuminuria by captopril in insulin dependent diabetics with nephropathy. Br Med J 1988; 297: 1086–1091.
[40] Parving H-H, Hommel E, Nielsen MD et al. Effect of captopril on blood pressure and kidney function in normotensive insulin dependent diabetics with nephropathy. Br Med J 1989; 299: 533–536.
[41] Björck S, Nyberg G, Mulec H et al. Beneficial effects of angiotensin converting enzyme inhibition on renal function in patients with diabetic nephropathy. Br Med J 1986; 293: 471–474.
[42] Pedersen MM, Christensen SE, Christiansen JS et al. Acute effects of the somatostatin analogue SMS 201–995 on kidney function in insulin-dependent diabetic patients. Diabetic Med 1990; 7: 304–309.
[43] Pedersen MM. Renal effects of an aldose reductase inhibitor (statil) during 6 months treatment in Type 1 (insulin-dependent) diabetic patients. Diabetologia 1989; 32: 516 A.
[44] Mogensen CE, Hansen W, Sommer S et al. Microalbuminuria: Studies in diabetes, essential hypertension, and renal diseases as compared to the background population. In: Grünfeld JP, ed. Actualités Néphrologiques de l'Hôpital Necker. Paris: Flammarion, 1990; 213–247.
[45] Mathiesen ER, Borch-Johnsen K, Jensen DV et al. Improved survival in patients with diabetic nephropathy. Diabetologia 1989; 32: 884–886.
[46] Hasslacher C, Borgholte G, Ritz E et al. Impact of hypertension on prognosis of IDDM. Diabete Metab 1989; 15: 338–342.
[47] Parving H-H, Hommel E. Prognosis in diabetic nephropathy. Br Med J 1989; 299: 230–233.
[48] The DCCT Research Group. Are continuing studies of metabolic control and microvascular complications in insulin-dependent diabetes justified? N Engl J Med 1988; 318: 246–250.

[49] Spiro RG. Pathogenesis of diabetic glomerulopathy: a biochemical view. In: Mogensen CE, ed. The Kidney and Hypertension in Diabetes Mellitus. Boston: Martinus Nijhoff Publishing, 1988; 117–130.
[50] Deckert T, Feldt-Rasmussen B, Borch-Johnsen K et al. Albuminuria reflects widespread vascular damage. The Steno hypothesis. Diabetologia 1989; 32: 219–226.
[51] Anderson S. Pathogenesis of diabetic glomerulopathy: hemodynamic factors. In: Brenner BM, Stein JH, eds. The Kidney in Diabetes Mellitus. Churchil Livingstone Inc., 1989; 67–85.
[52] Luetscher JA, Kraemer FB. Microalbuminuria and increased plasma prerenin. Prevalence in diabetics followed up for four years. Arch Intern Med 1988; 148: 937–941.
[53] Carr S, Mbanya J-C, Thomas T et al. Increase in glomerular filtration rate in patients with insulin-dependent diabetes and elevated erythrocyte sodium-lithium countertransport. N Engl J Med 1990; 322: 500–505.
[54] Townsend JC. Increased albumin excretion in diabetes (review). J Clin Path 1990; 43: 3–8.
[55] Cook J, Daneman D, Spino M et al. Angiotensin converting enzyme inhibitor therapy to decrease microalbuminuria in normotensive children with insulin-dependent diabetes mellitus. J Pediatr 1990; 117: 39–45.

Pharmacology of eye care in diabetes

P. M. Sullivan, E. M. Kohner

Introduction

The management of diabetic eye disease was revolutionised by the advent of photocoagulation in the early 1970s. As a result pituitary ablation, hitherto the only effective treatment, became obsolescent. Many drugs have been advocated for the treatment of retinopathy, especially in its early stages, but none have been shown to have a major clinical effect comparable to that of photocoagulation or pituitary ablation. The current role of drugs in the diabetic eye clinic is therefore confined to the assessment of diabetic eye disease, the palliative treatment of thrombotic glaucoma, and the treatment of coincidental eye disease such as chronic open angle glaucoma. After a brief discussion of the pharmacology of mydriatic agents (ie drugs used to dilate the pupil) the prospects for effective pharmacological treatment of diabetic retinopathy will be considered. Some of the agents discussed have chapters of this book devoted to them and the reader is referred to these for details of their general pharmacology.

Drugs in the assessment of diabetic retinopathy

Mydriasis is essential for the assessment and treatment of diabetic retinopathy. In diabetics it is best accomplished by putting one drop each of a muscarinic antagonist (such as 0.5% tropicamide) and an α_1 adrenergic receptor agonist (such as 10% phenylephrine) in the lower lid fornix while the patient looks upwards. Most patients' pupils will be dilated after 30 minutes and will remain so for one to two hours. Cyclopentolate, which produces muscarinic blockade lasting approximately 24 hours, is an alternative to tropicamide. The synergistic effect of a muscarinic antagonist (to block cholinergic receptors on the constrictor pupillae) and an α_1 agonist (to stimulate adrenergic receptors on the dilator pupillae) is particularly important. Diabetics do not dilate well with tropicamide alone and may have denervation hypersensitivity to phenylephrine secondary to pupillary autonomic neuropathy [1]. Side effects of mydriasis include blurred vision (patients should be warned not to drive with dilated pupils) and angle closure glaucoma. The latter is an exceedingly rare complication of dilating drops : in twenty years experience in a busy retinopathy clinic we have only seen it once. The possibility should not deter physicians from examining the fundus properly. As, however, it is a cause of general concern it will be dealt with in some detail.

Angle closure occurs in eyes with shallow anterior chambers – ie. the edge of the iris is close to the edge of the cornea. A shallow anterior chamber is best detected on a slit lamp, but may be inferred with a pen torch. If a pen torch is shone obliquely across the pupil in an eye with a shallow anterior chamber the central iris casts a shadow over the peripheral iris. There may be a family history of acute glaucoma. Dilatation of the pupil in such eyes allows the peripheral iris to come in contact with adjacent cornea (angle closure) and the drainage route of aqueous is blocked. The resulting increase in intraocular pressure leads to a painful red eye with profoundly reduced vision. Eyes at high risk of angle closure may be dilated with phenylephrine alone (as its action can be reversed by thymoximine 0.5%) and the two eyes examined on separate occasions [2]. Chronic open angle glaucoma, in which patients have no history of sudden painful visual loss, is not associated with angle closure and does not contraindicate routine mydriasis Systemic absorption of phenylephrine from the nasolacrimal duct may lead to cardiac tachyarrythmias, hypertension and reflex bradycardia. 2.5% phenylephrine is recommended rather than the 10% solution in the elderly and it is contraindicated in patients on tricyclic antidepressants or monoamine oxidase inhibitors.

Patients often ask for, and receive, 'reversing drops' after mydriasis to constrict their pupils and restore accommodation. The most commonly used is the muscarinic agonist pilocarpine, given to counter the effect of tropicamide. In a study on the effectiveness of pilocarpine compared to saline eye drops after mydriasis, pilocarpine was found to confer no benefit on a number of parameters including pupil size and amplitude of accomodation [3].

Drugs in the treatment of background diabetic retinopathy

Although diabetes affects every part of the eyc, most therapeutic interest is directed towards the retina. New vessels don't always disappear after photocoagulation and conditions such as ischaemic maculopathy are particularly unresponsive so that diabetic retinopathy is still an important cause of visual loss and blindness. Drug therapy offers the prospect of earlier and possibly more effective intervention, and the visibility of the retinal vessels affords a unique opportunity to study the effects of drugs in microangiopathy.

Table 1 Drugs used or proposed for the treatment of diabetic retinopathy

Class of drug	Examples
A. Treatment of background retinopathy	
NSAIDS and antiplatelet agents	Aspirin, dipyridamole glicazide, sulindac ticlopidine
Rheological agents	Calcium dobesilate, dextran Sulphate, diethylamine chromocarb, buflomedil
Aldose reductase inhibitors	Ponalrestat, Sorbinil
Free radical scavengers	Vitamin C and E
Lipid lowering agents	Clofibrate HMG CoA inhibitors
Antihypertensives	Captopril
Improved glycaemic control	CSII, MII, intraperitoneal insulin
Miscellaneous	Mecobalamin, Divascan Sodium etidronate Trapidil, Naftidurofyl Various androsterones
B. Treatment of proliferative retinopathy	
Growth hormone antagonism	Somatostatin and analogues
Promotion of collateralisation	Metformin

It is generally accepted that retinal capillary closure, which occurs even in early retinopathy is a critical change leading to sight threatening events such as neovascularisation and macular ischaemia [4]. The pathogenesis of capillary closure is not known, but a number of mechanisms have been proposed and the drugs which have been used to treat retinopathy may be classified according to the putative mechanism with which they interfere (see Table 1). Some drugs may act against two of the mechanisms, for example many aldose reductase inhibitors are also potent free radical scavengers.

The drugs in Table 1 have been claimed to have a therapeutic effect on the basis of published clinical trials, many of which have been unsatisfactory for a number of reasons. Many trials have studied small numbers of patients over relatively short periods of time. Given the natural history of early diabetic retinopathy, where changes occur over a period of years, such experiments are at best pilot studies. Many studies have only used functional assessment of the retina, rather than assessing morphological severity of retinopathy. In some cases there is no control group, poor 'masking' of patients and assessors, poor or no randomisation between the treatment and control groups, or the assessment of retinopathy severity has not been precise enough.

In designing or interpreting the relevance of a clinical trial of the effect of a drug in diabetic retinopathy, in addition to the generally accepted guidelines for good clinical trial design, a number of additional points have to be considered. Firstly, at what stage of retinopathy has treatment been started? Trials of very early intervention (eg before retinopathy develops) may make it more feasible to alter the course of the disease, but since progression is very slow and variable at this stage the trial should last longer. The methods used to assess retinopathy also have to be considered (Table 2). Morphological assessment of the severity of diabetic retinopathy may be based on grading of retinal photographs and fluorescein angiograms. Ophthalmoscopic examination does not allow sufficiently sensitive assessment of retinopathy severity. The Wisconsin '191' system is the gold standard of retinal photograph assessment and consists of scoring severity of a number of retinal lesions against standard photographs in 7 standard areas of the retina. An overall retinopathy severity score is then assigned to each eye which is prognostic of the probability of progression to more severe retinopathy [5]. Fluorescein angiograms, in which fluorescein is used as an intravascular contrast agent to show microvascular detail, may be quantitatively analysed. Microaneurysm counting is reproducible [6] and correlates well with severity of retinopathy [7]. Recent work has shown that microaneurysm counts are of prognostic significance [8]. Assessment of area of retinal non perfusion is also reproducible and has prognostic significance but requires consistently high quality angiograms.

A number of functional tests have been used during drug trials in diabetic retinopathy. The most commonly used, vitreous fluorophotometry is a reproducible technique to assess the integrity of the blood retinal barrier. Abnormal

Table 2 Methods of assessing diabetic retinopathy in clinical trials

A. Morphological severity of retinopathy	
1. Ophthalmoscopy	(subjective and unreliable)
2. Grading retinal photographs	(Hammersmith or Wisconsin)
3. Fluorescein angiography	– microaneurysm turnover
	– non perfused area
B. Functional assessment	
1. Visual function	– visual acuity
	– contrast sensitivity
2. Vitreous fluorophotometry	
3. Electroretinography	

fluorescein penetration of the blood retinal barrier reflects the severity of retinopathy, especially in the macular area [9]. A number of drugs seem to have a beneficial effect in diabetic retinopathy using this technique but, unless a beneficial effect on retinal morphology is also demonstrated, such drugs should not be used to treat retinopathy. This technique has the advantage of being easily combined with fluorescein angiography.

Whichever method of assessment is used, studies in which some form of external assessment is employed, such as the use of a fundus photograph reading centre, are likely to enjoy more credibility than those where all the analysis is carried out by the investigators.

Anti platelet drugs

In 1964 it was reported that diabetics with rheumatoid arthritis on long term salicylates had a lower than expected incidence of retinopathy [10]. Subsequently platelets from diabetic patients with retinopathy were shown to have enhanced aggregability in vitro [11,12] although shortened platelet survival in vivo has not been confirmed [13] and the pathogenic significance of these changes is therefore unclear. So intense was the interest aroused by this work that two large well conducted studies were set up to see whether aspirin had a therapeutic role in diabetic retinopathy. Viewed in the light of current knowledge on the pharmacology of thromboxane synthetase inhibition, both of these studies used relatively large doses of aspirin.

The Early Treatment of Diabetic Retinopathy Study was a large scale prospective study of the effect of photocoagulation and aspirin in diabetic retinopathy. Three thousand seven hundred and eleven patients with moderately severe background retinopathy were studied [14]. Patients were randomised to either aspirin 650 mg/day or placebo. Retinopathy was assessed by grading retinal photographs. There was no significant difference between the groups in the development of high risk characteristics after up to 7 years of follow up (Frederick Ferris, personal communication). The results for the subgroups with milder retinopathy have not been reported.

The DAMAD study [15] was a masked multicentre, binational study lasting 3 years. 475 patients entered the study, of whom 420 had 3 sets of gradeable fluorescein angiograms at the end of the study. Patients with mild retinopathy were stratified into type I and type II and separately randomised to 3 groups : aspirin and persantin (1g aspirin/day and 225 mg persantin/day), aspirin alone (1g/day) or placebo. Progression of retinopathy was assessed from microaneurysm counts on fluorescein angiograms. There was a statistically significant but very small (approximately one microaneurysm per year) reduction in the rate of yearly increase in the number of microaneurysms in the two treatment groups, which were not significantly different from each other, compared to the control group. Interestingly progression of microaneurysm count was related to ophthalmoscopically assessed retinopathy deterioration, showing that this technique reflected the overall severity of retinopathy.

The fact that two such carefully planned studies gave an apparently contradictory result illustrates some of the problems of drug trials in retinopathy. Overall, patients in the ETDRS had more severe retinopathy at baseline and were therefore less likely to respond to treatment. The difference in quantification of retinopathy may also be important : microaneurysm counting is a sensitive technique which might be expected to detect subtle changes that would not be detected by colour photographic grading.

A number of other drugs have been used as antiplatelet agents in diabetic retinopathy. The TIMAD study group found that ticlopidine slowed down the mean yearly increase in microaneurysm count, but the effect was small [16], similar to that found in the DAMAD study.

The sulphonylurea gliclazide has been reported to reduce platelet microthrombi in experimental animals and to be an effective antiretinopathy drug [17] but no well designed clinical trials have been published to support its clinical usefulness. A large prospective study suggested a beneficial effect in diabetic patients with and without retinopathy [18]. Only 37% of patients completed 39 months treatment and the gliclazide group had a higher proportion of non insulin dependant diabetics than the control group. A recent review of the pharmacology of gliclazide [19] concluded that further evidence was required to confirm a sustained clinical benefit unique to gliclazide.

Rheological therapy

Increased whole blood viscosity due to decreased red cell deformability has been described in diabetics, especially in those with retinopathy [20, 21]. Increased viscosity may also result from dehydration and haemoconcentration during ketoacidosis. The most widely advocated rheological agent in diabetic retinopathy is calcium dobesilate which increases red cell deformability and reduces whole blood viscosity [22]. Although the drug has been claimed to have a useful anti retinopathy effect a number of prospective clinical trials have not confirmed this [23, 24].

Aldose reductase inhibitors

The similarity between human diabetic retinopathy and galactosaemic retinopathy in dogs [25], in which aldose reductase has been implicated [26], gave impetus to the study of aldose reductase inhibitors (ARI) in retinopathy. Aldose reductase is found in retinal pericytes [27], where its activation by high intracellular glucose concentration could account for the early pericyte loss [28] seen in diabetic retinopathy. Since pericyte loss precedes clinically apparent diabetic retinopathy aldose reductase inhibition is most likely to be effective if given early in the course of, or before the onset of, diabetic retinopathy. The long term effects of ARI in preventing diabetic – like retinopathy in galactosaemic dogs has been investigated by a group at the NIH [29] and in Wisconsin [30]. Kador's group found that ARI inhibited pericyte ghost and microaneurysm formation for up to 36 months of galactose feeding. Engerman however has found that sorbinil treated dogs had similar retinopathy at 42 months to galactosaemic dogs on placebo. Methodological differences between the two groups make direct comparison difficult but it seems that aldose reductase inhibition delays but does not prevent galactosaemic retinopathy.

Sorbinil has been found by Cunha Vaz to slow progression of abnormal blood retinal barrier permeability in human diabetics with no or minimal retinopathy [31], though the study was a short one (six months) and no statistically significant effect on retinal morphology was reported. Sorbinil was also assessed in a large as yet unreported multicentre study in the USA. A large masked placebo controlled multicentre study in England on the effect of Ponalrestat studied 98 patients with mild background retinopathy (5–75 microaneurysms in a 20° field around the fovea). The retinal assessment included seven field colour photography of both eyes with Wisconsin grading, fluorescein angiography with semi automated microaneurysm counting and vitreous fluorophotometry. The treatment and control groups were similar at baseline. There was no significant difference between the treatment and placebo groups after two years [32], although this may merely indicate the need for a trial of earlier intervention. Furthermore, Ponalrestat in the doses used probably did not have reach therapeutic concentrations in the retinal pericytes.

Antihypertensive agents

The role of hypertension in the pathogenesis of diabetic retinopathy has not been fully established. It is a risk factor for the prevalence of diabetic retinopathy in some studies [33] and may also increase the incidence of retinopathy [34]. A small uncontrolled prospective study suggested that initiation of antihypertensive treatment stabilises the blood retinal barrier in hypertensive diabetics [35]. Angiotensin converting enzyme (ACE) inhibitors were used in every patient except one, raising the question of whether the improvement in blood retinal barrier permeability is attributable to a specific effect of ACE inhibition or to the drop in blood pressure. It has been suggested that ACE inhibitors have a unique beneficial effect in diabetic nephropathy not shared by other antihypertensives as they lower intraglomerular pressure by dilating the efferent arterioles. In the retina the existence of such an effect is at present purely speculative and it is equally possible that precapillary sphincter dilatation could subject the retinal capillaries to potentially damaging high intravascular pressures. A number of clinical trials are now under way to clarify the effect of antihypertensive treatment and ACE inhibition on retinal blood flow, blood retinal barrier permeability and progression of retinopathy.

Effect of improved glycaemic control

The Job study [36] instituted microaneurysm turnover as a measure of retinopathy deterioration and was a landmark in the therapy of retinopathy. This study showed that patients on more physiological regimes using multiple insulin injections had slower progression of microaneurysm counts (an increase of 5 per year) than a control group (which increased by 12 per year). These figures were used in the design of subsequent clinical trials which interestingly showed much slower rates of progression (1.5 per year) in the control groups. This striking reduction in the rate of progression of retinopathy is probably due to generally improved glycaemic control, especially in IDD patients. This is partially attributable to the development of the new techniques for insulin administration.

The first large scale prospective study on therapy of NIDD patients and retinopathy was the University Group Diabetes Program (UGDP). This study found no difference in the incidence of retinopathy between groups treated with diet only, insulin and oral agents [37]. The study was unsatisfactory in a number of ways : the initial difference in control between treatment groups was not sustained for the duration of the study and retinopathy was assessed using only a single colour photograph of the macular area. Maneschi et al [38] studied NIDD patients with no retinopathy at diagnosis and found that the patients who progressed to retinopathy over 5–10 years of follow up had significantly higher blood glucose throughout and a higher HbA1 at their last assessment. Nathan found high HbA1 to be an independent risk factor for retinopathy in a cross sectional study of NIDD [39]. In this study retinopathy was more common in patients treated with insulin but this was probably a spurious relationship as the two were not independently related. In Teuschers 8 year prospective study however both high initial blood glucose and insulin usage were independent risk factors for the development of retinopathy [40]. This does not necessarily indicate a causal relationship between insulin usage and development of retinopathy: it may reflect a tendency for patients to be started on insulin when retinopathy is diagnosed or for older patients to be managed by their general practitioners (primary care physicians) using oral agents. The United Kingdom Prospective Diabetes Study, in which 5000 NIDD patients are randomly allocated to different forms of therapy and have careful photographic retinopathy assessment over several years of follow up, is currently in progress and should clarify how these patients should be controlled.

What is the situation in IDD patients? These patients are all on insulin, does control matter in this group? It is in this group that the advances in treatment and monitoring of control have made the biggest difference. In the Wisconsin epidemiological study prevalence of both ‘any retinopathy’ and proliferative retinopathy were related to the blood glucose control [41]. Glycaemic control at baseline had a predictive value for the subsequent development of retinopathy [42], as was the case in Teuschers study [40] and uncontrolled studies have demonstrated the value of good control for many years [43, 44, 45]. It was therefore disappointing and surprising when 3 randomised controlled clinical trials showed an initial deterioration in retinopathy when control was improved using continuous subcutaneous insulin (CSII) [46, 47, 48]. The features that deteriorated most were microaneurysms, haemorrhages, cotton wool spots, and intraretinal microvascular abnormalities. The Oslo group [48] suggested that the transient deterioration was a consequence of a rapid improvement in control leading to reduced blood flow through the already damaged retinal vessels and retinal ischaemia. In the long term however the results suggested that the CSII group deteriorated less than the controls [49], though this trend was not statistically significant. Riechard studied the effect of improved control over 18 months using multiple injections [50] and found that nearly twice as many control patients deteriorated as those on intensified treatment. Rapid improvement in control may also be responsible for the frequently seen deterioration of retinopathy during pregnancy, especially in unplanned pregnancies with poor control at presentation [51]. The Diabetes Control and Complications Study, which is following some 1400 patients prospectively, will determine the effect of good control and possibly also the degree of control which one should aim at. In this study both CSII and multiple injections are used to achieve tight control.

Further improvements in the management of retinopathy may well come with the advent of the new 'designer' insulins discussed in chapter 5. These new preparations should allow us to achieve a level of glucose control which will prevent complications while avoiding hypoglycaemia.

Lipid lowering agents

Hypercholesterolaemia is associated with the presence of retinal exudates [52] and the development of severe diabetic retinopathy [53]. A well designed one year study in 56 patients showed that clofibrate could reduce the area of retinal exudates but did not benefit visual loss due to diabetic maculopathy [54]. A new generation of antihyperlipidaemic drugs, the HMG-CoA inhibitors, are effective in lowering LDL cholesterol in diabetics but have yet to be assessed in diabetic retinopathy.

Inhibition of non enzymatic glycosylation

Non enzymatic glycosylation may be important in the pathogenesis of diabetic retinopathy. There have been no reports of the effect of aminoguanidine, which inhibits the formation of advanced glycosylation end products, on retinopathy. Bendazac lysine seemed to have a beneficial effect on the blood retinal barrier in a small uncontrolled pilot study [55], although the mechanism was not apparent at the time. It now appears that Bendazac may inhibit non enzymatic glycation of protein in vivo [56] and further studies are in progress on this drug.

Drug treatment of proliferative diabetic retinopathy

The observation that proliferative diabetic retinopathy improved after hypophysectomy [57], especially with complete suppression of growth hormone secretion [58], lead to the suggestion that growth hormone might play a role in new vessel formation. The action of growth hormone is known to be mediated by somatomedins such as IGF-1. Infusion of somatostatin or octreotide (a long acting somatostatin analogue) suppresses growth hormone and IGF-1 secretion in normal subjects and has been claimed to improve the visual acuity in preproliferative retinopathy. More recently it has been shown however that neither octreotide infusion nor oral agents completely suppress

24 hour growth hormone secretion in diabetics [59, 60] and the rationale of clinical usefulness of these agents seems doubtful.

Metformin has been shown to prevent neovascularisation following experimental branch vein occlusion in the minipig by inducing collateralisation and reducing retinal ischaemia [61]. This interesting observation warrants further investigation with clinical trials in patients with preproliferative retinopathy, since these patients have widespread retinal ischaemia but photocoagulation can ethically be withheld until the appearance of new vessels.

Drug treatment of other diabetic ocular complications

Cataract

Cataract is a common cause of visual impairment in diabetics. It can be effectively treated surgically, but there is still some interest in the possibility of drug therapy, especially if it can be administered topically. Juvenile cataract is an uncommon acute complication of poor control. It may be a true 'sugar cataract' – that is, it may form because of the osmotic effects of sorbitol accumulation in the lens. It is reversible, in its early stages at any rate, by improved glycaemic control.

The cause of adult diabetic cataract is unknown, although oxidative stress, non enzymatic glycosylation and conjugation with urea breakdown products (in diabetics with renal failure) have all been implicated [62]. A number of drugs are currently being clinically evaluated. These include aldose reductase inhibitors, which may be acting as free radical scavengers, and Bendazac Lysine.

Keratopathy

Several corneal epithelial abnormalities have been reported in diabetes, including a tendency to develop spontaneous corneal erosions and delayed corneal reepithelialisation after eye trauma and surgery. Experimental work in galactosaemic rats has suggested that sorbitol accumulation may be responsible and there is a case report in which persistent diabetic keratopathy responded to sorbinil eye drops [63].

Thrombotic glaucoma

Rubeosis iridis (new vessels on the iris) may lead to fibrous adhesion of the peripheral iris to the cornea immediately in front of it, blocking the path of aqueous drainage through the iridocorneal angle so that glaucoma develops. This condition requires vigorous treatment which may include panretinal photocoagulation, retinal cryoablation and passage of a drainage tube into the anterior chamber. Medical management is largely palliative as conventional glaucoma therapy is relatively ineffective in this situation. Topical cycloplegics (eg atropine 1% once daily) reduce painful ciliary spasm and topical steroids (eg 0.1% dexamethasone four hourly) reduce any associated inflammation [64].

References

[1] Huber MJE, Smith SA, Smith SE. Mydriatic drugs for diabetic patients. British Journal of Ophthalmology 1985; 69: 425–427.

[2] Mapstone R. Dilating dangerous pupils. British Journal of Ophthalmology 1977; 61: 517–524.

[3] Nelson ME, Orton HP. Countering the effects of mydriatics – does it benefit the patient? Archives of Ophthalmology 1987; 105 (4): 486–489.

[4] Kohner EM. Diabetic retinopathy. British Medical Bulletin 1989; 45: 148–173.

[5] Klein BEK, Davis MD, Segal P et al. Diabetic retinopathy: assessment of severity and progression. Ophthalmology 1984; 91: 10–17.

[6] Baudoin C, Maneschi F, Quentel G et al. Quantitative evaluation of fluorescein angiograms: microaneurysm counts. Diabetes 1983; 32: 8–13.

[7] Kohner EM, Sleightholm MA. Does microaneurysm count reflect the severity of diabetic retinopathy? Ophthalmology 1986; 93: 586–590.

[8] Klein R, Meuer S, Moss SE et al. The relationship of retinal microaneurysm counts to the 4 year progression of diabetic retinopathy. Archives of Ophthalmology 1989; 107: 1780–1785.

[9] Plehwe WE, Sleightholm MA, Kohner EM. Does vitreous fluorophotometry reflect severity of early diabetic retinopathy? British Journal of Ophthalmology 1989; 73: 255–260.

[10] Powell ED, Field RG. Diabetic retinopathy and rheumatoid arthritis. Lancet 1964; 2: 17–18.

[11] Heath H, Brigden WD, Canever JV et al. Platelet adhesiveness and aggregation in relation to diabetic retinopathy. Diabetologia 1971; 7: 308–315.

[12] Bensoussan D, Levy-toledano S, Passa P et al. Platelet hyperaggregation and increased plasma level of Von Willebrand factor in diabetics with retinopathy. Diabetologia 1975; 11: 307–312 .

[13] Porta M, Peters AM, Cousins SA et al. A study of platelet relevant parameters in patients with diabetic microangiopathy. Diabetologia 1983; 25: 21–25.

[14] Rand LI. The early treatment diabetic retinopathy study. In: Friedman EA, L'Esperance FA, eds. Diabetic Renal Retinal Syndrome Volume 2. Brooklyn, New York 1981.

[15] The Damad Study Group. Effect of aspirin and aspirin plus dipyridamole in early diabetic retinopathy. Diabetes 1989; 38: 491–498.

[16] Perlemuter L, Baudoin C, Quentel G ct al. Effect of an antiplatelet agent, ticlopidine, in early diabetic retinopathy. Diabetes Research and Clinical Practice 1988; 5(suppl 1): 69.

[17] Lesobre B. Diabetic retinopathy – effects of gliclazide. In: Rathery M, ed. Journees Annuelles de Diabetologie De L'Hotel- Dieu. Paris: Flammarion Medicine-Sciences, 1983.

[18] Regnault AF. Prognosis of non proliferative diabetic retinopathy during treatment with gliclazide. In: Keen H, ed. Gliclazide and the treatment of diabetes. London: Academic Press Ltd, 1979.

[19] Holmes B, Heel RC, Brogden RN et al. Gliclazide. A preliminary review of its pharmacodynamic properties and therapeutic efficacy in diabetes mellitus. Drugs 1984; 27: 301–327.

[20] Barnes AJ, Locke P, Saidde PR et al. Is hyperviscosity a treatable component of diabetic microvascular disease ? Lancet 1977; 2: 789–791.
[21] McMillan DE, Utterback NG, LaPuma J. Reduced erythrocyte deformability in diabetes. Diabetes 1978; 27: 895–901.
[22] Barras JP, Michal M. Effect of calcium dobesilate on blood viscosity in patients with diabetic microangiopathy. Vasa 1986; 15: 200–205.
[23] Larsen H-W, Sander E, Hoppe R. The value of calcium dobesilate in the treatment of diabetic retinopathy: a controlled clinical trial. Diabetologia 1977; 13: 105–109.
[24] Stamper RL, Smith ME, Aronson SB et al. The effect of calcium dobesilate on nonproliferative diabetic retinopathy: a controlled study. Ophthalmology 1978; 85: 594–606.
[25] Engerman R, Kern TS. Experimental galactosaemia produces a diabetes – like retinopathy. Diabetes 1984; 39: 92–96.
[26] Kador PF, Akagi Y, Teribayashi H. Prevention of pericyte ghost formation in retinal capillaries of galactose fed dogs by aldose reductase inhibitors. Archives of Ophthalmology 1988; 106: 1099–1102.
[27] Akagi Y, Kador PF, Kuwabara T. Aldose reductase localisation in human retinal cells. Investigative Ophthalmology and Visual Science 1983; 24: 1516–1519.
[28] Addison DJ, Garner A, Ashton N. Degeneration of intramural pericytes in diabetic retinopathy. British Medical Journal 1: 264–266.
[29] Kador PF, Akagi Y, Takahasi Y et al. Prevention of retinal vessel changes associated with diabetic retinopathy in galactose-fed dogs by aldose reductase inhibitors. Investigative Ophthalmology and Visual Science 1989 (suppl.); 30: (3) 139.
[30] Engerman RL, Kern TS. Retinal vasculature in sorbinil-treated galactosaemic dogs. Investigative Ophthalmology and Visual Science 1989 (suppl.); 30 (3): 139.
[31] Cunha-Vaz JG, Mota C, Leite E. Effect of sorbinil on the blood-retinal barrier in early diabetic retinopathy. Diabetes 1986; 35: 574–578.
[32] Caldwell G, Brown F, Kohner EM et al. Statil in diabetic retinopathy. In preparation.
[33] Klein R, Klein BE, Moss S et al. The Wisconsin Epidemiologic study of diabetic retinopathy III. Prevalence and risk of diabetic retinopathy when age at diagnosis is over 30 years. Archives of Ophthalmology 1984; 102: 527–532.
[34] Knowler WC, Bennet PU, Ballantine E. Increased incidence of retinopathy in diabetics with elevated blood pressure: a six year follow up study in Pima Indians. New England Journal of Medicine 1980; 302: 645–650.
[35] Parving H-H, Larsen M, Hommel E et al. Effect of antihypertensive treatment on blood retinal barrier permeability to fluorescein in hypertensive Type I (insulin dependant) diabetic patients with background retinopathy. Diabetologia 1989; 32: 440–444.
[36] Job D, Eschwege E, Guyot-Argenton et al. Effect of multiple daily insulin injection on the course of diabetic retinopathy. Diabetes 1976: 463–469.
[37] The University Group Diabetes Program. Effect of hypoglycaemic agents on vascular complications in patients with adult onset diabetes. Diabetes 1982; 31 (suppl. 5): 17–20.
[38] Maneschi F, Cassar J, Lowy C et al. Development of diabetic microangiopathy and diabetic control, a study in non insulin dependent diabetics. Diabète et Metabolisme (Paris) 1981; 7: 181–187.
[39] Nathan DM, Singer DE, Godine JE et al. Retinopathy in older Type II diabetics: association with glucose control. Diabetes 1986; 35: 797–801.
[40] Teuscher A, Schnell H, Wilson PWF. Incidence of diabetic retinopathy and relationship to baseline plasma glucose and blood pressure. Diabetes Care 1988; 11: 246–257.
[41] Klein R, Klein BE, Moss S et al. The Wisconsin Epidemiologic study of diabetic retinopathy II. Prevalence and risk of diabetic retinopathy when age at diagnosis is less than 30 years. Archives of Ophthalmology 1984; 102: 520–526.
[42] Klein R, Klein BE, Moss S et al. Glycosylated haemoglobin predicts the incidence and progression of diabetic retinopathy. Journal of the American Medical Association 1984; 260: 2864–2871.

[43] Miki E, Fukuda M, Kuzuya T et al. Relationship of the course of retinopathy to control of diabetes, age and therapeutic agents in diabetic Japanese patients. Diabetes 1969; 18: 773–780.
[44] Pirart J. Diabète et complications degeneratives; presentation d'une étude prospective portant sur 4400 cas observes entre 1949–1973. Diabète et Metabolisme 1977; 3: 97–107.
[45] Rand LI, Krolewski AS, Aiello LM et al. Multiple factors in the prediction of risk of proliferative retinopathy. New England Journal of Medicine 1985; 313: 1433–1438.
[46] Lauritzen T, Frost-Larsen K, Larsen HW et al. Effect of one year near normal blood glucose levels on retinopathy in insulin dependent diabetes. Lancet 1983; 1: 200–204.
[47] The Kroc Collaborative Study Group. Blood glucose control and the evolution of diabetic retinopathy and albuminuria. New England Journal of Medicine 1984; 311: 665–672.
[48] Dahl-Jorgensen K, Brinchmann Hansen O, Hansen R et al. Rapid tightening of blood glucose control leads to transient deterioration of diabetic retinopathy in IDD, the Oslo study. British Medical Journal 1985; 290: 811–815.
[49] The Kroc Collaborative Study Group. Diabetic retinopathy after two years of intensified insulintreatment. Journal of the American Medical Association 1988; 260: 37–41.
[50] Riechard P, Britz A, Cars I et al. The Stockholm diabetes intervention study 18 month results. Acta Med Scand 1988; 224: 115–122.
[51] Phelps RL, Sakol P, Metzger BE et al. Changes in diabetic retinopathy during pregnancy – correlation with regulation of hyperglycaemia. Archives of Ophthalmology 1986; 104: 1806–1810.
[52] Esmann V, Kundbaek K, Madsen PH. Types of exudates in diabetic retinopathy. Acta Medica Scandanavica 1963; 174: 375–380.
[53] Dornan TL, Carter RD, Bron AJ et al. Low density lipoprotein cholesterol: an association with the severity of diabetic retinopathy. Diabetologia 1982; 27: 167–170.
[54] Harrold BP, Marmion VJ, Gough KRG. A double blind controlled study of clofibrate in the treatment of diabetic retinopathy. Diabetes 1969; 18: 285–291.
[55] Nuzzi G, Venturini I, Bonacini M et al. Improvement of the blood-retinal barrier induced by Lysine: preliminary clinical observation in insulin dependant diabetics. Archives of Ophthalmology 1987; 105: 1165–1166.
[56] Bruno MR, Sensi M, Goccia GP et al. Inhibition of protein non enzymic glycation induced by Bendazac. Diabetes Research 1988; 9: 11–14.
[57] Lundbaek K, Malmros R, Anderson RC. Hypophysectomy for diabetic retinopathy: a controlled trial. In: Goldberg MF, Fine SL, eds. Symposium on the treatment of diabetic retinopathy, Airlie House, Warrington, Virginia. Washington DC: US Government Printing Office, 1969; 291–311.
[58] Wright AD, Kohner EM, Oakley NW et al. Serum growth hormone levels and the response of diabetic retinopathy to pituitary ablation. British Medical Journal 1969; 2: 346–348.
[59] Hyer SL, Sharp PS, Brooks RA et al. Failure to suppress growth hormone secretion after two weeks treatment with atropine or propantheline in diabetics with proliferative retinopathy. Acta Endocrinol Copenhagen 1988; 119: 61–68.
[60] Hyer SL, Sharp PS, Brooks RA et al. Continuous subcutaneous octreotide infusion markedly suppresses IGF-1 levels whilst only partially suppressing GH secretion in diabetics with retinopathy. Acta Endocrinologica 1989; 120: 187–194.
[61] Pournaras CJ, Strommer KN, Tsacopoulos M et al. Experimental branch vein occlusion in miniature pigs: effect of metformin on the evolution of ischaemic microangiopathy. Diabète et Metabolisme 1988; 14 (4): 580–587.
[62] Bron AJ, Cheng H. Cataract and retinopathy: screening for treatable retinopathy. In: PJ Watkins, ed. Clinics in Endocrinology and Metabolism 1986; 15: 971–999.
[63] Cogan DG. Aldose reductase and complications of diabetes. Annals of Internal Medicine 1984; 101: 82–91.
[64] Motolko M, Phelps C. The secondary glaucomas. In: Duane T (ed) Clinical Ophthalmology. PA: Harper and Row, 1983.

Prevention and treatment of neuropathy

D. A. Greene

Introduction

Importance

Diabetic neuropathy, the most frequent symptom-producing chronic complication of diabetes mellitus, causes pain and discomfort, limits exercise tolerance, contributes to limb-amputation and erectile impotence, and probably diminishes life expectancy in diabetic patients [1]. Although its frequency is difficult to deduce from existing data [2], diabetic neuropathy presents a major public health problem without a generally recognized effective treatment [1]. Thus diabetes accounts for at least 50% of all non-traumatic amputations in the United States [3], with neuropathy almost certainly the major contributing factor. In 1978 NIH Diabetes Data Group (NIH Publication 78-1468) cited prevalence figures for clinical or subclinical neuropathy ranging from 10–100%, with the highest estimates including sub-clinical manifestations of neuropathy such as slowing of nerve conduction. The cumulative incidence rate for *symptomatic* distal symmetric polyneuropathy in a population-based cohort of "maturity onset" diabetic patients was 4% after 5 years and 15% after 20 years, with a median time from diagnosis of diabetes to development of neuropathic symptoms of 9 years [2, 4]. Comparable data collected by Pirart [5] indicated an overall cumulative prevalence of symptomatic neuropathy in a referral-based cohort of patients over a 25 year period of 8% in patients with newly-diagnosed diabetes, and over 40% in patients after 20 years of diabetes [5]. These estimates of cumulative incidence are several-fold higher than those for vision-impairing retinopathy or end-stage renal failure, identifying diabetic neuropathy as the most common symptomatic chronic complication of diabetes.

Classification and description

Diabetic neuropathy is divided into two stages or classes: subclinical (class I) and clinical (class II) neuropathy (Table 1) [1]. Subclinical or "asymptomatic"

Table 1 Classification and staging of diabetic neuropathy

---

*Class I: subclinical neuropathy**

A. *Abnormal electrodiagnostic tests* (EDX)
   1. *Decreased nerve conduction velocity*
   2. *Decreased amplitude of evoked muscle or nerve action potential*

B. *Abnormal quantitative sensory testing* (QST)
   1. *Vibratory/Tactile*
   2. *Thermal warming/cooling*
   3. *Other*

C. *Abnormal autonomic function tests* (AFT)
   1. *Diminished Sinus arrythmia (beat-to-beat heart rate variation)*
   2. *Diminished sudomotor function*
   3. *Increased pupillary latency*

Class II: clinical neuropathy

A. *Diffuse neuropathy*
   1. *Distal symmetric sensorimotor polyneuropathy*
      a) Primarily small fiber neuropathy
      b) Primarily large fiber neuropathy
      c) Mixed
   2. *Autonomic neuropathy*
      a) Abnormal pupillary function
      b) Sudomotor dysfunction
      c) Genitourinary autonomic neuropathy
         (1) bladder dysfunction
         (2) sexual dysfunction
      d) Gastrointestinal autonomic neuropathy
         (1) gastric atony
         (2) gall bladder atony
         (3) diabetic diarrhea
         (4) hypoglycemic unawareness (adrenal medullary neuropathy)
      e) Cardiovascular autonomic neuropathy
      f) Hypoglycemic unawareness

B. *Focal neuropathy*
   1. *mononeuropathy*
   2. *Mononeuropathy multiplex*
   3. *plexopathy*
   4. *radiculopathy*
   5. *Cranial neuropathy*

---

* Neurological function tests are abnormal but no neurological symptoms or clinically detectable neurological deficits indicative of a diffuse or focal neuropathy are present. Class I "Subclinical Neuropathy" is further subdivided into Class Ia if an AFT or QST abnormality is present, Class Ib if EDX or AFT and QST abnormalities are present, and Class Ic if an EDX and either AFT or QST abnormalities or both are present.

diabetic neuropathy consists of peripheral nerve dysfunction such as slowed motor and sensory nerve conduction or elevated sensory perception thresholds that occur in the absence of clinical signs and/or symptoms of peripheral neuropathy (Table 1). There is currently no indication to treat sub-clinical neuropathy except that clinical surveillance for the development of signs or symptoms of clinical neuropathy should be intensified. Clinical diabetic neuropathy consists of the appearance of symptoms and/or clinically detectable neurological deficits conforming to one of the recognized syndromes of diabetic neuropathy superimposed on subclinical neuropathy (Table 1). These clinical syndromes have been grouped into the diffuse or focal types of diabetic neuropathy [1]. Although each syndrome has a characteristic presentation and clinical course, they may coexist in the same patient, complicating classification of individual cases [6]. Diffuse clinical diabetic neuropathy encompasses distal symmetric sensorimotor polyneuropathy and autonomic neuropathy. Distal symmetric polyneuropathy, the most commonly recognized form of diabetic neuropathy [2], features sensory deficits and symptoms that overshadow motor involvement [1]. Sensory deficits originate in the most distal portions of the extremities and progress proximally in a "stocking-glove" distribution [7], ultimately forming vertical bands of sensory impairment on the chest as distal portions of truncal nerves become involved [7]. The signs, symptoms and neurological deficits of distal symmetric polyneuropathy vary with the classes of nerve fibers that are involved: loss of large sensory and motor fibers being associated with diminished light touch and proprioception and muscle weakness, and loss of small fibers being associated with diminished pain and temperature perception, paresthesias, dysesthesias and/or neuropathic pain [1]. Diminished or absent deep tendon reflexes, most commonly the Achilles tendon reflex, may be an early indication of otherwise asymptomatic neuropathy. Undetected but more advanced neuropathy devoid of paresthetic or painful symptoms may first present with late complications such as ulceration or neuroarthropathy ("Charcot's joints") of the foot [1]. The other form of diffuse clinical diabetic neuropathy is diabetic autonomic neuropathy, which often but not always accompanies distal symmetric polyneuropathy and can impair virtually any sympathetic or parasympathetic autonomic function [1]. Diabetic cardiovascular autonomic neuropathy initially affects cardiac parasympathetic function diminishing the normal bradycardic responses to sleep and deep inspiration; with progression, sympathetic cardiac and peripheral vascular denervation interferes with normal cardiovascular response to exercise and hypersensitizes the heart to circulating catecholamines predisposing to tachyarrythmias and sudden death [1]. Gastrointestinal autonomic neuropathy, which can involve virtually the entire length of the gastrointestinal tract, underlies many of the otherwise nonspecific gastrointestinal symptoms that afflict the majority of diabetic patients [1]. Esophageal motility impairment and reflux, decreased vagally-mediated gastric acid secretion, and delayed gastric emptying produce anorexia, nausea, vomiting, early satiety and postprandial bloating and fullness [1]. Diabetic enteropathy encompasses the clinical syndromes of diabetic constipation, diabetic diarrhea and fecal incontinence, which all reflect widespread abnormalities in the intrinsic and extrinsic intestinal autonomic nervous system [1]. Diabetic genitourinary autonomic neuropathy includes retrograde ejaculation, neuropathic erectile impotence and diabetic cystopathy, all of which result from loss of coordination of autonomic innervation [1]. Neuropathic importance is generally but not always accompanied by other manifestations of diabetic neuropathy. Hypoglycemic unawareness refers to the diminished epinepherine response to hypoglycemia in chronic diabetes and is generally believed to be the result of autonomic neuropathy of the adrenal medulla, which can blunt the usual adrenergic warning signs of impending hypoglycemia [1]. Diabetic autonomic sudomotor dysfunction produces an asymptomatic distal anhydrosis in a stocking-glove distribution similar to that of distal symmetric polyneuropathy. This diminishes thermoregulatory reserve, predisposes to heatstroke and hyperthermia, and produces a compensatory central hyperhydrosis that is often bothersome to the patient [1].

The focal forms of diabetic neuropathy correspond to the distribution of single or multiple peripheral nerves ("mononeuropathy" and "mononeuropathy multiplex"), cranial nerves, regions of the brachial or lumbosacral plexuses ("plexopathy") or the nerve roots ("radiculopathy") [8]. They are relatively uncommon, of sudden onset, and generally but not always self-limited in diabetic patients, and tend to occur in older age groups [8]. The third cranial nerve is often affected, presenting with unilateral pain, diplopia and ptosis with pupillary sparing in a syndrome termed "diabetic ophthalmoplegia" [8]. Diabetic ophthalmoplegia may occur in the absence of other manifestations of diabetic neuropathy, and may be bilateral and/or recurrent. Radiculopathy presents as band-like thoracic or abdominal pain, that is often misdiagnosed as an acute intrathoracic or intraabdominal emergency [8]. "Femoral neuropathy" in diabetic patients often involves motor and sensory deficits at the level of the sacral plexus as well as the femoral nerve, with the relative excess of motor versus sensory involvement differentiating diabetic "femoral neuropathy" from that seen in other conditions [8]. Other mononeuropathies mimic the compression neuropathies seen in non-diabetic individuals such as carpal tunnel syndrome [2]. In summary, distal symmetric polyneuropathy and autonomic neuropathy are common, diffuse, and generally progressive disorders, while the focal neuropathies are rare, sudden in onset, often self-limited, and occur primarily in older patients with diabetes. Generally accepted therapeutic approaches to these various forms of diabetic neuropathy are generally palliative, syndrome-specific, and involve both pharmacologic and other forms of intervention. General preventative measures such as improved glycemic control, though recommended by many, have not yet been proven by long-term prospective clinical trials. Other more specific preventive therapies based on putative underlying etiopathogenetic mechanisms are presently considered experimental, although some, such as the use of aldose reductase inhibitors, are now appearing in clinical practice in some countries.

Pathophysiology

A widening array of clinical and experimental evidence suggest that diabetic neuropathy is a secondary consequence of insulin deficiency and/or hyperglycemia (Table 2) [5, 9–31], but the specific pathophysiologic mechanism(s) linking altered metabolism with nerve damage in diabetes remains controversial (Table 3). Additional pathogenetic variables above and beyond hyperglycemia and insulin deficiency must also be operative since clinical neuropathy is not universally found in patients with very poorly controlled diabetes of long duration [32, 33], and clinical neuropathy assumes widely differing forms in individual patients [1, 27, 33]. Nevertheless, active investigation of possible mechanism(s) by which hyperglycemia and/or insulin deficiency destroy elements of the peripheral nervous system is the conceptual basis for

Table 2 Evidence supporting a pathogenetic role for hyperglycemia and/or insulin deficiency in diabetic neuropathy

1. Correlation between the cumulative prevalence of clinical neuropathy and the duration and severity of hyperglycemia in both insulin-dependent and non-insulin dependent diabetes [5, 13].
2. The presence of diabetic neuropathy in secondary forms of diabetes such as pancreatectomy, non-alcoholic pancreatitis and hemachromatosis [15].
3. Correlation between indices of glycemia and sub-clinical neuropathy both before and following acute changes in metabolic control [12–25].
4. Biochemical, functional and morphological similarities between human diabetic neuropathy and that occurring in animal models where the peripheral nerve changes can be directly attributed to insulin deficiency and hyperglycemia [26].
5. Anecdotal reports of clinical improvement in diabetic neuropathy following institution of improved metabolic control [28–31].

Table 3 The differential diagnosis of diabetic neuropathy

I. Distal symmetrical polyneuropathy

- A. Metabolic
  1. Diabetes mellitus
  2. Uremia
  3. Folic acid/cyanocobalamin deficiency
  4. Hypothyroidism
  5. Acute intermittent porphyria
- B. Toxic
  1. Alcohol
  2. Heavy metals (lead, mercury, arsenic)
  3. Industrial hydrocarbons
  4. Various drugs
- C. Infectious or inflammatory
  1. Sarcoidosis
  2. Leprosy
  3. Periarteritis nodosa
  4. Other connective-tissue diseases (e. g. systemic lupus erythematosus)
- D. Other
  1. Dysproteinemias and paraproteinemias
  2. Paraneoplastic syndrome
  3. Leukemias and lymphomas
  4. Amyloidosis
  5. Hereditary neuropathies

II. Pains and paresthesias without neurologic deficit

- A. Early small-fiber sensory neuropathy
- B. Psychophysiologic disorder (e. g. severe depression, hysteria)

III. Autonomic neuropathy without somatic component

- A. Shy-Drager syndrome (progressive autonomic failure)
- B. Diabetic neuropathy with mild somatic involvement
- C. Riley-Day syndrome
- D. Idiopathic orthostatic hypotension

IV. Diffuse motor neuropathy without sensory deficit

- A. Guillain-Barre syndrome
- B. Primary myopathies
- C. Myasthenia gravis
- D. Heavy-metal toxicity

V. Femoral neuropathy (sacral plexopathy)

- A. Degenerative spinal-disc disease (e. g. Paget's disease of the spine)
- B. Intrinsic spinal-cord-mass lesion
- C. Equina cauda lesions
- D. Coagulopathies

Table 3 (continued)

VI.	Cranial neuropathy
	A. Carotid aneurysm
	B. Intracranial mass
	C. Elevated intracranial pressure
VII.	Mononeuropathy multiplex
	A. Vasculidites
	B. Amyloidosis
	C. Hypothyroidism
	D. Acromegaly
	E. Coagulopathies

several putative new therapeutic approaches to the prevention and treatment of diabetic neuropathy [1, 11, 34].

There are currently four distinct but not mutually exclusive and possibly interrelated metabolic hypotheses for the pathogenesis of diabetic neuropathy: the "sorbitol-myo-inositol-(Na,K)-ATPase hypothesis", the "hypoxia-ischemia" hypothesis, the "non-enzymatic glycation" hypothesis and the "insulin-neurotrophism-axonal transport hypothesis".

The "sorbitol-myo-inositol-(Na,K)-ATPase hypothesis"

Detailed analysis of the biochemical factors contributing to the acutely reversible slowing of nerve conduction in short-term diabetic animals (and by analogy newly-diagnosed diabetes in man) have given rise to the "sorbitol-myo-inositol-(Na,K)-ATPase hypothesis". The similar slowing of nerve conduction velocity in newly-diagnosed insulin deficient diabetic subjects and laboratory animals is rapidly improved by insulin replacement that normalizes blood glucose [12, 13, 19–21, 25, 35–40]. In animals, this conduction slowing is unaccompanied by fixed alterations of peripheral nerve structure such as axonal degeneration or segmental demyelination [37, 41, 42] (although subtle reversible structural alterations occur at the node of Ranvier [35]) implicating acute metabolic disturbances in axons, Schwann cells and/or their endoneurial environment [7, 9, 36, 37, 43–45]. As has been recently reviewed [1, 26, 27, 34], studies in acutely diabetic animals have linked early functional defects such as slowing of nerve conduction and axonal transport to metabolism of excess nerve glucose via the polyol pathway, and the development of secondary alterations in nerve myo-inositol and phosphoinositide metabolism that

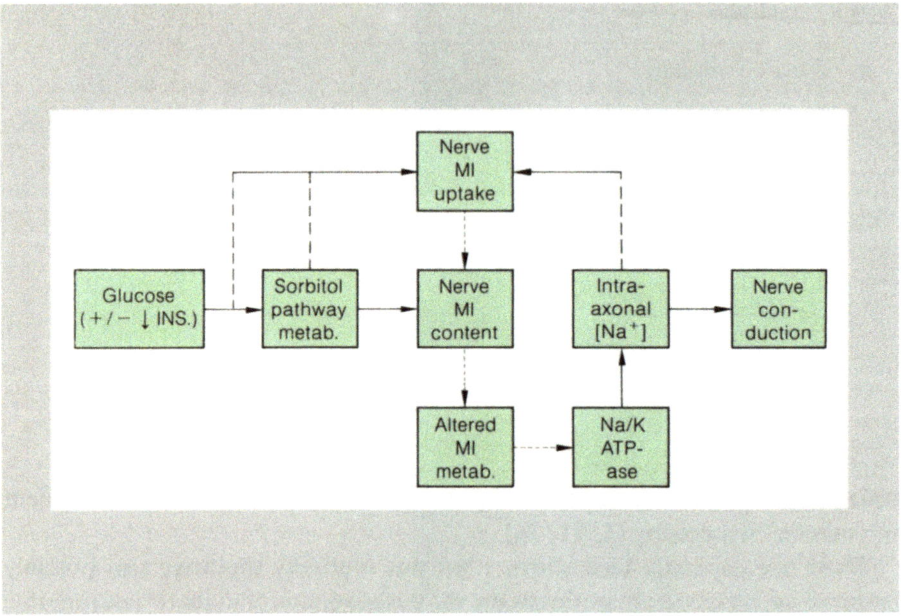

Fig. 1 The myo-inositol depletion hypothesis.

adversely affect nerve (Na,K)-ATPase activity (Fig. 1). Moreover, as discussed below, these early biochemical and functional changes are associated with subtle structural alterations at the node of Ranvier such as nodal swelling, that progress in chronic animal diabetes to lesions that have been identified in human diabetic nerve, such as axo-glial dysjunction [1, 26, 27]. Some [46–50], but not all [51], of the fragmentary biochemical data on diabetic human nerve samples support the major aspects of this biochemical hypothesis, although their interpretation is complicated by the severe structural and compositional alterations in diabetic human nerve, patients selection, post-mortem changes, and the possible presence of compensatory biochemical pathways in chronic diabetes.

The "hypoxia-ischemia hypothesis"

This hypothesis is derived from limited metabolic studies in chronically diabetic animals and in man, and from histopathological studies of nerve biopsies and autopsy material [1]. The clinical and histopathological features of the rare focal syndromes of diabetic neuropathy suggest an acute ischemic element [8]. Endoneurial vascular abnormalities such as basement membrane thickening and reduplication, endothelial cell swelling and proliferation, and platelet aggregation resulting in vessel occlusion have been noted in sural nerve biopsies [52, 53] and at autopsy [54–58] in diabetic distal symmetric polyneuropathy, but these findings are non-specific and occur in other neuropathies as well. A quantitative increase in these vascular abnormalities and focal loss of myelinated fibers in older neuropathic diabetic subjects has been interpreted to suggest hypoxic or ischemic damage [52–54]. A possible microvascular basis of diabetic neuropathy is further supported by faulty regulation of the microcirculation and oxygen delivery in peripheral nerve in diabetic animals demonstrated by Low and coworkers [59] who also reported that exposure of normal rats to chronic hypoxia slows conduction velocity, at least in the highly specialized tail nerve [60, 61], and that exposure of normal or chronically diabetic rats to hyperbaric oxygen produces metabolic and functional changes in the peripheral nervous system some of which may be interpreted as a selective partial reversal of abnormalities produced by the diabetic state [62–64]. Newrick and colleagues [65] also recorded low intra-neural oxygen tension in 11 severely neuropathic diabetics compared with 3 non-diabetic individuals and 1 newly-diagnosed non-neuropathic diabetic. These exciting and provocative observations suggest that endoneurial hypoxia probably occurs in chronic advanced human diabetic neuropathy, but whether this is a cause or effect of the neuropathy remains unknown (for instance, nerve fibrosis was so severe in one neuropathic patient that the oxygen electrode could not gain access to the nerve). The ischemia-hypoxia hypothesis, and its possible relationship to other pathogenetic mechanisms is summarized in Fig. 2.

The "non-enzymatic glycation hypothesis"

As discussed in Chapter 16, nonenzymatic glycation occurs in a variety of tissue proteins as a result of increased ambient glucose concentration, in some instances leading to altered protein function. Of significant interest is the discovery that brain tubulin may be nonenzymatically glycated in vitro and in vivo, with dramatic alteration in its self-assembly and solubility characteristics [66]. Glycation of peripheral nerve tubulin might well have important consequences on both fast and slow axonal transport, and on the physical characteristics of the axon cylinder. The fact that, under some circumstances, fructose, a product of polyol pathway activity, is more effective in nonenzymatic glycation than glucose, suggests a possible pathogenetic convergence between the polyol and glycation hypotheses [67]. With time, glycated

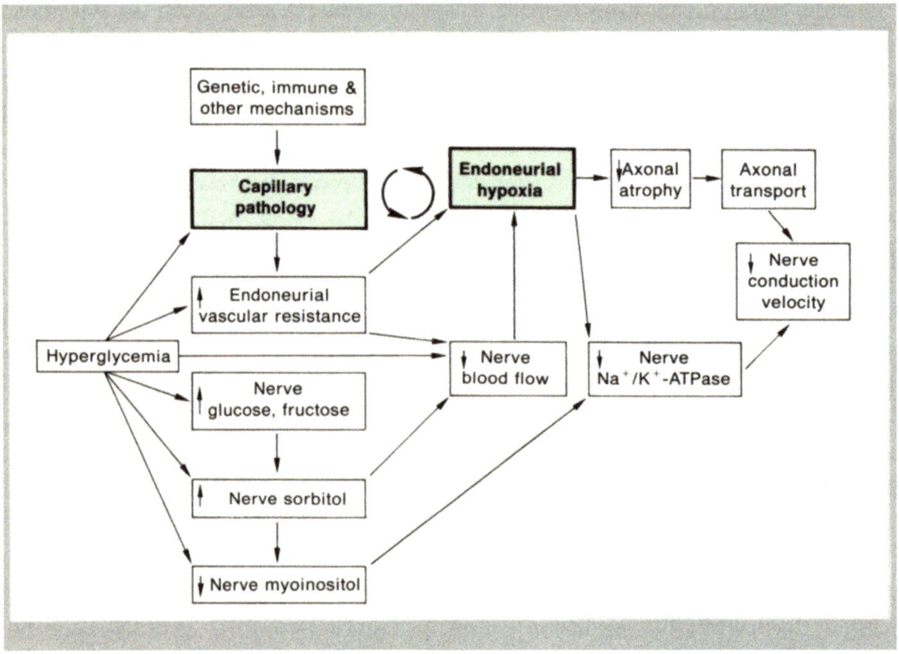

Fig. 2 Suggested pathogenesis of diabetic neuropathy [59].

Amadori products attached to proteins with slow metabolic turnover rates rearrange to form a series of chemically and possibly immunologically reactive "advanced glycosylation end-products" that promote covalent protein cross-linking, and activate cytokine production by macrophages [67]. Such products have been identified in peripheral nerve myelin, which has a slow rate of turnover, from diabetic humans [68]. Moreover, the presence of these products on myelin proteins can be reproduced by prolonged incubation of myelin with glucose metabolites, and appears to stimulate uptake of myelin by macrophages [68]. Whether the presence of these advanced glycosylation end-products on myelin or other long-lived proteins in peripheral nerve is of physiological or pathophysiological significance remains unknown, but represents an important area for future research, especially since pharmacologic agents that inhibit advanced glycosylation endproduct formation are currently under development [67].

The "insulin/neurotrophism/axonal transport hypotheses"

A variety of neurotrophic factors are necessary for normal growth and development, maintenance, and regeneration and repair of the nervous system. An impaired maturation of peripheral nerves has been suggested by Thomas and Sharma [69, 70] as an explanation of decreased myelinated fiber size and hence decreased nerve conduction velocity. The mechanism(s) underlying the characteristic axonal atrophy in experimental diabetes is not well understood, and most likely involves several factors such as decreased protein synthesis in the cell soma [71, 72], decreased axonal transport of structural proteins [66, 73, 74], as well as a continuous sequestration of axoplasm by the Schwann cell [75–77], some or all of which could reflect decreased neuronotrophism or neuronotropism. Diminished neurotrophism could be an important factor in the defects in axonal transport that have been described in diabetes [74, 78, 79], including the reduced antegrade transport of endogenous enzymes such as choline acetyltransferase and acetylcholinesterase [80–82] and structural protein such as neurofilaments and microtubules [73, 74, 80, 83]. Moreover, retrograde axonal transport which brings recycled axonal components and neurotrophic substances picked up in the periphery from the distal axon back to the perikaryon is decreased in streptozocin-diabetes [84, 85]. Moreover, a variety of neurotrophic peptides, including nerve growth factor [86, 87], enhance phosphoinositide turnover in neural tissue [88]. Thus, nerve growth factor accessability and action might be diminished in the peripheral nervous system in diabetes due to defective transport [84, 85] and post-receptor signal transduction [86, 87]. The neurite-promoting effects of insulin and insulin-like growth factors, but increasingly recognized as neuronotrophic agonists, can be duplicated by protein kinase C agonists, suggesting that they too are mediated by the phosphoinositide cascade [88]. Thus, insulin deficiency might impair neuronotrophism by diminishing the availabilty of and sensitivity to multiple neuronotrophic agonists in the peripheral nervous system, whose action are required not only for a regenerative response to injury, but also for maintenance of the integrity of peripheral nerve axons and Schwann cells. Observations consistent with diminished neurotrophism have been reported in experimental diabetes, including delayed regeneration after nerve transection [89]. One expression of this diminished neuronotrophic tone might well be impaired synthesis and centrifugal transport of axon-specific proteins by slow axonal transport. Additional factors, such as alterations in the endoneurial microenvironment, ischemia etc. might also blunt the ability of the peripheral nervous system to mount a regenerative response to injury in diabetes. Evidence for blunted regeneration in human diabetic neuropathy was recently suggested by studies of human sural nerve biopsies from patients with diabetic neuropathy following one year of treatment with an aldose reductase inhibitor that are reviewed below in the section on experimental interventions and therapies [90].

Present treatment modalities

Treatment of diabetic neuropathy is directed at its prevention, prophylaxis of its secondary complications, and palliation of symptoms arising from its somatic and autonomic neurological deficits and disfunction. Definitive therapy targeted at specific biochemical or cell biological processes thought to underly the neurological damage causing diabetic neuropathy, e. g. gangliosides or aldose reductase inhibitors, are recent additions to the therapeutic armamentarium available in only some countries, and are therefore discussed in the succeeding section on *Future therapies.*

Diagnosis

All therapeutic approaches require the proper diagnosis and classification of diabetic neuropathy as outlined in the Introduction and Table 1 [91]. Since neither the sub-clinical nor clinical manifestations of diabetic neuropathy are pathognomonic for the disease, other forms of peripheral neuropathy or diseases simulating peripheral neuropathy must be excluded by appropriate diagnostic tests [Table 3]; thus *diabetic neuropathy is a diagnosis of exclusion.*

Prevention

The strong evidence that hyperglycemia and/or insulin deficiency contribute to important biochemical, functional and structural abnormalities in peripheral nerve [9] implies that prudent diabetic control or pharmacological protection against the metabolic consequences of insulin deficiency and/or hyperglycemia should prevent, delay and/or ameliorate the development of clinical neuropathy [9]. Conclusive proof of this assertion awaits the completion and analysis of prospective long-term clinical trails such as the NIH-sponsored Diabetes Control and Complications Trial (DCCT) or the Neuropathy Component of the NIH-sponsored Sorbinil Retinopathy Trial, both of which assess the effect of metabolic intervention on the development of clinical diabetic neuropathy. Other putative risk factors for the development of diabetic neuropathy e. g. ethanol abuse etc. suggest additional strategies to prevent the development of the disorder [92, 93]. The presence of subclinical neuropathy should increase clinical surveillance for the development of clinical neuropathy, and should signal a re-evaluation of diabetic control and nutritional status, as well as exploration of other possible causes of peripheral nerve disease (Table 3). The appearance of occult sensory deficits unaccompanied by positive symptoms such as pain or paresthesias may predispose to secondary complications such as foot ulceration or Charcot's neuroarthropathy. Thus, a yearly clinical examination of sensation in the foot in otherwise asymptomatic patients is an essential component of health maintenance in diabetic patients.

Management of clinical diabetic polyneuropathy

The signs and symptoms of distal symmetrical polyneuropathy, and therefore its recognition and treatment, relate to the spectrum of nerve fiber involvement [94, 95]. While most cases involve both large and small fibers, predominantly large fiber loss may present as impaired balance, diminished proprioception and position sense, or simply absent or reduced vibration sense in the absence of subjective symptoms of pain, paresthesia or numbness. Late neuropathic complications such as Charcot neuroarthropathy or neuropathic ulceration may be presenting features in this form of diabetic neuropathy. Severe large fiber involvement with complete loss of position sense produces the sensory ataxia known as "pseudotabetic" diabetic neuropathy [94]. Primarily small fiber neuropathy may be asymptomatic, presenting with undetected trauma of the extremities (burns, acute abrasions and ulcerations of the hands or feet) due to insensitivity to pain. Alternatively, small fiber disease may give rise to subjective symptoms of numbness or feelings of "cold feet" or "dead feet," often in the presence of autonomic neuropathy. Most patients with diabetic polyneuropathy exhibit some elements of large and small fiber neuropathy including diminished deep tendon reflexes, especially the Achilles tendon reflex [94].

Improved control of hyperglycemia as treatment for clinically overt diabetic distal symmetric polyneuropathy has been recommended by many [16–18, 28, 29, 94]. Yet, there is no compelling basis on which to select among various alternatives of improved metabolic control for patients with distal symmetrical polyneuropathy. Prospective clinical trials, such as the Diabetes Control and Complications Trial, will hopefully resolve the role of intensive insulin treatment regimens in prevention and amelioration of distal symmetrical polyneuropathy [96]. As discussed below, various specific metabolic interventions based on discrete metabolic pathogenetic hypotheses for diabetic neuropathy have been attempted. The conflicting and/or marginal clinical responses most likely reflect the difficulty in assessing clinical response in distal symmetric polyneuropathy, but published evidence suggests that histological damage is improved by treatment with an aldose reductase inhibitor [97]. Although most patients with diabetic neuropathy experience minimal subjective symptoms, several kinds of spontaneous pain associated with diabetic polyneuropathy may require pharmacological intervention [94]. Typical mild neuropathic distal paresthesias or dysesthesias [94], exquisite cutaneous contact hypersensitivity to light touch, superficial and burning, shooting or stabbing, or bone-deep and aching or tearing pains, often more noticed at night, can be features of diabetic neuropathy, but pain becomes an overriding and disabling feature in a minority of cases. Muscle cramps, which begin distally and slowly ascend, are similar to those reported in other muscle denervation disorders [94]. Mild or severe pain may occur with primarily small myelinated nerve fiber involvement, in which case conduction velocity may be minimally impaired, vibration sensation may be intact, motor weakness may be absent, and if symptoms bring the patient to medical attention early in the course of the disease, sensory loss may be extremely subtle [98]. While severe painful symptoms in the absence of striking neurological deficit appears somewhat paradoxical, painfulness may reflect fiber regeneration [94], which may commence before degeneration is sufficiently severe to present marked sensory deficit. Most observers have concluded that troubling painful symptoms generally improve spontaneously within a matter of months [33, 94], but some others disagree with this view [29]. A variety of pharmacological agents have been recommended for the treatment of painful diabetic neuropathy, including standard analgesics, phenytoin (Dilantin) or carbamazepine (Tegretol) in anticonvulsive doses, and amitriptyline (Elavil) in sub-antidepressive doses (50 – 150 mg po at bedtime) either alone or in combination with fluphenazine (Prolixim) 1 mg three dimes a day [94]. Supporting well-controlled clinical trials are either generally unavailable [99] or negative [100], although a single double-blind cross-over clinical trial of carbamazine in doses up to 600 mg/day in 30 patients with painful diabetic neuropathy improved sensory symptoms more than placebo [101]. A placebo-controlled double-blind trial of stepwise addition to simple analgesics of tricyclic antidepressants with or without phenothiazines produced significant improvement in cases of painful peripheral symmetric neuropathy and in painful mononeuropathy, particularly in those cases where pain was most troublesome (Fig. 3) [102]. Depression, with associated anorexia, appears to interact very strongly with pain in diabetic neuropathy, and seems to exceed that which can be attributed entirely to the painful symptoms alone, suggesting that simultaneous antidepressant therapy might be efficacious [33]. One study suggests that painful

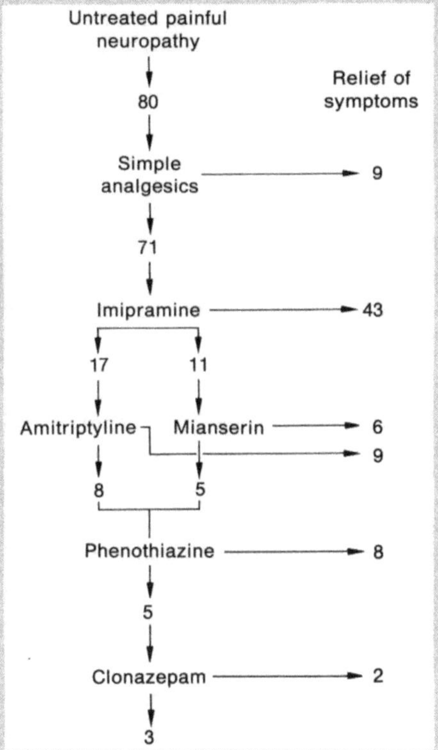

Fig. 3 Treatment of painful neuropathy [102].

diabetic neuropathy may constitute a depressive equivalent in a large proportion of patients referred for neuropathic therapy [103]. An exaggeration of this interaction probably constitutes the syndrome of diabetic neuropathic cachexia described by Ellenberg in 1974 [104]. This syndrome, reported in elderly male diabetics, combined severe weight loss with mild diabetes and painful neuropathy; weight loss was of sufficient magnitude (up to 60% of total body weight) to suggest an underlying malignancy [104]. Improved diabetic control, counselling, and amitriptyline plus fluphenazine have all been recommended in the therapy of this syndrome. For unclear reasons, spontaneous improvement and regain of weight may occur. Recently, the use of topical capsaicin, a naturally-occurring compound derived from red peppers that is said to selectively deplete substance-P from peripheral neurons, has been recommended for post-herpetic and post-mastectomy pain, and has been proposed as a treatment for painful diabetic neuropathy; promising controlled clinical trials have not yet been published as full-length articles in peer-reviewed journals however.

Management of complications of distal symmetrical polyneuropathy

These secondary mechanical and traumatic consequences of the sensorimotor denervation of diabetic polyneuropathy are largely preventable, and, as such, reflect inadequate clinical surveillance, patient-education, or patient compliance, especially that involving foot care and hygiene. Non-gangrenous diabetic foot ulceration occurs in the setting of diminished pain sensation, although diminished proprioception and muscle strength, and vascular factors may play contributing roles [33]. In the classic plantar ulcer, neurogenic atrophy of the intrinsic foot muscles and chronic flexion of the metatarsal-phalangeal joints shifts weight bearing to the unprotected metatarsal heads leading to callus formation. Subsequent liquification of the callus with fissuring, cracking and break-down of overlying skin due to sudomotor autonomic neuropathy, leads to formation of a central ulcer that is subject to infection (Fig. 4). More advanced architectural deformity due to neuroarthropathy (see below) or amputation produces plantar ulcers at alternative weight-bearing sites. Neuropathic foot ulcers at non-weight-bearing locations occur without callus formation due to abrasions unrecognized by the patient due to pain insensitivity [10]. The thin dorsal dermis of the foot may be abraided within hours, so that repeated self-examinations are mandatory with new foot wear or with prolonged walking or weight bearing on the insensitive foot. Prophylactic treatment of diabetic foot ulcers includes recognition of the insensitive foot, patient education, identification of abnormal weight-bearing and/or callus formation before ulceration occurs, and prescription of appropriate measures to reduce or readjust abnormal weight-bearing. With chronic plantar ulcers, a removable walking-cast that transfers weight-bearing to the upper leg is sometimes helpful, however, the casted leg must be examined for abrasions/ ulcerations at the new weight-bearing site. Complicating infection should be treated with antibiotics, including coverage for anerobic bacteria that may be difficult to culture from an open wound. In refractory cases, removal of the underlying metatarsal head, sometimes with amputation of the toe, may be necessary [33].

"Charcot" neuroarthropathy occurs when preserved motor function accompanies nociceptive impairment [105]. Diabetic neuroarthropathy involves the distal foot (tarsal-metatarsal or metatarsal-phalangeal joints) or the ankle

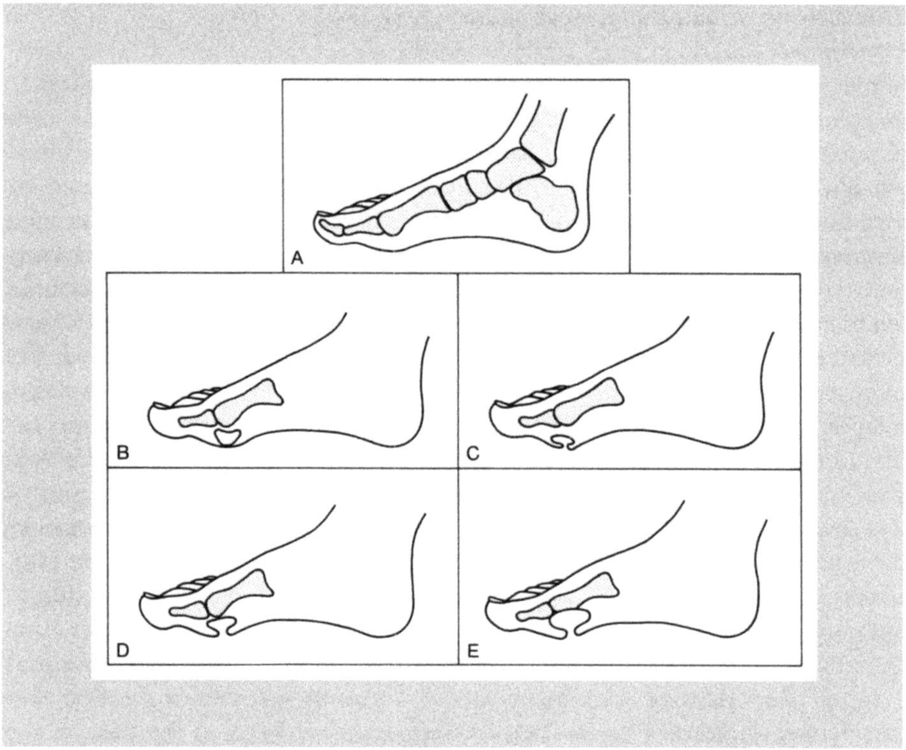

Fig. 4 The pathogenesis of diabetic ulcers [146].

[105]. Recent-onset diabetic neuroarthropathy presents as painless swelling and redness in the absence of fever or leukocytosis, but in the presence of clearly demonstrable distal symmetric sensory deficit. The differential diagnosis is usually cellulitis or osteomyelitis, depending upon the extent of radiographic bony destruction. Unhealed painless fractures are often evident radiographically, and a recent history of painless trauma is frequently illicited [105]. Advanced cases exhibit gross architectural distortion of the foot, with shortening and widening, at times progressing with multiple painless fractures accompanied by bone demineralization and reabsorption, so that the foot appears as "a bag of bones" [33]. As with other forms of neuroarthropathy, the pathogenetic mechanism is recurrent traumatic insults to the joint and surrounding bony structures unnoticed because of insensitivity to pain. Prophylactic measures include reinforced education in patients with insensitive feet, avoidance of prolonged weight-bearing, cushioned shoes, etc.

Management of autonomic neuropathy

Some but not all components of autonomic neuropathy are subject to pharmacological intervention as part of an overall treatment strategy for each type of autonomic neuropathy. *Gustatory sweating*, troubling profuse facial perspiration accompanying the ingestion of certain foods is best treated by avoidance of offending foods, but anticholinergic drugs have been used successfully in some cases [1]. *Neurogenic bladder*, which may reflect impairment of afferent and/or parasympathetic efferent innervation with or without bladder wall distention and sphincter involvement, requires detailed cystometric evaluation. Afferent involvement is treated by voluntary voiding, but parasympathetic agonists such as bethanechol (10–30 mg three times daily) may be helpful in some cases [106]. *Retrograde ejaculation* reflecting incoordination of the internal and external vesicle sphincters during ejaculation, produces infertility that is generally managed by artificial insemination of live sperm recovered from the post-coital urine [107], but sympathomemetics have been recommended [108, 109, 110]. *Erectile impotence* should be evaluated for pharmacological, vascular and endocrine causes, with that due to autonomic dysfunction treated either with commercially available suction devices [1] or penile protheses [111]. Injection of 30 mg of papaverine plus 1 mg of phentolamine into the corpus of the penis will induce erection that can be maintained for up to 2 hours with a rubber band at the base of the penis although ejaculation is prevented and priapism is a recognized risk [1]. Yohimbine, an alpha-2-adrenergic antagonist has also been recommended [1]. *Diabetic autonomic gastroparesis*, presents with post-prandial bloating, nausea or vomiting, or with "brittle" diabetes, is confirmed by radionuclide gastric emptying studies [111], and treated with frequent small feedings and metoclopramide, a dopamine antagonist, 10 mg 30 min before meals, with or without the parasympathetic agonist bethanechol [10–30 mg 30 min before meals) [1]. "*Diabetic diarrhea*" can be multifactorial [1]; bacterial overgrowth is treated with broad-spectrum antibiotics including ampicillin, tetracycline and metronidazole; bile-salt malabsorption with cholestyramine; in other cases, hypomotility has been treated with clonidine [1], and hypermotility with standard antidiarrheal agents such as loperamine [1] on an empiric basis. *Orthostatic hypotension* requires a diagnostic evaluation [1] to rule out hypovolemia or pharmacological causes, after which body stockings, plasma volume expanders such as a high salt diet or fludrocortisone, or autonomic drugs such as clonidine and neosynephrine spray [112, 113] may be used.

Management of focal neuropathies

Focal diabetic neuropathies often provide more of a diagnostic rather than a therapeutic challenge, since they are generally indistinguishable from focal neuropathies of other etiologies, and they are usually acute in onset and self-limited [1]. Mechanical, compressive and vascular etiologies should be excluded (Table 3). Motor weakness should be treated with appropriate physical therapy, pain with analgesics etc.

Future therapies

Aldose reductase inhibitors

Although large-scale long term therapeutic trials of aldose reductase inhibitors using both clinical and electrophysiological endpoints have been completed, the results have not yet appeared in full-length publications in peer-reviewed journals. One compound, Tolrestat, has been approved for treatment of diabetic neuropathy in several countries on the basis of large-scale clinical trials reported thus far only in abstract form [114]. Similar evidence of efficacy based on multi-center studies has been reported for another aldose reductase inhibitor, sorbinil [115–117], but this compound has been withdrawn from further studies because of safety issues. Other aldose reductase inhibitors are currently in various stages of development and testing. Existing published evidence does indicate that sorbinil improved median and peroneal motor and median sensory conduction velocity in patients with diabetes but without signs or symptoms of diabetic neuropathy [118]; and lowered nerve sorbitol levels, prevented further Wallerian degeneration, and stimulated nerve fiber regeneration in patients with clinically advanced diabetic neuropathy [97]. The clinical implications of these treatment effects remain to be established in fully-published controlled clinical trials. In an uncontrolled study with sorbinil in 11 patients with severely painful diabetic neuropathy, Jaspan et al. [119] reported relief of pain and improved autonomic function in sub-groups of the patients, but possible "placebo" effects or the influence of sub-group analysis could not be excluded in this preliminary report. Young et al. [120] reported improved pain, tendon reflex scores, and sural sensory potential amplitude but diminished scores of clinical sensory examinations in 15 neuropathic patients treated for 4 weeks with sorbinil in a double-blind crossover study, whereas similar studies with the same drug revealed no comparable improvement in 13 patients [121], or only an improvement in "overall subjective well-being" without confirmatory neurophysiological changes in 37 patients [121].

Myo-inositol

Oral myo-inositol supplementation to small groups of diabetic subjects with or without clinically-overt diabetic neuropathy [28, 122–125] have yielded inconclusive results [126]. A well-designed, large-scale, prospective, comprehensive therapeutic trial of myo-inositol supplementation in diabetic neuropathy using carefully defined endpoints that are both sensitive to a treatment response and thought to be clinically relevant has not been undertaken so that the myo-inositol hypothesis has never been tested clinically.

Gangliosides

Gangliosides are complex sphingosine-containing phospholipids normally found in great abundance in the nervous system. While there is no direct evidence that ganglioside metabolism is altered by diabetes, gangliosides reportedly increase nerve regeneration, nerve conduction velocity, axonal transport, and nerve fiber diameter in diabetic animals [127, 128]. These promising studies have been followed by a limited series of double-blind placebo controlled studies in diabetic human subjects of up to 6 months [129–132] which report modest improvement in sensory and motor nerve conduction velocities which in some instances are associated with improvement of neuropathic symptoms. Although the results are promising and need to be confirmed, the full potential therapeutic benefit of newly regenerated nerve fibers may not be fully realized in such short term trials and long term trials are needed to establish the potential efficacy of gangliosides in the treatment of diabetic neuropathy.

Isaxonine

Isaxonine also has been associated with an increase in nerve regeneration in peripheral neuropathy [134]. These newly generated nerve fibers are small, and, accordingly, there has not been an associated increase in nerve conduction velocity or amplitude in animals. Several uncontrolled studies suggest that isaxonine may be helpful in a neuropathy caused by alcohol, leprosy, and vincristine. One double-blind study in vincristine neuropathy [135], appeared to suggest a protective effect, but this drug is no longer in clinical trials because a small portion of patients developed hepatitis.

Vitamins

Several vitamins and other trophic agents have been used for the treatment of diabetic neuropathy but the rationale of using vitamins to treat diabetic neuropathy is not solidly based on the current view of the pathogenetic proceses thought to underlie diabetic neuropathy. The clinical trials of vitamin therapy for diabetic neuropathy have lacked rigorous placebo controls [134]. Because thiamine, pyridoxine and vitamin B_{12} deficiencies have been associated with peripheral neuropathy, these vitamins have been used empirically for the treatment of the neuropathy associated with diabetes. These drugs have not been studied in double-blind or placebo controlled clinical trials, precluding any unequivocal proof of efficacy. Despite the fact that diabetes and vitamin deficiencies may occur coincidentally, many of the clinical trials involving vitamin therapy have not excluded vitamin deficiencies in the diabetic patients involved in this study. There have been several conflicting clinical trials using thiamine for the treatment of diabetic neuropathy. Thompson [136] has reviewed the literature using thiamine as a therapeutic treatment of diabetic neuropathy, and found no biochemical basis for the claim that thiamine deficiency plays a role in the pathogenesis of diabetic neuropathy. A decrease in pyridoxine levels has been found in some [137] but not all clinical trials in diabetics with neuropathy [138]. Uncontrolled trials have indicated that there is a relief of symptoms associated with neuropathy [139] but controlled clinical trials [138, 140] have failed to show any statistically significant effect of pyridoxine. The streptozocin diabetic rat exhibits biochemical changes consistent with tissue vitamin B_{12} deficiency [141]. Furthermore, methylcobalamin therapy [142] has been associated with an increase in nerve conduction velocity in this animal model. In one study in human diabetic individuals, serum and nerve cobalamin were normal but a decrease in nerve methylcobalamin was reported [143]. Unfortunately, the "normal" control patients for this study were patients dying from end-stage heart disease. Studies of two months [144] or greater [145] have reported improvement in symptoms associated with diabetic neuropathy with therapy of methylcobalamin, but neither of these studies meet current criteria for randomized controlled clinical trials in that neither clinical nor objective measurements were subject to rigorous statistical analysis. As a result, it is not possible to determine whether vitamin B_{12} deficiency plays a pathogenic role and/or whether vitamin B_{12} therapy is helpful in the treatment of diabetic neuropathy.

References

[1] Greene DA, Sima AAF, Pfeifer MA. Pathophysiology of Diabetic Neuropathy. In: Rifkin H, Porte D, eds. Ellenberg and Rifkin's Diabetes Mellitus, Fourth Edition. New York: Elsevier Publishing Co., 1990; Chapt. 43.
[2] Melton LJ, Dyck PJ. Epidemiology. In: Dyck PJ, Thomas PK, Winegrad AI et al, eds. Diabetic Neuropathy. Philadelphia: WB Saunders, 1987; 27–35.
[3] The Physicians Guide to Type II Diabetes (NIDDM). Diagnosis and Treatment. The American Diabetes Association, 1984.
[4] Palumbo PJ, Elveback LR, Whisnant JP. Neurologic complications of diabetes mellitus: Transient ischemic attack, stroke, and peripheral neuropathy. Adv Neurol 1978; 19: 593.
[5] Pirart J. Diabetes mellitus and its degenerative complications: A prospective study of 4,400 patients observed between 1947 and 1973. Diabetes Care 1978; 1: 168–188, 252–263.
[6] Dyck PJ, Karnes J, O'Brian PC. Diagnosis, staging, and classification of diabetic neuropathy and associations with other complications. In: Dyck PJ, Thomas PK, Winegrad AI et al, eds. Diabetic Neuropathy. Philadelphia: WB Saunders, 1987; 36.
[7] Thomas PK, Brown MJ. Diabetic Polyneuropathy. In: Dyck PJ, Thomas PK, Winegrad AI et al, eds. Diabetic Neuropathy. Philadelphia: WB Saunders, 1987; 56.
[8] Asbury AK. Focal and multifocal neuropathies of diabetes. In: Dyck PJ, Thomas PK, Winegrad AI et al, eds. Diabetic Neuropathy. Philadelphia: WB Saunders, 1987: 45–55.
[9] Committee on Health Care Issues, American Neurological Association. Does improved control of glycemia prevent or ameliorate diabetic neuropathy? Ann Neurol 1986; 19: 288–290.
[10] Thomas PK, Ward JD, Watkins PJ. Diabetic Neuropathy. In: Keen H, Jarrett J, eds. Complications of Diabetes. London: Arnold, 1982; 109–136.
[11] Winegrad AI. Banting lecture 1986. Does a common mechanism induce the diverse complications of diabetes? Diabetes 1987; 36: 396–406.
[12] Gregersen G. Variations in motor conduction velocity produced by acute changes of the metabolic state in diabetic patients. Diabetologia 1968; 4: 273.
[13] Ward JD, Bowes CG, Fisher DJ et al. Improvement in nerve conduction following treatment in newly diagnosed diabetics. Lancet 1971; 1: 428.
[14] Terkidsen AB, Christensen NJ. Reversible nervous abnormalities in juvenile diabetics with recently diagnosed diabetes. Diabetologia 1971; 7: 113.
[15] Eng GD, Nellinton H, August GP. Nerve conduction velocity determination in juvenile diabetes. Mod Problem Paediat 1975; 12: 213.
[16] Gregersen G. Diabetic neuropathy: Influence of age, sex, metabolic control and duration of diabetes on motor conduction velocity. Neurology 1967; 17: 972.
[17] Graf RJ, Halter JB, Halar E et al. Nerve conduction abnormalities in untreated maturity-onset diabetes: Relation to levels of fasting plasma glucose and glycosylated hemoglobin. Ann Intern Med 1979; 90: 298.
[18] Graf RJ, Halter JB, Pfeifer MD et al. Glycemic control and nerve conduction abnormalities in noninsulin-dependent diabetic subjects. Ann Intern Med 1981; 94: 307–311.
[19] Holman RR, White VM, Orde-Peckar C et al. Prevention of deterioration of renal and sensory-nerve function by more intensive management of insulin-dependent diabetic patients. A two-year randomized prospective study. Lancet 1983; I: 204.
[20] Pietri A, Ehle A, Raskin P. Changes in nerve conduction velocity after six weeks of glycoregulation with portable insulin infusion pumps. Diabetes 1980; 29: 668.
[21] Service FJ, Rizza RA, Daube JR et al. Near normoglycaemia improved nerve conduction and vibration sensation in diabetic neuropathy. Diabetologia 1985; 28: 722.
[22] Steno Study Group. Effect of 6 months strict metabolic control on eye and kidney function in insulin-dependent diabetes with background retinopathy. Lancet 1982; I: 121.

[23] Gallai V, Agostini L, Rossi A et al. Evaluation of the motor and sensory conduction velocity (MCV, SCV) in diabetic patients before and after a three-day treatment with the artificial beta cell (Biostator). In: Canal N, Pozza G, eds. Peripheral Neuropathies. New Amsterdam: Elsevier/North-Holland Biomedical Press, 1978; 287.
[24] Service FJ, Daube JR, O'Brien PC et al. Effect of artificial pancreas treatment on peripheral nerve function in diabetes. Neurology 1981; 31: 1375.
[25] Troni W, Carta Q, Cantello R et al. Peripheral nerve function and metabolic control in diabetes mellitus. Ann Neurol 1984; 16: 178–183.
[26] Greene DA, Lattimer SA, Sima AAF. Pathogenesis of Diabetic Neuropathy: Role of Altered Phosphoinositide Metabolism. In: Nelson J, ed. CRC Critical Reviews in Neurobiology. Vol. 5, Issue 2, CRC Press, Inc., 1989; 143–219.
[27] Greene DA, Sima AAF, Pfeifer MA. Neuropathy. In: Mogensen CE, Standl E, eds. Prevention and Treatment of Diabetic Late Complications. Berlin: Walter de Gruyter, 1989; 93–149.
[28] Greene DA, Brown MJ, Braunstein SN et al. Comparison of clinical course and sequential electrophysiological tests in diabetics with symptomatic polyneuropathy and its implications for clinical trials. Diabetes 1981; 30: 139–147.
[29] Boulton AJM, Drury J, Clarke B et al. Continuous subcutaneous insulin infusion in the management of painful diabetic neuropathy. Diabetes Care 1982; 5: 386.
[30] Tolaymat A, Roque JL, Russo LS. Improvement of diabetic peripheral neuropathy with the portable insulin infusion pump. South Med J 1982; 75: 185.
[31] White NH, Waltman SR, Krupen T et al. Reversal of neuropathic and gastrointestinal complications related to diabetes mellitus in adolescents with improved metabolic control. J Pediatr 1981; 99: 41.
[32] Pirart J. Diabetic neuropathy: A metabolic or vascular disease? Diabetes 1965; 14: 1–9.
[33] Ellenberg M. Diabetic neuropathy: Clinical aspects. Metabolism 1976; 25: 1627–1655.
[34] Greene DA, Lattimer SA, Sima AAF. Perspectives in Diabetes: Are Disturbances of Sorbitol, Phosphoinositide, and Na^+-K^+-ATPase Regulation Involved in Pathogenesis of Diabetic Neuropathy? Diabetes 1988; 37: 688–693.
[35] Greene DA, Chakrabarti S, Lattimer SA et al. Role of sorbitol accumulation and myo-inositol depletion in paranodal swelling of large myelinated nerve fibers in the insulin-deficient spontaneously diabetic bio-breeding rat: Reversal by insulin replacement, an aldose reductase inhibitor and myo-inositol. J Clin Invest 1987; 79: 1479–1485.
[36] Greene DA, DeJesus PV, Winegrad AI. Effects of insulin and dietary myo-inositol on impaired peripheral motor nerve conduction velocity in acute streptozotocin diabetes. J Clin Invest 1975; 5: 1326.
[37] Jakobsen J. Early and preventable changes of peripheral nerve structure and function in insulin deficient diabetic rats. J Neurol Neurosurg Psychiatry 1979; 42: 509.
[38] Robertson DM, Sima AAF. Diabetic neuropathy in the mutant mouse [C57/BL/Ks (db/db)]. A morphometric study. Diabetes 1980: 25: 60.
[39] Tomlinson DR, Mayer JH. Reversal of deficits in axonal transport and nerve conduction velocity by treatment of streptozotocin diabetic rats with myo-inositol. Exp Neurol 1985; 89; 420.
[40] Mayer JH, Tomlinson DR. Prevention of defects of axonal transport and nerve conduction velocity by oral administration of myo-inositol or an aldose reductase inhibitor in streptozotocin-diabetic rats. Diabetologia 1983; 25: 433.
[41] Sharma AK, Thomas PK. Peripheral nerve structure and function in experimental diabetes. J Neurol Sci 1974; 23: 1.
[42] Brown MJ, Sumner AJ, Greene DA et al. Distal neuropathy in experimental diabetes mellitus. Ann Neurol 1980; 8: 118.
[43] Greene DA, Lattimer S, Ulbrecht J et al. Glucose-induced alterations in nerve metabolism: Current perspective on the pathogenesis of diabetic neuropathy and future directions for research and therapy. Diabetes Care 1985; 8: 290–299.

[44] Greene DA, Lattimer SA, Sima AAF. Sorbitol, phosphoinositides, and sodium potassium-ATPase in the pathogenesis of diabetic complications. New Engl J Med 1987; 316: 599–606.
[45] Clements RS. Diabetic neuropathy: new concepts of its etiology. Diabetes 1979: 28: 604.
[46] Mayhew JA, Gillon KRW, Hawthorne JN. Free and lipid inositol, sorbitol and sugars obtained post mortem from diabetic and control subjects. Diabetologia 1983; 24: 13–15.
[47] Ward JD, Baker RWR, Davis BH. Effect of blood sugar control on the accumulation of sorbitol and fructose in nervous tissue. Diabetes 1972; 21: 1173.
[48] Greene DA, Bril V, Lattimer SA et al. Correction of myo-inositol depletion in diabetic human sural nerve by treatment with an aldose reductase inhibitor. Diabetes 1987; 36 (supple 1): 86 A.
[49] Dyck PJ, Zimmerman BR, Vilen TH et al. Nerve glucose, fructose, sorbitol, myo-inositol and fiber degeneration and regeneration in diabetic neuropathy. New Engl J Med 1988; 319: 542–548.
[50] Brown MJ, Iwamori M, Kishimoto Y et al. Nerve lipid abnormalities in human diabetic neuropathy: a correlative study. Ann Neurol 1979: 5: 245–252.
[51] Dyck PJ, Sherman WR, Hallcher LM et al. Human diabetic endoneurial sorbitol, fructose and myo-inositol related to sural nerve morphometry. Ann Neurol 1980; 8: 590–596.
[52] Dyck PJ, Lais A, Karnes JL et al. Fiber loss is primary and multifocal in sural nerves in diabetic polyneuropathy. Ann Neurol 1986; 19: 425–439.
[53] Williams E, Timperley WR, Ward JD et al. Electron microscopic studies of vessels in diabetic peripheral neuropathy. J Clin Pathol 1980; 33: 462–470.
[54] Johnson PC, Doll SC, Cromey DW. Pathogenesis of diabetic neuropathy. Ann Neurol 1986; 19: 450–457.
[55] Vracko R. A comparison of the microvascular lesions in diabetes mellitus with those of normal aging. J Am Geriatr Soc 1982; 30: 201–205.
[56] Yasuda H, Dyck PJ. Abnormalities of endoneurial microvessels and sural nerve pathology in diabetic neuropathy. Neurology 1987; 37: 20–28.
[57] Dyck PJ, Karnes JL, O'Brien P et al. The spatial distribution of fiber loss in diabetic polyneuropathy suggests ischemia. Ann Neurol 1986; 19: 440–449.
[58] Fagerberg SE. Diabetic neuropathy, a clinical and histological study on the significance of vascular affection. Acta Med Scand 1959; 164: 1–97.
[59] Low PA, Tuck RR, Takeuchi M. Nerve micro-environment in diabetic neuropathy. In: Dyck PJ, Thomas PK, Asbury AK et al, eds. Diabetic Neuropathy. Philadelphia: WB Saunders, 1987; 266–278.
[60] Low PA, Schmelzer JD, Ward KK. The effects of endoneurial hypoxia on peripheral nerve function. Neurology 1985; 35: 292, Abstract.
[61] Low PA, Schmelzer JD, Ward KK et al. Experimental chronic hypoxic neuropathy: relevance to diabetic neuropathy. Am J Physiol 1986; 250: E 94–99.
[62] Low PA, Schmelzer JD, Ward KK et al. Effects of hyperbaric oxygenation on normal and chronic streptozotocin diabetic peripheral nerve. Neurology 1987; 27: 254, Abstract.
[63] Low PA, Tuck RR, Dyck PJ et al. Prevention of some electrophysiologic and biochemical abnormalities with oxygen supplementation in experimental diabetic neuropathy. Proc Natl Acad Sci USA 1984; 81: 6894–6898.
[64] Yao JK, Low PA. Improvement of endoneurial lipid abnormalities in experimental diabetic neuropathy by oxygen modification. Brain Res 1986; 362: 362–365.
[65] Newrick PG, Wilson AJ, Jakubowski J et al. Sural nerve oxygen tension in diabetes. Br Med J (Clin Res) 1986; 293: 1053–1054.
[66] Williams SK, Howarth NL, Devenny JJ et al. Structural and functional consequence of increased tubulin glycosylation in diabetes mellitus. Proc Natl Acad Sci USA 1982; 79: 6546–6550.
[67] Brownlee M, Cerami A, Vlassara H. Advanced glycosylation end products in tissue and the biochemical basis of diabetic complications. New Engl J Med 1988; 318: 1315–1321.

[68] Vlassara H, Brownlee M, Cerami A. Recognition and uptake of human diabetic peripheral nerve myelin by macrophages. Diabetes 1985; 34: 553–557.
[69] Sharma AK, Duguid IGM, Blanchard DS et al. The effect of insulin treatment of myelinated nerve fiber maturation and integrity on body growth in streptozotocin-diabetic rats. J Neurol Sci 1985; 67: 285.
[70] Sharma AK, Bajada S, Thomase PK. Influence of streptozotocin induced diabetes on myelinated nerve fiber maturation and on body growth in the rat. Acta Neuropath (Berl) 1981; 53: 257.
[71] Greene DA, Mackway AM. Decreased myo-inositol content and Na^+-K^+ATPase activity in the superior cervical ganglion of STZ diabetic rat, and prevention by aldose reductase inhibition. Diabetes 1986; 35: 1106.
[72] Thomas PK, Wright DW, Tzebelikos E. Amino acid uptake by dorsal root ganglia from streptozotocin-diabetic rat. J Neurol Neurosurg Psychiatry 1984; 47: 912.
[73] Medori R, Antilio-Gambetti L, Monaco S et al. Experimental diabetic neuropathy: impairment of slow transport with changes in axon cross-sectioned area. Proc Natl Acad Sci USA 1985; 82: 7716.
[74] McLean WG, Meiri KF. Slow axonal transport of protein in sciatic motor nerves during early experimental diabetes. J Physiol 1980; 301: 57 P.
[75] Sima AAF. Neuropathic and ocular complications in the BB-Wistar rat. In: Shafrir E, Renold AE, eds. Lessons from Animal Diabetes. London: John Libbey, 1984; 447.
[76] Sima AAF. Peripheral neuropathy in the spontaneously diabetic BB-Wistar rat. An ultrastructural study. Acta Neuropath (Berl) 1980; 51: 223.
[77] Spencer PS, Thomas PK. Ultrastructural studies on the dying-back process. II. The sequestration and removal by Schwann cells and oligodendrocytes of organelles from normal and diseased axons. J Neurocytol 1979; 3: 763.
[78] Medori R, Gambetti P, personal communication.
[79] Jakobsen J, Sidenius P. Decreased axonal transport of structural proteins in streptozotocin diabetic rats. J Clin Invest 1980; 66: 292.
[80] Masiori P, Vitadello M, Bianchi et al. Impaired axonal transport of acetylcholinesterase in the sciatic nerve of alloxan-diabetic rats: effect of ganglioside treatment. Diabetologia 1986; 29: 254.
[81] Mayer JH, Tomlinson DR. Axonal transport of cholinergic transmitter enzymes in vagus and sciatic nerves of rats with acute experimental diabetes mellitus: correlation with motor nerve conduction velocity and effects of insulin. Neuroscience 1983; 9: 951.
[82] Vitadello M, Couraud J-Y, Hassig R et al. Axonal transport of acetylcholinesterase in the diabetic mutant mouse. Exp Neurol 1983; 82: 143.
[83] Vitadello M, Filliatreau G, Dupont JL et al. Altered axonal transport of cytoskeletal proteins in the mutant diabetic mouse. J Neurochem 1985; 45: 860.
[84] Jakobsen J, Brimijoin S, Skan K et al. Retrograde axonal transport of transmitter enzymes, fucose-labeled protein and nerve growth factor in streptozotocin-diabetic rats. Diabetes 1981; 30: 797.
[85] Schmidt RE, Modert CW, Yip HK et al. Retrograde axonal transport of intravenously administered ^{125}I-nerve growth factor in rats with streptozotocin-induced diabetes. Diabetes 1983; 32: 654.
[86] Calker DV, Heumann R. Nerve growth factor potentiates the agonist-stimulated accumulation of inositol phosphates in PC-12 pheochromocytoma cells. European J Pharm 1987; 135: 259.
[87] Contreras ML, Guroff G. Calcium-dependent nerve growth factor-stimulated hydrolysis of phosphoinositides in PC12 cells. J Neurochem 1987; 48: 1466.
[88] Ishii DN, Recio-Pinto E. Role of insulin, insulin-like growth factors, and nerve growth factor in neurite formation. In: Raizada MK, Phillips MI, LeRoith D, eds. Insulin, IGF's and Their Receptors in the Central Nervous System. New York: Plenum Pub., 1987; 315.

[89] Longo FM, Powell HC, Lebeau J et al. Delayed nerve regeneration in streptozotocin diabetic rats. Muscle and Nerve 1986; 9: 385.
[90] Chan K-FJ. Ganglioside-modulated protein phosphorylation in myelin. J Biol Chem 1987; 262: 2415.
[91] American Diabetes Association. Report and recommendations of the San Antonio conference on diabetic neuropathy. Diabetes 1988: 37(7): 1000 – 1004.
[92] The DCCT Research Group. Factors in the development of diabetic neuropathy: baseline analysis of neuropathy in the feasibility phase of the Diabetes Control and Complications Trial (DCCT). Diabetes 1988; 37: 476 – 481.
[93] Gadia MT, Natori N, Ramos LB et al. Influence of height on quantitative sensory, nerve conduction, and clinical indices of diabetic peripheral neuropathy. Diabetes Care 1987; 10: 613 – 616.
[94] Brown MJ, Greene DA. Diabetic Neuropathy: Pathophysiology and Management. In: Asbury AK, Gilliat RW, eds. Neurology, Peripheral Nerve Disorders: A Pracital Approach. Boston: Butterworths, 1984; 126.
[95] Levy DM, Abraham RR, Abraham RM. Small- and large-fiber involvement in early diabetic neuropathy: a study with the medial plantar response and sensory thresholds. Diabetes Care 1987; 10: 441 – 447.
[96] Eliasson SG. Nerve conduction changes in experimental diabetes. J Clin Invest 1964; 43: 2353.
[97] Sima AAF, Bril V, Nathaniel V et al. Regeneration and repair of myelinated fibers in sural nerve biopsy specimens from patients with diabetic neuropathy treated with sorbinil. New Engl J Med 1988; 319: 548 – 555.
[98] Brown MJ, Martin JR, Asbury AK. Painful diabetic neuropathy. A morphometric study. Arch Neurol 1976; 33: 164 – 171.
[99] Davis JL, Lewis SB, Gerich JE et al. Peripheral diabetic neuropathy treated with amitriptyline and fluphenazine. J Amer Med Assn 1977; 238: 2291 – 2292.
[100] Saudek CD, Werns S, Reidenberg MM. Phenytoin in the treatment of diabetic symmetrical polyneuropathy. Clin Pharm Therapeut 1977; 22: 196 – 199.
[101] Rull JA, Quibrera R, Gonzalez-Millan H et al. Symptomatic treatment of peripheral diabetic neuropathy with carbamazine (Tegretol): double blind crossover trial. Diabetologia 1969; 5: 215 – 218.
[102] Young RJ, Clarke BF. Pain relief in diabetic neuropathy: the effectiveness of imipramine and related drugs. Diabetic Medicine 1985; 2: 262 – 266.
[103] Turkington RW. Depression masquerading as diabetic neuropathy. J Amer Med Assn 1980; 243: 1147 – 1150.
[104] Ellenberg M. Diabetic neuropathic chachexia. Diabetes 1974; 23: 5 – 9.
[105] Sinha S, Munichoodappa CS, Kozak GP. Neuro-arthropathy (Charcot joints) in diabetes mellitus: clinical study of 101 cases. Medicine 1972; 51: 191 – 210.
[106] Ellenberg M. Sexual function in diabetic patients. Ann Intern Med 1980; 92; 331.
[107] Walters D, Kaufman MS. Sterility due to retrograde ejaculation of semen: report of pregnancy achieved by autoinsemination. Am J Obstet Gynecol 1959; 78: 274 – 275.
[108] Hosking DJ, Bennett T, Hampton JR. Diabetic autonomic neuropathy. Diabetes 1978; 27: 1043 – 1054.
[109] Andaloro VA, Dube A. Treatment of retrograde ejaculation with brompheniramine. Urology 1975; 5: 520 – 522.
[110] Budd HA. Brompheniramine in treatment of retrograde ejaculation. Urology 1975; 6: 131.
[111] Peterson HP, Best JD, Berger R et al. Attitudes of diabetic men after implantation of semirigid penile prostheses. Diabetic Care 1985; 8: 156.
[112] Robertson D, Goldberg MR, Hollister AS et al. Clonidine raises blood pressure in severe idiopathic orthostatic hypotension. Am J Med 1983; 74: 193.
[113] Robertson D, Wade D. Management of severe idiopathic orthostatic hypotension with phenylephrine nasal spray. Clin Res 1980; 92: 308.

[114] Boulton AJM, Atiea J, De Leeuw IH et al. The efficacy and safety of the aldose-reductase inhibitor tolrestat in the treatment of chronic sensorimotor diabetic neuropathy. 25th Annual Meeting of the European Association for the Study of Diabetes. EASD Abstracts 1989; 469 A.
[115] The Sorbinil Neuropathy Group. Clinical response to Sorbinil treatment in diabetic neuropathy. Diabetes 1989; 38: 14 A.
[116] Greene DA, Porte D, Bril V et al. Clinical response to sorbinil treatment in diabetic neuropathy. EASD Abstracts 1989; 493 A.
[117] Jaspan J, Malone J, Nikolai T et al. Clinical response to Sorbinil (S) in painful diabetic neuropathy (DN). Diabetes 1989; 38: 14 A.
[118] Judzewitsch RG, Jaspan JB, Polonsky KS et al. Aldose reductase inhibition improves nerve conduction velocity in diabetic patients. N Engl J Med 1983; 308: 119.
[119] Jaspan J, Maselli R, Herold et al. Treatment of severely painful diabetic neuropathy with an aldose reductase inhibitor: relief of pain and improved somatic and autonomic nerve function. Lancet 1983; 2: 758.
[120] Young RJ, Ewing DJ, Clarke BF. A controlled trial of sorbinil, an aldose reductase inhibitor, in chronic painful diabetic neuropathy. Diabetes 1983; 32: 938.
[121] Lewin IG, O'Brien IAD, Morgan MH et al. Clinical and neurophysiological studies with the aldose reductase inhibitor sorbinil in symptomatic diabetic neuropathy. Diabetologia 1984; 26: 445.
[122] Clements RS, Vourganti B, Kuba T et al. Dietary myo-inositol intake and peripheral nerve function in diabetic neuropathy. Metabolism 1979; 28: 477.
[123] Gregersen G, Bertelsen B, Harbo H et al. Oral supplementation of myo-inositol: effects on peripheral nerve function in human diabetics and on the concentration in plasma, erythrocytes, urine, and muscle tissue in human diabetics and normals. Acta Neurol Scand 1983; 67: 164.
[124] Gregersen G, Børsting H, Theil P et al. Myo-inositol and function of peripheral nerves in human diabetics. A controlled clinical trial. Acta Neurol 1978; 58: 241.
[125] Salway JG, Finnegan JA, Barnett D et al. Effect of myo-inositol on peripheral nerve function in diabetes. Lancet 1978; 2: 1282.
[126] Gregersen G. Myo-inositol supplementation. In: Dyck PJ, Asbury AK, Winegrad AI et al, eds. Diabetic Neuropathy. Philadelphia: WB Saunders, 1987; 188.
[127] Gorio A, Aporti F, Norido F. Gangliosides in treatment of experimental diabetic neuropathy. In: Rapport MM, Gorio A, eds. Gangliosides in Neurological and Neuromuscular Function, Development and Repair. New York: Raven Press, 1981.
[128] Norido F, Canella R, Gorio A. Ganglioside treatment of neuropathy in diabetic mice. Muscle Nerve 1982; 5: 107.
[129] Pozza G, Saibene V, Comi G et al. The effect of ganglioside administration in human diabetic peripheral neuropathy. In: Rapport MM, Gorio A, eds. Gangliosides in Neurological and Neuromuscular Function, Development and Repair. New York: Raven Press, 1981.
[130] Abraham RR, Abraham RM, Wynn V. A double-blind placebo controlled trial of mixed gangliosides in diabetic peripheral and autonomic neuropathy. In: Gangliosides Structure, Function, and Biomedical Potential. Adv Exp Med Biol 1984; 174: 607.
[131] Fedele D, Crepaldi G, Battistin L. Multicenter trial on gangliosides in diabetic peripheral neuropathy. In: Ganglioside Structure, Function, and Biomedical Potential. Adv Exp Med Biol 1984; 174: 601.
[132] Horowitz SH. Ganglioside (Cronassial) therapy in diabetic neuropath. In: Ganglioside Structure, Function, and Biomedical Potential. Avd Exp Med Biol 1984; 174: 593.
[133] Naarden A, Davidson J, Harris L et al. Treatment of painful diabetic polyneuropathy with mixed gangliosides. In: Ganglioside Structure, Function, and Biomedical Potential. Adv Exp Med Biol 1984; 174: 581.

[134] LeQuesne PM. Trophic factors and vitamin therapy. In: Dyck PJ, Thomas PK, Asbury AK et al. Diabetic Neuropathy. Philadelphia: WB Saunders, 1987; 194–198.
[135] LeQuesne PM, Fowler CJ, Harding AE. A study of the effects of isazonine on vincristine induced peripheral neuropathy in man and regeneration following peripheral nerve crush in the rat. J Neurol Neurosurg Psychiatry 1985; 48: 93.
[136] Thompson RHS. Biochemical aspects of diabetic neuropathy. In: Cumings JN, Kremer M, eds. Biochemical Aspects of Neurological Disorders, 2nd Series. Oxford: Blackwell, 1965.
[137] McCann VJ, Davis RF. Serum pyridoxal concentration in patients with diabetic neuropathy. Aust NZ J Med 1978; 8: 259.
[138] Levin ER, Hanscom TA, Fisher M et al. The influence of pyridoxine in diabetic peripheral neuropathy. Diabetes Care 1981; 4: 606.
[139] Jones CL, Gonzalez V. Pyridoxine deficiency: A new factor in diabetic neurology. J Am Podiatry Assoc 1978; 68: 646.
[140] McCann VJ, Davis RE. Pyridoxine and diabetic neuropathy: a double-blind controlled study. Diabetes Care 1983; 6: 102.
[141] Bhatt HR, Linnell JC, Matthews DM. Can faulty Vitamin B_{12} (cobalamin) metabolism produce diabetic neuropathy? Lancet 1983; 2: 57.
[142] Kikkawa R, Hatanaka I, Kobayashi N et al. The effect of aldose reductase inhibitor (sorbinil) and methylcobalamin on peripheral nerve disorders in streptozotocin-diabetic rats. In: Goto Y et al, eds. Diabetic Neuropathy. Amsterdam: Excerpta Medica, 1982.
[143] Tanaka N, Yamazaki Y, Sakato H et al. Relation of partial deficiency of cobalamins to occurrence of diabetic neuropathy. In: Goto Y et al, eds. Diabetic Neuropathy. Amsterdam: Excerpta Medica, 1982.
[144] Yamada K, Goto Y, Takebe K. Treatment of diabetic peripheral neuropathy with methylcobalamin. In: Goto Y et al, eds. Diabetic Neuropathy. Amsterdam: Excerpta Medica, 1982.
[145] Sancetta SM, Ayres PR, Scott RW. The use of Vitamin B_{12} in the management of the neurological manifestations of diabetes mellitus, with notes on the administration of massive doses. Ann Intern Med 1951; 35: 1028.

Typical infections in diabetes and their treatment

J. Larkin

Introduction

The spectre of infection no longer appears to hang over diabetes with its previous menace. Whereas in the 1920s, more than 20% of diabetic deaths could be directly attributed to infection [1], nowadays the emphasis falls on the "late" vascular complications – as witness the previous volume in this series. There is, however, an almost unique "synergism" between diabetes and infection. Poorly controlled diabetes predisposes to infection, and this in turn can alarmingly upset metabolic control. This tight vicious circle puts the patient at risk on two fronts, and infection remains a potentially life-threatening complication in diabetes, where early recognition and institution of therapy are of paramount importance.

The association of diabetes and infection

With the growing medical dependence on clinical trials and statistical data, the anecdotal presumption of a link between diabetes and infection has come under critical appraisal. There seems to be controversy still, but often this is due to the analysts' syntax rather than viewpoint. Thus in 1980, two separate monographs on diabetes stated that "the increased frequency of infection in the diabetic is well known" [2] and that "infections are no commoner in well-controlled diabetics than in non-diabetics" [3]. Both authors are probably correct, and close scrutiny of the literature reveals that the better the metabolic control of diabetes, the more closely the incidence of infection will resemble that of the normal population [4, 5]. Thus the incidence of urinary tract infection will be found to be increased in diabetics [6,7] but not in those with good glycaemic control [8]. Skin infections are also more common in poorly controlled diabetes [9] but not in patients with mild disease [10]. A significant correlation has been shown between overall prevalence of infection and mean plasma glucose while uninfected [11].

Asymptomatic colonisation of the urinary tract [8], the nasal mucosa [12] and of the mouth (Candida) [13] seems to occur independently of glycaemic control. Such studies may exhibit positive-selection by studying patients at clinics. Boyko et al [14] failed to confirm increased nasal carriage when using other recruitment methods, and this may suggest that even colonisation is dependent on the severity of diabetes.

It is appealing to consider that colonisation may progress to clinical infection if poor control reduces the host's immunological defences. Acidosis has been shown to produce a reversible defect in phagocytic migration [15] and phagocytosis itself [16]. Intracellular bactericidal activity to S. aureus and E. coli is inversely related to glycaemic control [11], while antibody production [17] and cell mediated immunity [18] can be shown to vary with glucose levels. The immunological deficiencies are clearly not a problem only of long-duration diabetes as patients with newly-diagnosed disease may present with a fatal infection [19].

The trend for questioning long-held beliefs in medicine continues, but the "myths" often turn out to be true. Poorly controlled diabetes does predispose to infection. As prevention is proverbially better than cure, it follows that the first principle of treating infection in diabetes should be the pursuit of tight control of blood glucose concentrations in all diabetic patients.

General management of infections in diabetes

The "stress" response to infection seems specifically designed to upset glycaemic control. Plasma concentrations of the insulin-antagonistic hormones cortisol, ACTH, glucagon and growth hormone are all increased [20, 21]. Adrenergic production of catecholamines further increases the likelihood of hyperglycaemia and ketogenesis, while the general catabolic response to infection, with loss of body nitrogen and potassium, adds to the metabolic upset.

As a consequence of the above, insulin requirements during infection may be increased by at least 30% [21] – a well-known educational point for the patient, who often stops his insulin because of vomiting or anorexia. Patients with NIDDM may require the temporary introduction of insulin, perhaps for as long as several months e.g. with chronic foot infections.

General management of mild to moderately severe infections is based on three principles [1]:

a) Monitoring of blood glucose – the introduction of stix-testing now makes this feasible even in patients managed at home. The lability of glycaemic control in infection makes it mandatory.

b) Maintenance of reasonable calorie intake – with liquid diet supplementation if required.

c) Continuation of normal insulin requirements in the first instance, with daily assessment for possible changes in dosage.

Varying the insulin regimen from bd to tds [1] – with 10% of morning medium-acting moved to the evening, and the short-acting split into three doses – may be useful. Most patients requiring such manipulations should be managed in hospital, where insulin dosage can be matched to blood sugars. Many with incipient ketoacidosis will require intra-venous insulin, fluid and calories. As with all cases of ketoacidosis, it is the frequent monitoring of blood sugar, potassium and clinical parameters allied to appropriate responses which is more important than rigid adherence to a preset regimen of treatment.

Antibiotic therapy should follow standard principles – obtaining specimens for microscopy and culture before commencing "best-guess" therapy based on knowledge of likely culpable organisms and their sensitivities (Table 1) [22]. Specific treatment may then be commenced according to results.

Table 1 Sensitivities of common organisms to standard antibiotics [22, 47]

Antibiotic	Sensitive	Variable	Notably resistant
Penicillin	1, 3, 5, 12	2, 6, (5)	7, 11
Ampi/amoxycillin	1–3, 5, 9, 12	6, 7, (5)	4
(+ clavulanate)	1–9, 11, 12		10
Cloxacillin	1, 3, 4, 5		2, 6, 7
Carbeni/ticarcillin	(1), 3, 5, 6, 9, (10)	7, 8, 11, 12	2, 4
Imipenem	1, 3–12	2	
2nd, 3rd generation cephalosporins	1, 3–9	10, 11, 12	2
Nalidixic acid	7, 8, 9		1–4, 10
Trimethoprim	1–4, 8	5–7	10–12
Cotrimoxazole	1–9		10–12
Clindamycin	1, 3, 4, 11, 12		2
Metronidazole	11, 12	7	
Chloramphenicol	1, 3–9, 11, 12	2	10
Aminoglycosides	3–10		1, 2, 11, 12
Nitrofurantoin	1–5, 7	8, 9	10
Ciprofloxacin	1–10	11	12

1. Strep. (pyogenes, pneumoniae)
2. Strep. faecalis
3. Staph. (penicillin sensitive)
4. Staph. (penicillin resistant)
5. Neisseria
6. H. influenzae
7. E. coli
8. Klebsiella
9. Proteus
10. Ps. aeruginosa
11. Bacteroides frag.
12. Other anaerobes

Table 2 Infections associated with diabetes

	Disease	Organism	% Associated with diabetes	Treatment	Mortality
Definite association	Mucormycosis	Mucoraceae fungus	Rhinocerebral 60 – 85% Others 20 – 30%	Radical surgery + amphoteracin B	15 – 50%
	Malignant external otitis media	Ps. aeruginosa	> 90%	Moderate surg. debridement + combination antibiotic	20%
	Emphysematous Pyelonephritis	Coliforms, Klebsiella	> 90%	Nephrectomy + antibiotic	20 – 32%
	Emphysematous Cholecystitis	Clostridia	38%	Cholecystectomy + antibiotic	25%
	Necrotising fasciitis	beta-haem Strep A (B) polymicrobial	50 – 75%	Extensive debridement + specific antibiotic	35% (12 – 60%) increased in DM
	Foot ulcer infections	Polymicrobial (Staph. Enterococc.)	?	Specific antibiotic often + surgery	?
Probable association	Candidiasis	Candida (albicans)	2 – 3 times normal incidence	Nystatin, Clotrimazole Amphoteracin B	–
	UTI	Coliforms + others	4 times normal incidence	Trimethoprim, short course amoxycillin	–
	Tuberculosis	Myco. tuberculosis	?	Rifampicin, isoniazid ethambutamol	?
Possible association	Furunculosis, Pneumonia (Klebsiella, Staph.), Influenza, Post-op sepsis, Periodontal disease, Histoplasmosis, Blastomycosis, Coccidiodomycosis.				

Specific infections

"Exclusive" to diabetes

The infections associated with diabetes are many and varied (Table 2). A few rare diseases occur almost exclusively in diabetic or otherwise immunocompromised hosts. These present difficult diagnostic and management problems, and I will deal with them first.

Mucormycosis

Mucormycosis is extremely rare in Northern Europe, but cases may arrive from Mediterranean countries or America [19]. It is an aggressive fungal infection caused, paradoxically, by organisms of the family Mucoraceae, often found in mouldy bread. In the past, almost all sufferers had diabetes mellitus, usually with ketoacidosis [23] but more recently patients with leukaemia and other immunocompromised subjects have developed the disease [24]. Rhinocerebral mucormycosis has maintained a more marked association with diabetes than other forms of the disease (e. g. pulmonary, cutaneous and disseminated) [24].

The classical presentation of rhinocerebral mucormycosis is of headache, facial pain and lethargy in a patient with slowly resolving ketoacidosis [25]. Examination (Fig. 1) may reveal cellulitis, bloodstained nasal discharge and on the palate a characteristic black eschar caused by haemorrhagic necrosis [26, 19]. The organism invades blood vessels, causing an arteritis. Facial nerve palsies, convulsions and hemiplegia may be late complications [19].

Mortality was greater than 90% [23] until the advent of combined radical surgery and amphoteracin B therapy. This has brought the survival rate to between 50% [27] and 85% [25], the latter perhaps being an overoptimistic estimate.

Confirmation of diagnosis is possible by direct microscopy of adequate biopsy samples (not nasal mucus!) showing the broad, sparsely-septate hyphae with right-angled branching of Rhizopus, Mucor or Absidia species. Treatment, however, should be initiated on clinical grounds alone. Survival may thus be improved, although the morbidity from the surgical procedures is often collosal.

Amphoteracin B remains the antifungal of choice, in vitro sensitivity testing being of little value. The lack of evidence for any efficacy of flucytosine, miconazole, clotrimazole and griseofulvin has been discussed by Wong & Armstrong [28]. They recommend a 1mg. test dose of amphoteracin B over one hour, followed by escalating doses of 5, 10, 20 and 40 mg. given at 6-hourly intervals as 4–6 hour infusions. Maintenance therapy of 1 $mgkg^{-1}$ daily is usually then possible. Fevers and chills should be preventable by antihistamines. Impairment of renal function may necessitate reduction of dosage if serum creatinine goes above 250 $umolL^{-1}$, while anaphylaxis following the test dose may require careful reintroduction of the drug at minimal dosing under intensive care facilities.

The above is a particularly aggressive approach, and successes have been achieved with more benign regimens when surgical debridement has appeared particularly successful [25]. The importance of prompt, aggressive surgical intervention and control of the underlying diabetes cannot be overstated, one mild case having responded to treatment of the ketoacidosis alone.

Recent attempts at improving survival include the use of hyperbaric oxygen to reduce tissue hypoxia and acidosis, and perhaps make use of its fungicidal action [29]. The largest series to date [30] avoided major toxicity using 100% oxygen at 2 ATA for 2 hour spells 12 hourly. The results in 6 patients, though

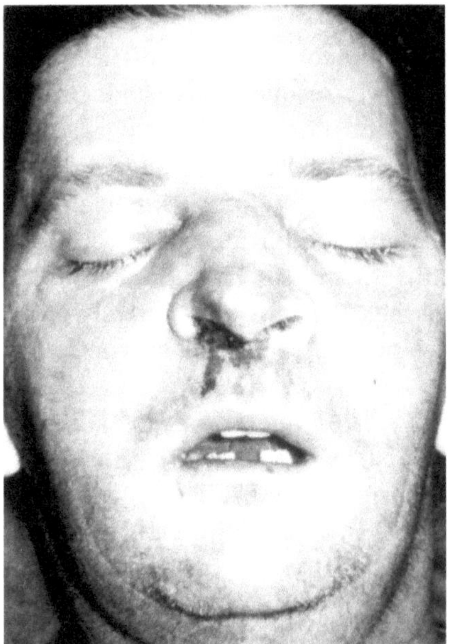

Fig. 1 Patient with rhinocerebral mucormycosis showing periorbital and perinasal swelling and discolouration, with bloodstained nasal discharge (and eschar on palate); courtesy John Wiley & Sons.

promising, were simply compared with historical controls and this modality remains experimental.

A mention should be made of pulmonary mucormycosis which classically presents as pulmonary infarction, though a more insidious onset is common [26]. Haemoptysis may be very severe. Chest radiograph shows patchy infiltration with consolidation and possible cavity formation. Treatment is with surgery (lobectomy or segmental resection) and amphoteracin B.

Malignant external otitis

Malignant external otitis is probably the most acceptable name [31] for this deep-seated ear infection, almost invariably caused by Pseudomonas aeruginosa, and almost exclusively occurring in diabetic patients. As with mucormycosis, the infection can spread directly or through the invasion of blood vessels causing extensive necrosis of cartilage, bone and soft tissues and also palsies of cranial nerves. The facial nerve is most commonly (50%) involved as it exits the stylomastoid foramen, but others may follow. These palsies may resolve with the disease, although their presence worsens prognosis [32]. Presentation is usually that of a chronic ear infection with pain (often unrelenting) and purulent discharge unresponsive to standard topical and oral therapy [33]. It is not well associated with ketoacidosis or poorly controlled diabetes, but a possible link with recent ear-irrigation procedures has been noted (Pseudomonas sp. may be present in tap water) [32]. Examination may reveal inappropriately extensive tenderness and swelling, particularly of the auricle itself, while the ear canal may feature granulation tissue or polyps.

Leucocytosis is unusual, and the only consistent laboratory abnormality is a raised Erythrocyte Sedimentation Rate, which may be useful for monitoring progress [32]. Conventional radiology may be late in showing soft tissue changes and boney erosions, while isotope scans are sensitive, but not specific. Computerised tomography is useful to define extent of disease, but lacks sensitivity for diagnostic purposes.

Aggressive surgical debridement was initially considered as mandatory in the treatment of the disease [31], but with combined use of an aminoglycoside and carbenicillin, local excision of granulation tissue with curettage of any abscess cavity has been found to be sufficient unless granulation recurs [32, 33].

The newer aminoglycosides such as tobramycin and amikacin may be preferred over gentamicin as they are respectively more active against Pseudomonas sp. and less likely to encounter resistant organisms. Nephrotoxicity and ototoxicity are also less likely with the newer drugs. Tobramycin is used in doses similar to gentamicin, dependent on age, weight and renal function. Typically, 1 – 3 mg/kg every 8 h. will produce appropriate blood levels. Peak concentrations > 12mg/l and trough levels > 2mg/l are more often associated with toxicity, the trough levels being the more important [34].

Similarly, the ureidopenicillins azlocillin (5 g 8-hourly or 300 mg/kg/day) and piperacillin (4 g 6-hourly or 300 mg/kg/day) should now be preferred to carbenicillin. Dosage of these drugs should be decreased (by increasing dosage intervals) if creatinine clearance is < 40 ml/min. Maximum dose of piperacillin for patients on dialysis is 6g. daily. If the patient is allergic to penicillins, ceftazidine or ciprofloxacin may be substituted.

Antibiotic therapy is recommended to last 4 – 8 weeks. Recent trials of the oral quinolone ciprofloxacin, possibly in combination with rifampicin [32] are very promising and may herald a further improvement in management.

Emphysematous pyelonephritis and cholecystitis

The serious implications of 'renal emphysema' were first noted in 1898 [35]. Having excluded trauma, surgery and fistulae, the main causes are emphysematous pyelonephritis and emphysematous pyelitis. The latter is associated with urinary obstruction, but the former, where gas is seen in the renal parenchyma on X-ray, is > 90% associated with diabetes mellitus [36].

The disease presents with nausea, vomiting, and abdominal or loin pain. Fever and localised tenderness over the affected kidney are very common (80%). Occasionally a tender mass may be palpable. There is usually a leucocytosis and a raised serum creatinine, while pyuria is present in 95 – 100% of cases. Culture of urine will often grow gas-forming coliforms (63% of cases have E. coli [36]) but other organisms, including Klebsiella, have been reported.

Plain radiography of the abdomen will usually give the diagnosis, but CT-scan should follow a "negative" X-ray if clinical suspicion is present [37]. Intravenous or retrograde pyelograms may be useful to delineate any obstruction, but the risks in dehydrated diabetic patients need to be considered. Ultrasound is rarely useful.

Many patients will require nephrectomy, but much can be said for assessing the extent of the disease with computerised tomography, and treating with drainage, appropriate I – V antibiotics and management of the diabetes in the initial phase. The necessity for nephrectomy can then be assessed [37]. Initial antibiotics should include an aminoglycoside, and possibly clindamycin, but definitive therapy may be based on urine and blood cultures. Mortality from this disaease is 20 – 30%. Early diagnosis is essential, and must be suspected in diabetic patients with tardy improvement of UTI or pyelonephritis.

Emphysematous cholecystitis, characterised by gas in the gall bladder lumen or wall, is a rare disease which may present as an acute abdomen with pneumoperitoneum [38]. More commonly, symptoms will be similar to those of conventional cholecystitis with right upper quadrant pain, fever and leucocytosis. Males are more commonly affected than females. Approximately half of cases are caused by Clostridia species and treatment is with intravenous antibiotics (initially broad-spectrum + anti-Clostridia) and early cholecystectomy, though the use of a defunctioning cholecystostomy has been suggested. Mortality remains around 15% [39].

Necrotising fasciitis

The terminology of this potentially lethal infection has long raised difficulties. "Meleney's Gangrene" was first described in 1924 [40], but Fournier gave an earlier account (1883) [41] of a fulminating gangrene of the genitalia, and his name still applies to similar disease in the perineum. Necrotising fasciitis is an aggressive infection of the fascial planes under the skin which may be caused by a single organism (usually beta-haemolytic streptococcus group A) or mixed anaerobes (Bacteroides) and facultative anaerobes (Enterobacteracea, non-A Streptococcus) [42]. "Synergistic necrotising cellulitis" is caused by aerobic and anaerobic organisms (eg Enterobacteraceae and Clostridia) and is a slower process which invades muscle as well as fascial planes. Necrotising fasciitis may be acute and fulminating, or follow a subacute course where the prognosis is improved. Histologically, inflammation, patchy necrosis and haemorrhage are present in both, with intravascular thrombi more prominent in the fulminant cases [43].

The patient may present after a minor injury, burn, insect bite or surgical procedure with swollen, red tender skin. Pain may be prominent, but is not universal. As the underlying subcutaneous necrosis progresses, the skin becomes dusky, usually anaesthetic, with blue-grey patches and fluid-filled blisters [44]. Systemic illness supervenes after 4–7 days as the affected area becomes gangrenous and later suppurative. Crepitus is usually [44] but not always [45] absent. Radiography, particularly CT scanning, may show gas in the soft tissues. Incisional biopsy plus frozen section may give a quick diagnosis and reduce mortality [46].

At surgery, a blunt probe will often go easily between tissue planes, undermining the skin. This sign is an indication for extensive debridement using several long incisions [42]. Intravenous antibiotics should be commenced before bacteriological culture and sensitivities are available, but should then be altered according to this information, penicillin G often being introduced once Streptococcus is identified. Suggestions for initial therapy vary. Clindamycin alone covers most of the usual organisms [42, 47] but combinations include an aminoglycoside plus either chloramphenicol [42] or metronidazole and a cephalosporin [45]. Hyperbaric oxygen has not been shown to help. Mortality remains around 30% and is higher in diabetic patients (> 50%). A dubious link has been suggested between a fulminant course and the use of non-steroidal anti-inflammatories [48] but it seems more likely that early antibiotic use by the General Practioner may predispose to the more chronic course.

The most important factor affecting prognosis in these rare, potentially fatal infections, is awareness. Any diabetic patient with an unexplained illness, or slow recovery from infection or ketoacidosis, should be carefully appraised with these diseases in mind. Combined management from medical, surgical and bacteriological teams is required to institute a) control of diabetes b) full debridement and c) appropriate, aggressive antimicrobial therapy.

Common infections

Foot infections

There are many reasons why the diabetic foot should be particularly susceptible to infection. Autonomic and peripheral nerve dysfunction may make it dry and prone to injury, while poor vascular supply delays healing. The infection may progress from a foot ulcer to cellulitis, osteomyelitis, necrotising fasciitis or abscess. More than 30% of diabetic hospital admissions may be due to foot infections.

Specimens for culture should be taken from the depths of the infection, avoiding contamination from the ulcer or other open lesions, as superficial organisms will only identify with those from deep sources in 25% of cases [49]. A bone biopsy, however, may not be advisable to exclude osteomyelitis when clinical findings are equivocal. Untainted specimens are difficult to obtain, and osteomyelitis may be precipitated when not already present. It is better to repeat X-ray examination after two weeks, while continuing antibiotic therapy.

Staphylococcus is the most common organism (60%) but most infections are polymicrobial (70%). Aerobes include Streptococcus, Proteus, Klebsiella and Serratia, while Peptostreptococcus and Bacteroides are the main anaerobes. Antibiotic therapy thus depends on results from appropriate cultures.

For "best-guess" therapy, Wheat [49] suggests cefoxitin or latamoxef (Moxalactam) for mild to moderate disease, and cefoxitin, ampicillin (vs. enterococcus) and an aminoglycoside for severe infections. The new carbapenem penicillin, imipenem sodium (I–V 1–2 g daily in 3–4 doses) has an impressive range of sensitivities and covers all the likely bacteria [49]. The exciting potential of this drug is threatened by indiscriminate use, but these infections may be a genuine indication, particularly if there are any contraindications to other regimens.

Surgical debridement is often important in diabetic foot infections. Amputation is required in a surprising number of cases, up to half of those requiring admission. Scher and Steele [50] recently reviewed their experience of 65 amputations for infection, usually following a plantar ulcer. Partial and total ("Guillotine transmalleolar") foot amputations were successful in a significant number of patients, with below-knee amputation a satisfactory fall-back procedure. Open stumps healed more quickly than closed.

Infection of the diabetic foot covers a wide spectrum of disease. Patients need to be alerted to the importance of foot care, and the need to seek specialist attention at the earliest stage of any foot injuries or ulcers.

Candidiasis

Infection with Candida species ("thrush", "moniliasis"), both oral and vaginal, has long been associated with diabetes [7, 11]. It is a common presentation of the disease, and exclusion of diabetes is mandatory in any patient with recurrent problems. Oral colonisation with Candida may occur in up to 50% of the normal population, but a recent survey [13] confirmed a marked increase in diabetics (75%) vs. matched controls (35%). This did not appear to relate to glucose control, but the situation with invasive disease may differ.

Most patients with oral candidiasis have the 'pseudomembranous' form with painless curdlike plaques, and occasionally painful inflammation at the angle of the mouth. Vaginal thrush may present with pruritis and discharge, sometimes with pain on micturition or intercourse. There may be an erythematous rash on the surrounding perineum, or even discrete pustules on the inner thighs. Males may develope circinate balanitis, and bladder invasion can occasionally occur following catheterisation.

Candida is sensitive to most antifungals. Appropriate treatment for oral thrush is nystatin suspension, though amphoteracin lozenges may be useful. More severe infections, involving the pharynx or oesophagus may respond to oral fluconazole. Vaginal thrush also responds to nystatin, best used as a pessary on fourteen consecutive nights. Clotrimazole has the advantage of requiring a shorter course – either of three daily doses or a single 500 mg vaginal pessary – but is more expensive. Systemic candidiasis is rare and requires intravenous amphoteracin B. Dosage requirements of this drug may be reduced by adding flucytosine. Bladder thrush may respond to daily irrigation with amphoteracin B 50 ug/l for five days [51].

Recurrence of Candidal infection is common in diabetic patients. The suggested importance of excess glucose for growth of the fungus is debatable, but avoidance of glycosuria may help deter infection. Antibiotics for minor infections should be as narrow-spectrum as possible to minimise overgrowth of yeast colonisation.

Urinary tract infection (UTI)

Reasons for frequent UTIs in diabetic patients include increased exposure to catheterisation (now reduced) and an insensitive and poorly functioning neurogenic bladder. Review of clinical and post-mortem studies suggests an increased incidence [7] and an increased frequency of asymptomatic bacteruria has been recently confirmed [52]. Most UTIs still respond to amoxycillin or cotrimoxazole. Risk of Candidal overgrowth might be lessened by substituting trimethoprim for cotrimoxazole, or using single dose amoxycillin (3 g) which is as effective as conventional therapy of UTI, but not of pyelonephritis [53]. Other options include nitrofurantoin and nalidixic acid which reaches effective concentrations only in the urine. A recent survey linked UTI with spermicide and diaphragm use, and blamed early relapses on a vaginal reservoir [53]. Treating asymptomatic bacteruria is often frowned upon, but a good case can be made for this in diabetic patients. Chronic therapy e.g. with trimethoprim may also be considered in those patients particularly susceptible to recurrence.

Other infections

Other infections purported to be associated with diabetes range from simple periodontal disease [54] to potentially serious post- operative infections [55, 56]. Some pneumonias (e.g. Klebsiella) may be more common, but pneumococcus does not appear to be so [4]. A tendency to more severe disease, however, may indicate a use for vaccination [57] although the efficacy of other vaccines is reduced in diabetes [58].

Antibiotics: toxicity and interactions

The details of administration and possible toxic effects of any unfamiliar drug should always be checked before commencing therapy. Predictable and idiosyncratic reactions to antibiotics have recently been reviewed [59]. Of the drugs mentioned in this chapter, the penicillins will most often cause hypersensitivity reactions, ranging from simple rash and fever to bronchospasm, vasculitis or anaphylaxis. There is cross-reactivity with all of the penicillins, which should be remembered when considering such drugs as imipenem or carbenicillin. Ten percent of these patients will also be hypersensitive to cephalosporins. Amongst the penicillins, ampicillin is particularly likely to cause diarrhoea (amoxycillin may not). Carbenicillin occasionally causes platelet dysfunction, and a bleeding tendency can also occur with the cephalosporin latamoxef, where low prothrombin and platelets may coincide.

The ototoxicity and nephrotoxicity of aminoglycosides are caused by accumulation damage to the cochlear sensory cells and proximal tubule cells respectively. Since back-diffusion is facilitated by low trough levels, it is failure of these to go below e.g. 2 mg/l for gentamicin which predisposes to tissue damage. The renal problems are usually reversible, but the hearing loss is often permanent [34]. Both problems are less common with tobramycin or amikacin than with gentamicin. These drugs may also cause neuromuscular blockade, and should be avoided in myasthenia gravis. They should also be avoided in pregnancy as they can injure the eighth cranial nerve of the foetus.

Chloramphenicol may supress marrow function in a dose-dependent fashion or cause idiosyncratic aplastic anaemia. The latter is rare (1:30,000) and does not preclude the use of the drug in serious infections. Other drugs to cover anaerobic organisms include metronidazole which may cause a dose-dependent peripheral neuropathy, and clindamycin which has fallen from grace because of a significant incidence of pseudomembranous colitis. While this potentially serious condition, caused by Clostridium difficile, is also associated with other antibiotics – including tetracycline and ampicillin – the link with clindamycin and lincomycin is most obvious. Most cases respond to vancomycin or metronidazole, but avoidance of clindamycin is suggested where options exist.

Ciprofloxacin often causes diarrhoea, as do the other quinolones. Convulsions have also been reported and the drug is not advised in pregnancy. Nitrofurantoin and nalidixic acid can both cause false positive glycosuria (if testing is for reducing substances) but this should rarely present a problem as should the frequently quoted inhibitory interaction between the two [22].

Table 3 *Drug interactions with antibiotics*

Antibiotic	Other drug	Type of interaction	Effect
Aminoglycosides	Amphoteracin B Cephalosporins	Additive	Increased nephrotoxicity
	Diuretics	Decreased excretion	Increased nephro/ototoxicity
Amphoteracin B	Steroids	Additive	Hypokalaemia
	Digoxin	Hypokalaemia	Digoxin toxicity
Cephalosporins	Oral contraceptive	Intestinal hurry Decreased deconjugation	Contraceptive failure
Chloramphenicol	Sulphonyl ureas	Enzyme inhibition	Hypoglycaemia
	Warfarin	Enzyme inhibition	Overanticoagulation
	Anticonvulsants	Opposing enzyme effects	Anticonvulsant toxicity or antibiotic failure
Ciprofloxacin	Theophylline	Enzyme inhibition	Theophylline toxicity
Erythromycin	Anticonvulsants Digoxin Theophylline Warfarin	Enzyme inhibition	Toxicity of other drug
Metronidazole	Anticonvulsants Warfarin	Enzyme inhibition	Toxicity of other drug
Penicillins	Oral contraceptive	Decreased deconjugation	Contraceptive failure
Rifampicin	Antacids	Decreased absorption	Antibiotic failure
	Chloramphenicol Ketoconazole Oral contraceptive Anticonvulsants Steroids, Digoxin Theophylline, Warfarin	Enzyme induction	Decreased effect of other drug

Rare acute reactions to the former include a pneumonitis, while in the longer term a sensorimotor neuropathy may occur [22].

Drug 'interactions' involving antibiotics resemble those of other drug groups. Most follow logically from knowledge of the drugs' basic pharmacology. Enzyme inducers (e.g. rifampicin) will decrease the activity of the same lipid-soluble drugs (chloramphenicol, oral contraceptives, anticonvulsants, theophylline, warfarin) as will have their actions enhanced by enzyme inhibitors (chloramphenicol, erythromycin, metronidazole). Recently a marked increase in theophylline concentrations has been shown in patients given ciprofloxacin. Drugs causing intestinal hurry (penicillins, cephalosporins, quinolones) may decrease others' absorption, while some (particularly ampicillin) may specifically inhibit deconjugation of hormones by bacteria, decreasing enterohepatic recirculation and causing failure of the contraceptive pill. Exhaustive lists of interactions can be found elsewhere [59] but the main ones relevant to this chapter are found in Table 3.

The future

Hopefully, as glycaemic control in the diabetic population continues to improve, the incidence of infection will also continue to decrease. Home glucose monitoring is enhancing this trend, while the effect of other innovations, such as insulin infusion pumps, is yet to be assessed. No doubt technological advances will also bring new problems – a recent case of resistent peritonitis caused by Serratia in a diabetic patient on chronic ambulatory peritoneal dialysis [60] is unlikely to be the last such novelty.

Newer antibiotics such as ciprofloxacin and imipenem may further improve 'best-guess' therapy, but their future usefulness depends on a degree of propriety in their use today. In the meantime, the important thing is to be aware of the possibility of infection in any ill diabetic patient and to be ready to take swift and appropriate action.

References

[1] Alberti KGMM, Hockaday TDR. Diabetes Mellitus. In: Weatherall DJ, Ledingham JGG, Warrell DA, eds. Oxford Textbook of Medicine. Oxford, New York, Toronto: Oxford Univ. Press, 1983; 9.38–9.39.

[2] Galloway JA. Chronic complications of diabetes. In: Diabetes Mellitus, 8th edition. Indianapolis, Indiana USA: Lilly Research Labs, 1980.

[3] Ireland JT. Chapter 7. Diabetic Coma, Ketoacidosis and other forms of severe metabolic decompensation including lactic acidosis and hyperosmolar states. In: Ireland JT, Thomson

WST, Williamson J, eds. Diabetes today. Aylesbury, England: HM+M publications, 1980; 84–104.
[4] Casey JI. Host defense and infections in diabetes mellitus. In: Ellenburg M, Rifkin H, eds. 3rd edition. New York: Medical Examination Publishing Co, 1983; 667–678.
[5] Larkin JG, Frier BM, Ireland JT. Diabetes and Infection. Postgrad Med J 1985; 61: 233–237.
[6] Robbins SL, Tucker AW. The cause of death in diabetes, a report of 307 cases. New Eng J Med 1944; 231: 865–868.
[7] Wheat LJ. Infection and diabetes mellitus. Diabetes Care 1980; 3: 187–197.
[8] Sjucs S, Cserhati I, Csapo G et al. The relation between diabetes mellitus and infections of the urinary tract. Am J Med Sciences 1960; 240: 186–191.
[9] Farrer SM, MacLeod CM. Staphylococcal infections in a general hospital. Am J Hygiene 1960; 72: 38–58.
[10] Welborn TA, Curnous DH, Wearne JT et al. Diabetes detected by blood sugar measurements after a glucose load. Med J Australia 1968; 2: 778–786.
[11] Rayfield EJ, Ault MJ, Kensch GT et al. Infection and diabetes: the case for glucose control. Am J Medicine 1982; 72: 439–450.
[12] Smith JA, O'Connor JJ, Willis AT. Nasal carriage of Staphylococcus aureus in diabetes mellitus. Lancet 1966; II: 776- 777.
[13] Bartholomew GA, Rodu B, Bell DS. Oral candidiasis in patients with diabetes mellitus: a thorough analysis. Diabetes Care 1987; 10: 607–612.
[14] Boyko EJ, Lipsky BA, Sandoval R et al. NIDDM and prevalence of nasal Staphylococcus aureus colonisation. Diabetes Care 1989; 12: 189–192.
[15] Perillie PE, Nolan JP, Finch SC. Studies of the resistance to infection in diabetes mellitus: local exhudative cellular response. J Lab Clin Medicine 1962; 59: 1008–1015.
[16] Bybee JD, Rogers DE. The phagocytic activity of polymorphonuclear leukocytes obtained from patients with diabetes mellitus. J Lab Clin Med 1964; 64: 1–13.
[17] Ludwig H, Eibl M, Schernthaner G et al. Humoral immunodeficiency to bacterial antigens in patients with juvenile onset diabetes mellitus. Diabetologia 1976; 12: 259–261.
[18] McCuish AC, Urbaniak SJ, Campbell CJ. Phytohemaglutinin transformation and circulating lymphocyte subpopulations in insulin-dependent diabetic patients. Diabetes 1974; 23: 708–712.
[19] Larkin JG, Butcher IG, Frier BM et al. Fatal Rhinocerebral mucormycosis in a newly diagnosed diabetic. Diabetic Med. 1986; 3: 266–268.
[20] Beisel WR. Metabolic response to infection. Ann Rev Med 1975; 26: 9–19.
[21] Rayfield EJ, Cornow RT, Reinhard D et al. Effects of acute endotoxaemia on glucoregulation in normal and diabetic subjects. J Clin Endocrinol & Metab 1977; 45: 513–521.
[22] Mandell GL, Douglas RG jun, Bennett JE. Principles and Practice of Infectious Diseases (2nd edition). New York, Chichester, Brisbane, Toronto, Singapore: John Wiley & Sons 1985.
[23] McBride RA, Corson JM, Dammin GJ. Mucormycosis. Am J Medicine 1960; 28: 832–846.
[24] Marchevsky AM, Bottone EJ, Geller SA et al. The changing spectrum of disease, etiology and diagnosis of mucormycosis. Human Pathology 1980; 11: 457–464.
[25] Pillsbury HC, Fischer ND. Rhinocerebral mucormycosis. Arch Otolaryngol 1977; 103: 600–604.
[26] Lehrer RI (Moderator). Mucormycosis. Ann Int Med 1980; 93: 93–108.
[27] Abramson E, Wilson D, Arky RA. Rhinocerebral phycomycosis in association with diabetic ketoacidosis. Ann Int Med 1967; 66: 735–742.
[28] Wong B, Armstrong D. Clinical manifestations and management of mucormycosis in the compromised patient. In: Warnock DW, Richardson MD (eds) Fungal infections in the compromised patient. Chichester: Wiley & Sons, 1982; 161–163 and 176–179.
[29] Robb SM. Reactions of fungi to ten atmospheres of pressure of oxygen. J Gen Microbiol 1966; 45: 17–29.

[30] Ferguson BJ, Mitchell TG, Moon R et al. Adjunctive hyperbaric oxygen for treatment of rhinocerebral mucormycosis. Rev Inf Diseases 1988; 10: 551 – 559.
[31] Chandler J. Malignant External Otitis. Laryngoscope 1968; 78: 1257 – 1294.
[32] Rubin J, Yu VL. Malignant external otitis. Insights into pathogenesis, clinical manifestations, diagnosis and therapy. Am J Med 1988; 85: 391 – 398.
[33] Zaky DA, Bentley DW, Lowy K et al. Malignant external otitis: a severe form of otitis in diabetic patients. Am J Med 1976; 61: 298 – 302.
[34] Sande MA, Mandell GL. Antimicrobial agents – the aminoglycosides. In: Gilman AG, Goodman LS, Rall TW et al., eds. The Pharmacological basis of therapeutics. New York, Toronto, London: McMillan, 1985; 1150 – 1169.
[35] Kelly HA, McCallum WG. Pneumaturia. JAMA 1898; 31: 375 – 381.
[36] Evanoff GV, Thompson CS, Foley R et al. Spectrum of gas within the kidney. Am J Med 1987; 83: 149 – 154.
[37] Hussein MH, Rotellar C, Mackow RC et al. Emphysematous Pyelonephritis. Am J Med 1988; 84: 176 – 177. (letter)
[38] Radin DR, Halls JM. Emphysematous cholecystitis presenting with pneumoperitoneum. Am J Radiol 1987; 149: 1175 – 6.
[39] Ruby ST, Gladstone A, Treat M et al. Emphysematous cholecystitis. JAMA 1983; 249: 248 – 9.
[40] Meleney FL, Haemolytic Streptococcus gangrene. Arch Surg. 1924; 9: 317 – 364.
[41] Fournier JA. Gangrene foudroyante de la verge. La Semaine Medicale (Paris) 1883; 3: 345 – 347.
[42] Janevicius RV, Hann SE, Batt MD. Necrotizing Fasciitis. Surg Gynaecol Obstet. 1982; 154: 97 – 102.
[43] Barker FG, Leppard BJ, Seal DV. Streptococcal necrotising fasciitis: comparison between histological and clinical features. J Clin Pathol 1987; 40: 335 – 341.
[44] Riefler J III, Molavi A, Schwartz D et al. Necrotizing fasciitis in adults due to Group B Streptococcus. Arch Int Med 1988; 148: 727 – 729.
[45] Lamerton AJ. Fournier's Gangrene: non-Clostridial gas gangrene of the perineum and diabetes mellitus. J Roy Soc Med 1986; 79: 212 – 216.
[46] Stamenkovic I, Lew PD. Early recognition of potentially fatal necrotizing fasciitis: the use of frozen section biopsy. New Eng J Med 1984; 310: 1689 – 1693.
[47] Finch R. Antibacterial chemotherapy. Medicine International 1988; 52: 2146 – 2154.
[48] Rimailho A, Riou B, Richard C et al. Fulminant Necrotizing Fasciitis and Non-Steroidal Anti-Inflammatory Drugs. J Infectious Dis 1987; 155: 143 – 146.
[49] Wheat LJ, Allen SD, Henry M et al. Diabetic foot infections. Bacteriological analysis. Arch Int Med 1986; 146: 1935 – 1940.
[50] Scher KS, Steele FJ. The septic foot in patients with diabetes. Surgery 1988; 104: 661 – 666.
[51] Bennet JE. Candidiasis. In: Isselbacher KJ, Adams RA, Braunwald E et al., eds. Principles of Internal Medicine 9th edition. Tokyo: McGraw-Hill. 1982.
[52] Keane EM, Boyko EJ, Reller LB et al. Prevalence of asymptomatic bacteruria in subjects with NIDDM in San Luis Valley of Colorado. Diabetes Care 1988; 11: 708 – 712.
[53] Stamm WE, Hooton TM, Johnson JR et al. Urinary tract infections: from pathogenesis to treatment. J Infectious Dis 1989; 159: 400 – 406.
[54] Finestone AJ, Boornzy SR. Diabetes mellitus and periodontal disease. Diabetes 1967; 16: 336 – 340.
[55] Cruse PJ. Surgical wound sepsis. Can Med Assoc J 1970; 102: 251 – 258.
[56] Ariyan S, Halasz NA. The incidence of postoperative gram negative shock in diabetics. Am J Med Science 1967; 254: 808 – 815.
[57] Editorial. Pneumococcus infection in diabetes mellitus: is this a justification for immunisation? J Am Med Assoc 1980; 243: 2301 – 3.

[58] Diepersloot RJA, Bouter KP, Beyer WEP et al. Humoral immune response and delayed type hypersensitivity to influenza vaccine in patients with diabetes mellitus. Diabetologia 1987; 30: 397–401.
[59] Brodie MJ, Munday AS. Toxicity of and interactions with antibacterial agents. Medicine International 1988; 52: 2155–2163.
[60] Connacher AA, Old DC, Phillips G et al. Recurrent peritonitis caused by Serratia marescens in a diabetic patient receiving continuous ambulatory peritoneal dialysis. J Hosp Infection 1988; 11: 155–160.

Drug administration in relation to pregnancy and diabetes

L. Mølsted-Pedersen, S.O. Skouby, P. Damm

Introduction

The clinical condition of diabetes and pregnancy has had a brief history. Practically speaking, it was born with the advent of insulin treatment in the twenties, matured in the forties, and has since developed into an important clinical problem. In addition, the combination of pregnancy and diabetes has posed a multitude of scientific problems involving internal medicine, endocrinology, obstetrics, pediatrics, genetics and other disciplines [1].

Generally, prescription of drugs during pregnancy must be performed with the utmost care. Diabetes mellitus implies a continuous use of insulin or hypoglycemic agents. During pregnancy, betasymphatomimetic drugs and glucocorticoids may be used in order to treat preterm labor and prevent respiratoy distress in premature infants.

In the past decade there has been considerable improvement in the management and outcome of pregnancy in women with diabetes. Important factors include strict control of maternal blood glucose *before* and during pregnancy as a result, careful planning of pregnancy is essential. The main stress in this survey on drug administration in relation to diabetes and pregnancy will be laid on oral contraceptives.

Insulin species and insulin antibodies

The dramatic improvement of diabetic pregnancies over the past decade is, as mentioned in the introduction, based on improved blood glucose control but appropriate time of delivery and improved neonatal care have also been of great importance.

Daily multiple insulin injections are recommended during pregnancy and in the western countries human insulin is readily available in most formulations. Most patients, however, still use highly purified porcine or bovine insulins. Insulin antibodies, which may be produced in mothers treated with insulin have been shown to cross the placenta [2, 3]. With regard to fetal-maternal interactions, insulin antobodies could probably transport insulin across the placenta and release insulin in the fetus, bind endogenous insulin released from fetal islets, or affect fetal islets directly with alterations in insulin release or damage the fetal islet [4–6]. It is therefore logical to treat pregnant women with insulin formulations of minimum antigenicity. Switching from beef/pork to pure pork insulin [7] or changes to human insulin in insulin dependent diabetics [9] leads to a reduction in antibody levels in the newborn. Thus it is recommended to use human insulin preparations in pregnancy when necessary or to change to human insulin before conception in insulin dependent diabetic women.

Oral hypoglycemic agents

Recorded experiences with oral hypoglycemic drugs in diabetic pregnancy have so far been scanty and somewhat confusing. In the latest overview [9] and textbook [10], oral hypoglycemic agents are not recommended for use during pregnancy. In regard to the sulphonylureas, the main reason for this negativ attitude is the fact that these drugs are transferrred across the placenta [11]; theoretically they might stimulate islet growth and increase insulin activitiy in the newborn and thereby aggravate a possible neonatal hypoglycemia.

Biguanides represented by metformin do not cross the placenta, and animal work seems to indicate that these drugs are safe to use during pregnancy [12]. A few case reports of severe prolonged neonatal hypoglycemia following continuous sulphonylurea treatment of the mother during pregnancy has been published [13, 14]. By adding up the published figures from Cape Town [15, 16], Aberdeen [17, 18] and Copenhagen [19, 20] a total of 130 diabetic mothers have been treated with sulphonylureas (chlorpropamide, tolbutamide and glibenclamide) and 80 with metformin during pregnancy and no cases of severe prolonged neonatal hypoglycemia have been recorded in these studies.

There might be a place for oral hypoglycemic compounds in a few selected diabetic pregnant women in the last half of pregnancy, but it is clear that these drugs should still only be used to treat pregnant women in the course of controlled studies which are designed to carefully evaluate the benefits of the therapy.

Beta-sympathomimetics and glucocorticosteroids

Pregnancies complicated by diabetes are associated with an increased risk of spontaneous preterm labor and delivery. Since a significant correlation exists between neonatal complications and/or later cerebral dysfunction and preterm delivery [21], measures to effectively treat preterm labor deserve particular attention.

The most popular treatment modality to suppress preterm labor during the last 15 years has been the beta-symphatomimetic drugs of which ritodrine, salbutamol and terbutaline are the most commonly used. It is now well established that intravenous administration of these drugs causes an elevation of plasma glucose and insulin concentrations in normal women and increased insulin requirements in diabetics [22].

For nearly the same period of time, corticosteriods have been used with increasing frequency in an attempt to prevent respiratory distress syndrome (RDS) in premature infants. As corticosteroids are known to produce insulin resistance [23], their administration in combination with beta-symphatomimetic drugs to women in preterm labor is potentially hazardous in those patients with any degree of carbohydrate intolerance.

Significant maternal and fetal adverse effects of the above mentioned regimen in diabetic pregnancies have been described [24]. However, maintenance of blood glucose concentration within acceptable limits is possible if the effects of the beta-symphatomimetic infusion are anticipated [25]. This may be achieved by starting an insulin infusion or by giving an intramuscular insulin injection at the same time as the tocolytic treatment is initiated. Blood glucose should be monitored hourly throughout the period of administration of the beta-symphatomimetic agent and the insulin dose adjusted according to blood glucose concentration.

The diabetogenic potential of glucocorticosteroids has been well described since the 1950's [26]. Glucocorticosteroids act by promoting gluconeogenesis in peripheral tissues and the liver, as well as through inhibition of peripheral utilization of glucose [27].

The diabetogenic effect of beta-symphatomimetics could not be explained by inhibition of insulin secretion or stimulation of glucagon secretion. The drug seems to exert a direct cellular effect which is augmented with the severity of diabetes [28]. Treatment with intravenous beta-symphatomimetics should be performed under close surveillance of plasma glucose, standard bicarbonate and plasma potassium, especially in diabetics.

Antihypertensive drugs

Both pregnancy-induced hypertension (preeclampsia) and chronic hypertension occur with a significant higher incidence in diabetic than in non-diabetic pregnancies [29]. In pregnancy the decision to treat elevated blood pressure is more complex and controversial than outside pregnancy. This is because of the relatively short duration of the problem and the need to consider a second patient, the fetus. In this respect it is important to realize that virtually all drugs prescribed to pregnant women reach the fetus [30] and that the teratogenecity of all antihypertensives remains practically unknown, since drug trials have generally included gravidas only when they are beyond the first trimester.

Even minimally elevated blood pressure during pregnancy increase the perinatal mortality [31], and drug therapy seems to have a beneficial effect on this condition [32]. The possible fetal benefits of antihypertensive treatment must be weighed carefully against possible adverse effects on the offspring.

One major concern specific to the use of antihypertensive drugs during pregnancy is that uteroplacental blood flow can be influenced by several vasoconstrictors and that circulating levels of endogenous pressor hormones may be markedly augmented following excessive drug-induced decrements in maternal arterial pressure [33].

In our clinic the antihypertensive treatment in diabetic pregnancy rely on a few drugs with a well-documented history of efficacy and safety.

If preeclampsia or severe hypertension occurs beyond the 36th gestational week, a point at which fetal pulmonary maturity has generally occured, delivery is the therapy of choice following control of elevated blood pressure. In case of further acute increase in blood pressure (i. e. >170/100 mmHg) hydralizine is given i. v. in a constant infusion of 0.5 – 10 mg/hr or 5 mg i. m. every 20 – 40 minute. This direct vasodilator, which is the most frequently used agent to treat severe hypertension near term or during labour and delivery, has a long story of proven effectiveness [34].

In chronic hypertension in pregnancy our agent of choice is methyldopa 500 – 2000 mg in 2 – 4 divided doses. Methyldopa also has a long history of effective use in pregnancy, it has been extensively studied and has a well-documented record of safety so therefore we prefere this agent for the treatment of chronic hypertension during both diabetic and non-diabetic gestation [35].

Labetalol, a beta-blocker with some alpha-adrenoreceptor activity, has been claimed to be superior to other agents in the treatment of hypertension in pregnancy. However Sibai et al [36] found that labetalol treatment was associated with a higher incidence of growth retardation when compared with no drug therapy. Thus, this drug requires further study before its use for hypertension in pregnancy can be recommended.

Contraception in diabetic women

Theoretically there is no difference in the methods available to diabetic and non-diabetic women, but the state of disease alters the risk-benefit ratio that is normally taken into consideration when contraceptive advice is given.

Hormonal contraception

The most widely used contraceptive method today is the combination-type oral contraceptive (OC) containing an estrogen and progesteron steroid. They are also recognized as the most effective with a Pearl-index of 0 – 1. During the last 20 years the information concerning the risks and benefits of these hormonal compounds has accumulated rapidly and has revealed that the intake influences a series of organ and metabolic systems apart from the main target, namely the pituitary/ovarian system. Initially, changes in glucose, lipid and protein metabolism were demonstrated after ingestion of compounds contianing 50 micrograms of estrogen.

During recent years it has become evident, that many of the undesired metabolic effects may be reduced by lowering the dosage of estrogen and the progesteron [37]. Therefore, a distinction should be made between preparations containing 50 micrograms or more of ethinylestradiol and a high progesteron content (high dose OC) and the new low-dose preparations with 35 micrograms or less estrogen and a reduced amount of progesteron (low-dose OC).

Although metabolic alterations are not synonymous with metabolic disease, they should be followed carefully, especially in women with a pre-existing risk factor such as diabetes. The change in carbohydrate and lipid metabolism in non-diabetics and diabetic women following intake of OCs will therefore be reviewed in detail.

a) The pharmacological profile of sex steroids in oral contraceptives: Today, the general concept is that the influence on glucose metabolism of combined sex steroid products is mainly caused by the progesteron components although artificial estrogens may act synergistically [38 – 40].

The estrogens used in contraceptive compounds marketed today are either ethinylestradiol or mestranol. Unconjugated ethinylestradiol is the active substance in both compounds. Following oral administration, the bioavailability of ethinylestradiol is about 40% due to a first pass effect in the liver [41]. Ethinylestradiol undergoes enterohepatic recirculation and reabsorption. Approximately 30% of a given dose can be discovered in the feces and the fecal/urine ratio is about 2:3. The half-life in plasma varies from 6 to 20 hours and the elimination occurs mainly by hydroxylation and conjugation to sulphate or glucuronide [42].

Genuine or non-alkylated estrogens, 17-β-estradiol and estriol are not used in commercially available contraceptive compounds, whereas they have been used extensively for substitution therapy in climacteric women [43]. Compared with artificial estrogens, higher dosages of estradiol must be used in oral compounds due to higher rates of metabolism in the gut wall and first-pass effects of the liver. Production of microcrystalline forms improves the absorption [44]. Estradiol is cleared rapidly from the circulation and has a half-life of about 1 hour and passes through the enterohepatic circulation. Most of it is metabolized to estrone and/or conjugates; the excretion occurs mainly in the urine [27].

In contrast to the artificial estrogens used in oral commercially available contraceptives, ethinylestradiol and mestranol, the progestagens are represented by a variety of steroid formations with marked differences in their pharmacodynamic responses and classified as estranes, gonanes and pregnanes. Most of the progestational components used in the combined contraceptive pills are 17-α-ethinyl derivates of the reduced form of testosterone (19-nortestosterone) and these derivates constitute the estranes and gonanes. Progestagens of the estrane type are converted to norethisterone after oral intake [42]. The gonanes differ from other 19-nortestosterone products in having a beta-ethyl group at carbon-13 instead of the one-carbon chain unit present in the other products, thus the parmacokinetic properties are markedly different.

For many years, the gonanes have been represented in oral contraceptives only by norgestrel and its active component the dextroisomer levonorgestrel. But during recent years new types of progestogens of the gonane type e.g. desogestrel, gestodene and norgestimate have succeeded the widely used norgestrel/levonorgestel in the combined type of oral contraceptives.

The bioavailability of estranes is approximately 60% [46] whereas no first-pass effect seems to occur after intake of the gonanes. The half-life of estranes varies from 5 to 14 hours compared to 10 to 24 hours for the gonanes [42]. Both are eliminated by conjugation to sulphates and glucuronides, whereas hydroxylation is unusual.

Pregnanes are derivatives of 17-hydroxyprogesterone and include chlormadinone, megestrol, medroxyprogesterone and cyproterone acetate. Today, cyproterone acetate, which possesses specific antiandrogen properties, is the only pregnane used in OCs and so far only to a very limited extent.

The biological activity of the different progesterones is normally measured by the delay of menses test or endometrial subnuclear vacuolization. According to these tests, levonorgestrol is roughly 10 to 20 times as potent as norethisterone [47].

b) Mechanism of action: The sex steroid hormones enter the cells readily because of their small size and lipid solubility. The effects on target organs can be subdivided into direct and receptor mediated. Apart from the intended effects on the pituitary/ovarian system and the endometrium, both direct and receptor-mediated effects occur in various other parts of the body including the liver, pancreas and kidney.

The direct effects show a dose-response relation and usually decline within the first 3 months after the beginning of oral intake due to enzyme induction [48]. The receptor mediated effects occur as a result of the steroid binding to the cytoplasmatic receptor protein [49, 50]. The hormone/receptor complex is activated and transferred across the nuclear membrane to the nucleus where it binds to nuclear DNA. Transcription and synthesis of mRNA occur and the RNA is transported to the ribosomes and finally proteins are synthesised in the cytoplasma. The receptor mediated effects increase with dose, but level off when the dose becomes high. The cellular response to a hormone stimulus is dependent on the stability of the hormone/receptor complex and on the binding of the steroid/receptor complex to the DNA molecule. Thus, small changes in the steroid configuration may result in marked differences in the hormone response [51].

c) Oral contraceptives and glucose metabolism: Today, it is well-established that the intake of oral contraceptives may decrease glucose tolerance and cause a rise in insulin levels in healthy non-diabetic women. Such changes have become evident in both intravenous and oral glucose tolerance tests [52]. A possible decreased insulin sensitivity at the cellular level in peripheral tissues has been suggested as the mechanism behind the altered glucose metabolism [53, 54]. Despite these adverse effects on glucose tolerance, no risk of developing clinical diabetes has been found in epidemiological studies [55] even in women who had used OCs for 10 years or more [56]. However, in women with previous gestational diabetes an overall incidence of 44% of deterioration of glucose tolerance has been registered during intake of older "high dose" OCs [57, 58].

Only a limited number of studies have been published on the effect of low-dose OCs on glucose metabolism. Generally, two types of products have been investigated, both containing 30 or 35 micrograms estrogen combined with either an estrane (e. g. norethisterone) or a gonane (e. g. levonorgestrol). There has been conflicting evidence concerning the effects of these compounds on glucose tolerance. It has been postulated [59, 60] that products containing levonorgestrol are associated with more marked alterations of glucose and/ or insulin levels than products containing norethisterone, but not all investigations support these findings [61]. We have previously reported the effects of a monophasic preparation of 30 micrograms ethinylestradiol and 150 micrograms levonorgestrel [62]. In healthy non-diabetic women no changes in fasting glucose, insulin or glucagon values or in glucose tolerance where observed after 2 and 6 months.

Women with previous gestational diabetes and normal body weight had significantly elevated glucose values before treatment compared to non-diabetic controls. After hormonal intake for 6 months the insulin response to oral glucose increased significantly, but no deterioration of glucose tolerance was observed. The glucagon response was similar in the women with previous gestational diabetes (GDM) and in the controls [62]. These findings are in accordance with the observations made in a small number of women with borderline abnormal glucose tolerance before intake of a monophasic low-dose ethinylestradiol/norethisterone preparation [59].

The strategies used to reduce the metabolic side effects of oral contraceptives have included reduction of steriod dose, development of new steroids, and combinations of reduced steroid dosages and different adminstration regimes. The triphasic approach is a response to this view using the lowest possible dose of both hormones without a concomitant unacceptable uterine bleeding pattern [63]. When compared to the most widely used low-dose monophasic ethinylestradiol/levonorgestol combination, the ethinylestradiol ratio is 1.08 during one 3-week treatment period with the triphasic preparation whereas the levonorgestrol ratio is only 0.61. We have therefore examined the influence of such a triphasic compound on glucose tolerance in normal women and in women with previous gestational diabetes (GDM) during a 6-month treatment period [64]. Before treatment the women with previous GDM had significantly elevated fasting glucose levels and impaired OGTT when compared to the controls. However, in both groups the glucose, insulin and glucagon responses to oral glucose remained unchanged during the treatment. No progressive effects of glucose tolerance were observed from the triphasic compound in either group after a 12-month follow-up period.

In both the women with previous GDM and the normal women the triphasic preparation resulted in a significantly lower insulin response to oral glucose than the low-dose monophasic estradiol/levonorgestrol preparation (Table 1).

Table 1 Insulin areas (min × nmol/l) (mean ± SEM) calculated from glucose tolerance tests performed in women with previous gestational diabetes (GDM) (n = 10) and in normal women (n = 10) during intake of triphasic and monophasic low-dose oral contraceptives (ethinylestradiol and levonorgestrel)

Months	Normal		Previous GDM	
	Monophasic	Triphasic	Monophasic	Triphasic
0	53 ± 5	63 ± 17	49 ± 9	53 ± 5
2	55 ± 8	58 ± 6	53 ± 6	62 ± 5
6	65 ± 6*	60 ± 9	69 ± 11*	63 ± 5

* 0 vs 6 months; $P < 0.05$

d) Oral contraceptives in women with insulin dependent diabetes mellitus (IDDM) – Glycemic control and clinical effects: In insulin dependent diabetic women, there are several reports on undesirable side-effects of OC's. Osler and Wiese [65] found increased difficulties in diabetic control during treatment with traditional "high-dose" combined compounds. Steel and Duncan [66] found increased insulin requirements in 19% of diabetic women. No differences in the effects on insulin requirement were found between compounds containing only 50 micrograms ethinylestradiol versus low-dose compounds containing only 30 micrograms ethinylestradiol and a reduced amount of progesterone. These authors also reported a high incidence of severe clinical side-effects during intake of the combined compounds [67]. Rådberg et al. [68] investigated the effects of 50 micrograms ethinylestradiol plus 250 micrograms lynestrenol in women with IDDM. The insulin requirement increased by 7% without any change in body weight or blood glucose level. The clinical events were comparable to those observed in non-diabetic women.

Combined compounds containing natural or genuine estrogen for hormonal substitution in climacteric women produce less influence on glucose metabolism than compounds containing synthetic estrogen as in oral contraceptives [43]. We were therefore prompted to examine the clinical and biochemical effects on diabetes control of a monophasic oral contraceptive compound containing natural estrogen (4 milligrams estradiol plus 2 milligrams estriol and 3 milligrams norethisterone) [69]. Such a preparation has been reported previously to give effective suppression of ovulation and fewer metabolic side-effects compared with a compound containing artificial estrogen with identical progestational content [70, 71]. We observed no accidental pregnancies during the 12 month study period and the overall continuation rate of

60 compares well with the continuation rate normally found in non-diabetic women after administration of conventional types of OCs [72]. No difficulties were found with diabetes control and there were no significant changes in insulin requirement, 24-hour urinary glucose excretion, body weight or concentration of glycated hemoglobin (HBA_1C) after 12 months treatment.

From a pharmacological point of view, however, oral contraceptives with the lowest hormonal content appear to be the most attractive, despite different biochemical configurations. In women with IDDM we have therefore compared the influence of the non-alkylated estrogen/progesterone compound with the influence of (a) a low-dose monophasic ethinylestradiol/norethisterone combination, (b) progesterone-only treatment with norethisterone and (c) a triphasic ethinylestradiol/levonorgestrel combination.

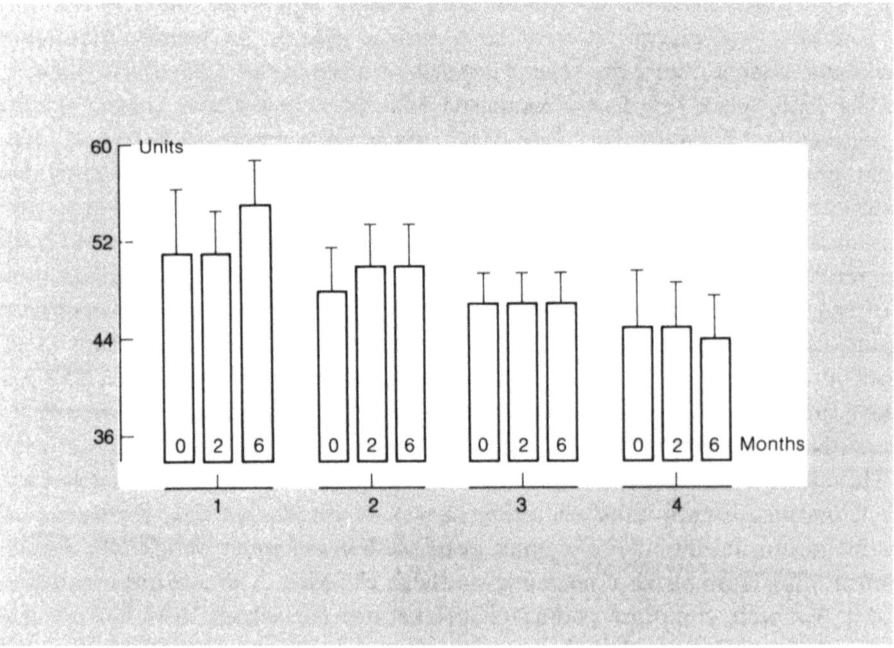

Fig. 1 24-hour insulin requirements in insulin dependent diabetic women during intake of four different OCs.
(with kind permission from the Editors of Carbohydrate metabolism in pregnancy and the newborn IV. Springer-Verlag, London 1989.)

1. 4 mg 17-β E_2 + 2 mg E_3 + 3 mg NE
2. 35 μg EE + 500 μg NE
3. 300 μg NE
4. Triphasis EE + LNG.
(days 1–6 : 30 μg EE + 50 μ LNG,
days 7–12: 40 μg EE + 75 μg LNG,
days 13–21: 30 μg EE + 125 μg LNG)

Measurements were performed on blood pressure, body weight, fasting plasma glucose, 24-hour insulin requirements, HBA_1C, total plasma cortisol and plasma free fatty acids (FFA) levels before and during hormonal intake for two and six months [73]. The patients in each treatment group were matched with regard to age, weight, duration of diabetes and socioeconomic status. No significant changes in body weight or blood pressure were recorded within or between the groups during treatment and none of the participants experienced noticeable difficulties with their diabetes control. Fasting plasma glucose, 24-hour insulin requirements (Fig. 1), HBA_1C levels (Fig. 2) and FFA concentrations (Fig. 3) were similar in all groups before and during treatment and no significant changes were observed within the groups during treatment. From this study it therefore appears that in insulin-dependent

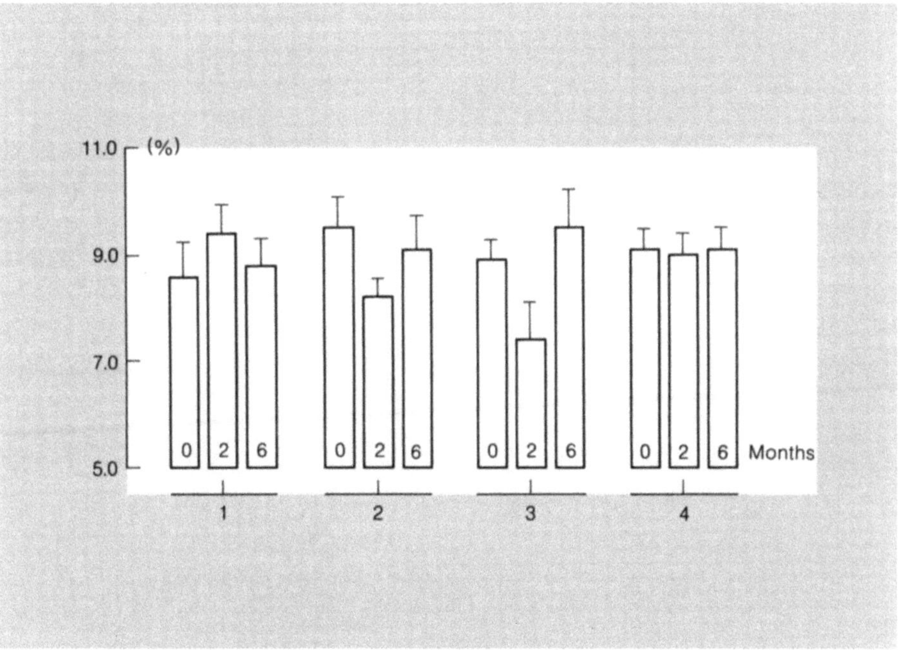

Fig. 2 Fasting HbA_1C in insulin dependent diabetic women during intake of four different OCs. (With kind permission from the Editors of Carbohydrate metabolism in pregnancy and the newborn IV. Springer-Verlag, London 1989.)

1. 4 mg 17-μ E_2 + 2 mg E_3 + 3 mg NE
2. 35 μg EE + 500 μg NE
3. 300 μg NE
4. Triphasic EE + LNG.
(days 1–6 : 30 μg EE + 50 μg LNG,
days 7–12: 40 μg EE + 75 μg LNG,
days 13–21: 30 μg EE + 125 μg LNG)

diabetic women, the metabolic control was equally good during administration of the low-dose artificial oral contraceptives as compared with the non-alkylated estrogen/protesterone compound.

e) Lipid/lipoprotein metabolism: Substantial evidence has confirmed that oral contraceptives adversely influence lipid/lipoprotein metabolism [74, 75]. Hyperlipidemia characterised by increased low-density lipoprotein (LDL) and very-low-density lipoprotein (VLDL) and decreased high-density lipoprotein (HDL) has been demonstrated during intake of the combined type of OCs [74, 75], suggesting increased risk of atherosclerotic complications [76, 77]. There is evidence that during intake of OCs the risk of arterial disease is positively correlated to the estrogen/progestagen ratio [78].

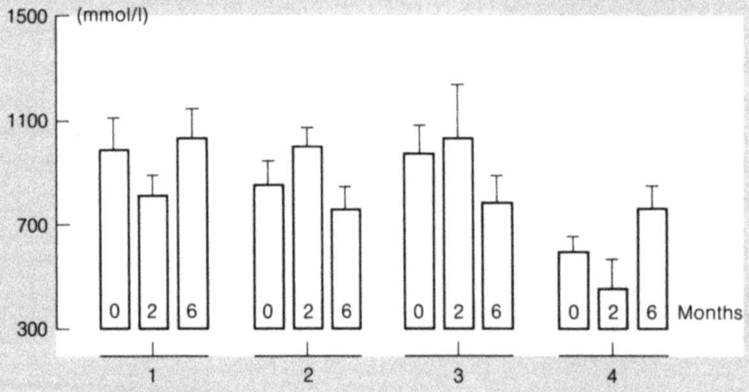

Fig. 3 Fasting FFA in insulin dependent diabetic women during intake of four different OCs. (With kind permission from the Editors of Carbohydrate metabolism in pregnancy and the newborn IV. Springer-Verlag, London 1989.)

1. 4 mg 17-β E_2 + 2 mg E_3 + 3 mg NE
2. 35 μg EE + 500 μg NE
3. 300 μg NE
4. Triphasic EE + LNG (days 1–6 : 30 μg EE + 50 μg LNG, days 7–12: 40 μg EE + 75 μg LNG, days 13–21: 30 μg EE + 125 μg LNG)

Only a few studies have been published on the effects of OCs on lipid metabolism in women with IDDM, NIDDM (non-insulin dependent diabetes mellitus) or in women predisposed to diabetes such as those with previous gestational diabetes (GDM). Using "high-dose" oral compounds an increase in triglyceride (TG) was found in women predisposed to diabetes [79] as in women with previous GDM [80]. In women with IDDM, Beck et al. [81] found no change in plasma TG concentration, but increased plasma cholesterol level during intake of combined "high-dose" compounds.

We examined [64] the effect of the triphasic ethinylestradiol/levonorgestrel compound on plasma levels of TG, FFA, total cholesterol, HDL cholesterol LDL cholesterol and VLDL cholesterol in women with previous GDM and in normal women. Investigations were performed prior to the hormonal intake and after treatment for 2 and 6 months. Plasma FFA, lipoproteins and the HDL cholesterol/total cholesterol ratio remained unchanged in both groups.

In the atherosclerotic-prone women with IDDM it is of special interest to examine abnormalities in plasma lipid/lipoprotein levels following intake of OCs. In the comparative trial of the influence on glycemic control of four different contraceptive compounds already described [73], we therefore also included measurements on the influence of different compounds on lipid/lipoprotein levels. No differences were found between the norethisterone only preparation and the non-alkylated estrogen/norethisterone and the triphasic ethinylestradiol/levonorgestrel combinations whereas intake of monophasic ethinylestradiol/norethisterone preparation resulted in small but significant increases in plasma TG and VLDL cholesterol levels.

f) Conclusion: Oral compounds of the "low-dose" triphasic type with reduced estrogen/progestagen ratio and the combined steroid compounds containing "natural estrogen" (estradiol-estriol/norethisterone) may be administered as effective and acceptable contraceptives in women with IDDM without any concomitant adverse effect on the diabetic control or lipid/lipoprotein metabolism. Treatment with low-dose norethisterone alone, as "mini-pills" appears to be an appropriate alternative to both the non-alkylated estrogen/norethisterone combination and the triphasic ethinylestradiol/leveonorgestrel preparations. On the other hand the monophasic low-dose ethinylestradiol/norethisterone combination results in small but significant changes in lipid/lipoprotein levels which appear unfavorable from a clinical point of view.

Administration of a low-dose steroid compound containing the new gestagens gestoden or desogestrel causes no changes in the lipid/lipoprotein metabolism known to increase the risk of developing cardiovascular disease in non-diabetic women [82]. Ongoing investigations of these compounds in IDDM women seems promising (unpublished).

Intrauterine contraceptive device (IUD)

For many women the intrauterine contraceptive device is the only acceptable alternative contraceptive to hormonal compounds. The Pearl index is 1.5–2 for the newer copper releasing models. The general risk factors for this method should however not be ignored. For all users, pelvic inflammations occur 2–3 times as frequently as in non-users and even in nulli-gravidae the risk is reported to be increased six-fold [83]. Moreover the risk of ectopic pregnancy is doubled. Despite the theoretical risk of such complications, IUD's have been applied on a wide-scale to women with diabetes because the method, from a metabolic point of view, is preferable to oral contraceptives. Wiese [84] for example, used a Lippes loop in 118 insulin-dependent diabetic women. After 12 and 24 months he found the accidental pregnancy rate and the continuation rate at the same level as in non-diabetic women. The removal rate because of bleeding and/or pain was equal in diabetic and non-diabetic women.

Since a few years ago, however, the efficacy of the IUD's in diabetic women has been disputed [66], and a possible relation between composition of the corrosion products and the efficacy has been suggested [85]. We have, however, in the early eighties investigated the clinical performance of a copper IUD model in 105 insulin-dependent diabetic women and 119 non-diabetic controls. The events and overall efficacy rates were compared by life-table analysis and no difference in accidental pregnancy rate, removal rate or total continuation rate could be demonstrated [86]. In our center in Copenhagen the IUD method is therefore still considered as a reliable and acceptable contraceptive agent in diabetic women.

References

[1] Pedersen J. The pregnant diabetic and her newborn. Munksgaard, Copenhagen 1977; 15–16.

[2] Spellacy WN, Goetz FC. Insulin antibodies in pregnancy. Lancet 1963; II: 222–224.

[3] Jørgensen KR, Deckert T, Mølsted-Pedersen L et al. Insulin antibody and glucose in plasma of newborn infants of diabetic women. Acta Endrocrinol (Copenh) 1966; 52: 154–167.

[4] Heding LG, Persson B, Stangenberg M. B-cell function in newborn infants of diabetic mothers. Diabetologia 1980;: 19: 427–32.

[5] Baumann WA, Yalow RS. Transplacental passage of insulin complexed to antibody. Proc Natl Acad Sci USA 1981; 78: 4588–4580.

[6] Deckert T. The immunogenecity of new insulins. Diabetes 1985; 34 (suppl 2): 94–96.

[7] Mylvaganam R, Stowers JM, Steel JM et al. Insulin Immunogenecity in Pregnancy: Maternal and Fetal Studies. Diabetologia 1983; 24: 19–25.

[8] Chertow BS, Baranetsky NG, Sivitz WI et al. The effects of human insulin antibody formation is pregnant diabetics and their newborns. Obstet Gynecol 1988; 72: 724–728.

[9] Vaughan NSA. Prescribing in pregnancy. Treatment of diabetes in pregnancy. Br Med J 1987; 294: 558–560.
[10] Coustan DR. Management of gestational diabetes. In: Reece EA, Coustan DR, eds. Diabetes mellitus in pregnancy. Principles and practice. New York: Churchill Livingstone, 1988; 443.
[11] Adams PAJ, Schwartz R. Diagnosis and treatment: Should oral hypoglycemic agents be used in pediatric and pregnant patients? Pediatrics 1968; 42: 819–823.
[12] Cohen Y, Costerousse O. Étude expérimentale du metabolisme du dimethylbiguanide marqué an carbon 14.4°. Med Hyg 1961; 145–148.
[13] Zuker P, Simon G. Prolonged symptomatic neonatal hypoglycemia associated with maternal chlorpropamide therapy. Pediatrics 1968; 42: 824–826.
[14] Kemball ML, McIver C, Milner RDG et al. Neonatal hypoglycaemia in infants of diabetic mothers given sulphonylurea drugs in pregnancy. Archi Dis Child 1970; 45: 696–701.
[15] Coetzee EJ, Jackson WPU. Metformin in management of pregnant insulin-independent diabetics. Diabetologia 1979; 16: 241–245.
[16] Coetzee EJ, Jackson WPU. Pragnancy in established non-insulin-dependent diabetics. S Afr Med J 1980; 58: 795–802.
[17] Sutherland HW, Stowers JM, Cormack JD et al. Evaluation of chlorpropamide in chemical diabetes diagnosed during pregnancy. Br Med J 1973; 3: 9–13.
[18] Stowers JM, Sutherland HW. The use of sulphonylureas biguanides and insulin in pregnancy. In: Sutherland HW, Stowers JM, Persson DWM, eds. Carbohydrate metabolism in pregnancy and the newborn. Edinburgh: Churchill Livingstone 1975; 205–220.
[19] Pedersen J, Mølsted-Pedersen L. Oral "antidiabetic" compounds in pregnancy. In: Camarini-Davalos R, Cole HS, eds. Early diabetes in early life. New York: Academic Press Inc, 1975; 487–494.
[20] Mølsted-Pedersen L. Unpublished.
[21] Petersen MB. Status at 4–5 years in 90 children of insulin-dependent diabetic mothers. In: Sutherland HW, Stowers JM, eds. Carbohydrate metabolism in pregnancy and the newborn IV. Berlin: Springer-Verlag 1989; 353–361.
[22] Borberg C, Gillmer MDG, Beard RW et al. Metabolic effects of beta-sympathomimetic drugs and dexamathasone in normal and diabetic pregnancy. Br J Obstet Gynaecol 1978; 85: 184–189.
[23] Landy HJ, Isada NB, McGinnis J et al. The effect of chronic steroid therapy on glucose tolerance in pregnancy. Am J Obstet Gynecol 1988; 159: 612–615.
[24] Mordes D, Kreutner K, Metzger W et al. Dangers of intravenous ritodrine in diabetic patients. JAMA 1982; 248: 973–976.
[25] Barnett AH, Stubbs SM, Mander AM. Management of premature labour in diabetic pregnancy. Diabetologia 1980; 18: 365–368.
[26] Fajans SS, Conn JW. An approach to the prediction of diabetes mellitus by modification of the glucose tolerance test with cortisone. Diabetes 1954; 3: 296–304.
[27] Gilman AG, Goodman LS, Rall TW, eds. Goodman and Gilman's the pharmacological basis of therapeutics. 7th ed. New York: Macmillan Publishing, 1985; 1467.
[28] Lenz S, Kühl C, Wang P et al. The effect of ritodrine on carbohydrate and lipid metabolism in normal and diabetic women. Acta Endocrinol 1979; 92: 669–679.
[29] Cousins L. Obstetric complications. In Reece EA, Coustan DR eds. Diabetes mellitus in pregnancy. Principles and practice. New York: Churchill Livingstone 1988; 455.
[30] Briggs GG, Freeman RK, Yaffe SJ. Drugs in pregnancy and lactation. A reference guide to fetal and neonatal risk, 2nd edition. Baltimore: Williams and Wilkins, 1986.
[31] Friedman EA, Neff RK. Pregnancy hypertension: a systemic evaluation of clinical diagnostic criteria. Littleton, MA: PSG Publishing Co, 1977.
[32] Fletcher AE, Bulpitt CJ. A review of clinical trials in pregnancy hypertension. In: Rubin PC eds. Hypertension in pregnancy. New York: Elsevier, 1988; 186.
[33] Barron WM, Murphy MB, Lindheimer MD. Management of hypertension during pregnancy. In: Laragh H, Brenner BM eds. Hypertension, Pathophysiology, diagnosis and management. New York: Raven Press 1990; 1809.

[34] Wallenburg HCS. Hemodynamics in hypertensive pregnancy. In: Rubin PC eds. Hypertension in pregnancy. New York: Elsevier, 1988; 66.
[35] Cocburn J, Moar VA, Ounsted M et al. Final report of study on hyptertension during pregnancy: the effects of specific treatment on the growth and development of children. Lancet 1982; II: 647 – 649.
[36] Sibai BM, Gonzales AR, Mabie WC et al. A comparision of labetalol plus hospitalization versus hospitalization alone in the management of preeclampsia remote from term. Obstet Gynecol 1987; 70: 323 – 327.
[37] Spellacy WN. Carbohydrate metabolism during treatment with estrogen, progestogen, and low-dose oral contraceptives. Am J Obstet Gynecol 1982; 142: 732 – 734.
[38] Spellacy WN, Buhi WC, Birk SA. Effects of norethindrone on carbohydrate and lipid metabolism. Obstet Gynecol 1975; 46: 560 – 563.
[39] Spellacy WN, Newton RE, Buhi WC et al. Lipid and carbohydrate metabolic studies after one year of megestrol acetate treatment. Fertil Steril 1976; 27: 157 – 161.
[40] Spellacy WN, Buhi WC, Birk SA. Carbohydrate and lipid metabolic studies before and after one year of treatment with ethynodiol diacetate in "normal" women. Fertil Steril 1976; 27: 900 – 904.
[41] Back DJ, Backenbridge AM, Crawford FE et al. An investigation of the pharmacokinetics of ethinylestradiol in women using radioimmunoassay. Contraception 1979; 20: 263 – 273.
[42] Orme ML'E, Back DJ, Backenbridge AM. Clinical pharmacokinetics of oral contraceptive steroids. Clinical Pharmacokinetics 1983; 8: 95 – 135.
[43] Larsson-Cohn U, Wallentin L. Metabolic and hormonal effect of post menopausal estrogen replacement treatment. Acta Endocrinol 1977; 86: 583 – 596.
[44] Martin PL, Burnier AM, Greaney MO. Oral menopausal therapy using 17-micronized estradiol. A preliminary study of effectiveness tolerance and patient preference. Obstet Gynecol 1972; 39: 771 – 774.
[45] Bolt HM. Metabolism of estrogens – natural and syntehtic. Pharmacol Ther 1979; 4: 155 – 181.
[46] Okerholm RA, Peterson FE, Keeley FJ et al. Bioavailability of norethindrone in human subjects. Eur J Clin Pharmacol 1978; 13: 35 – 39.
[47] Dorflinger JD. Relative potency of progestins used in oral contraceptives. Contraception 1985; 31: 557 – 570.
[48] Samsioe G. Direct hormonal effects. In: Sex steroids and lipid metabolism. Berlin: Schering AG 1985; 11 – 12.
[49] Muldoon TG. Regulation of steroid hormone receptor activity. Endocrin Rev 1980; 1: 339 – 364.
[50] King WJ, Greene GL. Monoclonal antibodies localized oestrogen receptor in nuclei of target cells. Nature 1984; 307: 745 – 747.
[51] Skouby SO. Oral contraceptives: effects on glucose and lipid metabolism in insulin-dependent diabetic women and women with previous gestational diabetes. Dan Med Bull 1988; 2: 157 – 167.
[52] Kalkhoff RK. Effects of oral contraceptive agents on carbohydrate metabolism. J Steroid Biochem 1975; 6: 949 – 952.
[53] De Pirro R, Fusco A, Bertoli A et al. Insulin receptors during the menstrual cycle in normal women. J Clin Endocrinol Metab 1978; 47: 1387 – 1389.
[54] Skouby SO, Andersen O, Sauerbrey N et al. Oral contraception and insulin sensitivity: In vivo assessment in normal women and in subjects with previous gestational diabetes. J Clin Endocrinol Metab 1987; 64: 519 – 526.
[55] Wingrave SJ, Kay CR, Vessy MP. Oral contraceptives and diabetes mellitus. Br Med J 1979; 1: 23 – 24.
[56] Hannaford PC, Kay CR. Oral contraceptives and diabetes mellitus. Br Med J 1989; 299: 1315 – 1316.

[57] Beck P, Wells SA. Comparison of the mechanisms underlying carbohydrate intolerance in subclinical diabetic women during pregnancy and during post partum oral contraceptive steroid treatment. J Clin Endocrinol Metab 1969; 29: 807–818.
[58] Szabo AJ, Cole HS, Grimaldi RD. Glucose tolerance in gestational diabetic women during and after treatment with a combination-type oral contraceptive. New Engl J Med 1970; 282: 646–650.
[59] Spellacy WN, Buhi WC, Birk SA. Carbohydrate metabolism prospectively studied in women using low-estrogen oral contraceptive for six months. Contraception 1979; 20: 137–148.
[60] Wynn V, Adams PW, Godsland I et al. Comparison of different combined oral contraceptive formulations on carbohydrate and lipid metabolism. Lancet 1979; I: 1045–1049.
[61] Sadik W, Kovacs L, Pretnar-Darovec A et al. A randomized double-blind study of the effects of two low-dose combined oral contraceptives on biochemical aspects Contraception 1985; 32: 223–236.
[62] Skouby SO, Mølsted-Pedersen L, Kühl C. Low dosage oral contraception in women with previous gestational diabetes. Obstet Gynecol 1982; 59: 325–328.
[63] Upton GV. The phasic approach to oral contraception: The triphasic concept and its clinical application. Int J Fertil 1983; 28: 121–140.
[64] Skouby SO, Kühl C, Mølsted-Pedersen L et al. Triphasic oral contraceptives: Metabolic effects in normal women and those with previous gestational diabetes. Am J Obstet Gynecol 1985; 153: 495–500.
[65] Osler M, Wiese J. Contraceptiòn in diabetic women. Acta Endocrinol (Copenh) 1974; Suppl 182: 87–94.
[66] Steel JM, Duncan LJP. Contraception for the insulin dependent diabetic woman: The view from one clinic. Diabetes Care 1980; 3: 557–60.
[67] Steel MJ, Duncan LJP. Serious complications of oral contraception in insulin dependent diabetics. Contraception 1978; 17: 291–295.
[68] Rådberg T, Gustafson A, Skryter A et al. Oral contraception in diabetic women. Diabetes control, serum and high density lipoprotein lipids during low-dose progesteron, combined oestrogen/progesteron and non hormonal contraception. Acta Endocrinol (Copenh) 1981; 98: 246–251.
[69] Skouby SO, Møller-Jensen B, Kühl C et al. Hormonal contraception in diabetic women: Acceptability, diabetes regulation and influence on ovarian function of a nonalkylated estrogen/progesteron compound. Contraception 1985; 32: 23–31.
[70] Lebech PE. Oral contraception with natural human oestrogen – differences between natural and artificial oestrogens. In: Haspels A, ed. Hormonal Contraception. Amsterdam: Excerp Med, 1977; 33–38.
[71] Samsioe G, Skryter A, Silverstolpe G. Oral contraception with a nonalkylated estrogen compound. Effects on lipid metabolism. Gynecol Obstet Invest 1983; 15: 275–282.
[72] Belsey MA, Hall PE, Parker RA et al. A randomized double-blind study of six combined oral contraceptives. Contraception 1982; 25: 231–241.
[73] Skouby SO, Mølsted-Pedersen, Bennet P. Oral contraceptives in diabetic women: Metabolic effects of four compounds with different estrogen/progestogen profiles. Fertil Steril 1986; 46: 858–864.
[74] Arntzenius AC, van Gent CM, Van der Voort H et al. Reduced high-density lipoprotein in women aged 40–41 using oral contraceptives. Lancet 1978; I: 1221–1223.
[75] Wallace RB, Hoover J, Barret-Connor E et al. Altered plasma lipid lipoprotein levels associated with oral contraceptive and oestrogen use. Lancet 1979; II: 111–115.
[76] Fotherby K. Oral contraceptives and cardiovascular disease. Contraception 1985; 31: 369–394.
[77] Kay CR. The Royal College of General Practioners' Oral Contraceptive Study: Some Recent Observations. Clin Obstet Gynaecol 1985; 11: 759–86.
[78] Kay CR. Progesterons and arterial disease. Evidence from the the Royal College of General Practioners Study. Am J Obstet Gynecol 1982; 142: 762–765.

[79] Hassing-Nielsen F. Serum triglyceride in women with and without a predisposition to diabetes during short-term adminstration of a combined oral-contraceptive. Acta Obstet Scand 1974; 53: 13–19.

[80] Rådberg T, Gustafson A, Skryter A et al. Metabolic studies in gestational diabetic women during contraceptive treatment: Effects on serum and high density lipoproteins lipids. Gynecol Obstet Invest 1982; 13: 17–29.

[81] Beck P, Arnett DM, Alsever RN et al. Effect of contraceptive steriods on arginine-stimulated glucagon and insulin secretion in women. II. Carbohydrate and lipid physiology in insulin-dependent diabetics. Metabolism 1976; 25: 23–31.

[82] Rubeck-Petersen K, Skouby SO, Dreisler A et al. Comparative trial of the effects on glucose tolerance and lipoprotein metabolism of two new oral contraceptives containing gestoden and desogestrel. Acta Obstet Gynecol Scand 1988; 67: 37–41.

[83] Weström L, Bengtsson LP, Mårdh PA. The risk of pelvic inflammatory disease in women using intrauterine contraceptive devices as compared to non-users. Lancet 1976; II: 221–224.

[84] Wiese J. Intrauterine contraception in diabetic women. Fertil Steril 1977; 28: 422–425.

[85] Gosden C, Steel JM, Ross A et al. Intrauterine contraceptive devices in diabetic women. Lancet 1982; I: 530–535.

[86] Skouby SO, Mølsted-Pedersen L. Intrauterine contraceptive devices for diabetics. Lancet 1982; I: 968.

Immunotherapy after renal and pancreas transplantation in diabetics

K. J. Berg, I. Brekke, J. Jervell

Introduction

The first attempt to treat diabetes by pancreas transplantation was made in 1966, when a pancreas and a kidney were transplanted simultaneously into a diabetic uremic patient [1]. Until a few years ago however, diabetic patients were considered a high risk group for organ transplantation. The conventional immunosuppressive regimen necessary to prevent rejection of the transplanted organs was poorly tolerated by diabetics, and renal as well as pancreatic transplantation were associated with high morbidity and mortality. Thus, only a small number of pancreas and/or kidney transplantations were performed world-wide. Better immunosuppressive therapy through the introduction of cyclosporine in the 1980s led to a remarkable improvement in both patient and graft survival [2, 3], and the results of renal transplantation in diabetics now equals those achieved in non-diabetics (see Table 1). Consequently, during the last decade uremic diabetic patients have gradually been

Table 1 Survival of diabetic uremic patients following kidney and pancreas transplantation at Rikshospitalet, Oslo 1983–89

	Survival %					
	Patient		Kidney graft		Pancreas graft	
	1 year	5 years	1 year	5 years	1 year	5 years
Group 1 (n = 41)	92	76	92	73		
Group 2 (n = 45)	81	45	78	43		
Group 3 (n = 46)	95	87	84	69	67	45

Group 1 = kidneys from living HLA non-identical donors
Group 2 = cadaveric kidney alone.
Group 3 = combined kidney and pancreas from cadaveric donor

accepted for renal transplantation on equal terms with non-diabetic uremic patients. Furthermore, more than 400 pancreas transplantations are now performed annually at more than 100 centres [4]. In some institutions combined pancreas and kidney transplantations have become the standard treatment for diabetic patients approaching end stage renal disease [5]. Approximately 85% of a world total of more than 2000 pancreatic transplantations so far have been performed in uremic diabetic patients simultaneously with a renal transplantation from the same donor. The remaining 15% were performed as pancreas transplantations alone, either in brittle diabetics or in diabetics who had previously received a renal transplant.

The best results in terms of pancreatic graft survival rates were achieved when both kidney and pancreas are transplanted simultaneously from the same donor. The success rate tends to be somewhat lower when the pancreas is given after a previous kidney transplantation. In the non-uremic recipient of a pancreas transplant alone, the success rate has been relatively low with a one-year graft survival of only 30–40%. Most pancreas transplantations are therefore performed simultaneously as combined kidney/pancreas transplantations in uremic diabetic patients. In these patients the potential hazard of immunosuppressive medication has already been accepted, and the 70–80% pancreas graft survival in these patients is approaching that of the renal transplant.

Pancreatic transplantation is being performed by various surgical techniques. Data from the transplant registry show no significant difference in graft and patient survival obtained using the different techniques [6]. Drainage of exocrine pancreatic secretion to the urinary bladder is, however, preferred by an increasing number of centres since fall in urine amylase secretion may be a help in diagnosing rejection episodes early [7].

Immunosuppression

The most common drugs used to prevent allograft rejection are azathioprine, glucocorticoids, usually prednisolone, and cyclosporine-A (CyA). The antimitotic drug mercaptopurine or its derivate azathioprine has been one of the main immunosuppressive drugs since the dawn of clinical organ transplantation. In most centres, this drug is still part of the basic triple drug immunosuppressive regimen together with steroids and CyA. Two mg/kg body weight azathioprine is usually given in the first postoperative week. Later, the dose is adjusted according to the white blood cell count, with a maintenance dose of 25–75 mg/day.

For about 2 decades, the combination of azathioprine and steroids represented the standard immunosuppressive regimen. In the pre-cyclosporine era steroids were given in high dosages. When combined with CyA and azathioprine (triple therapy), the dose may be drastically reduced. The initial post transplant dose of prednisolone of about 1.5 mg/kg/day is usually tapered to 20 mg/day after one week and further reduced to a maintenance dose of 7.5 – 10 mg/day.

The introduction of CyA to clinical organ transplantation in the early 1980s represented a major improvement in graft survival. CyA is at present an obligatory part of the basic immunosuppression protocols in the majority of transplant centres all over the world. In most centres the initial dose given is 5 – 10 mg/kg/day. The whole blood concentrations should be followed closely and the dosage adjusted accordingly to 50 – 150 ng/ml 2 months after transplantation and to 50 – 100 ng/ml after 6 months.

An increased frequency of rejection episodes in combined renal and pancreatic transplantation and the problems of diagnosing early pancreas graft rejection have led many centres to apply increased immunosuppression during the first critical 10 – 14 days after transplantation. This is achieved by adding a 4th immunosuppressive drug, for instance a polyclonal antilymphocyte (ALG) or antithymocyte globulin (ATG), or a monoclonal antibody like OKT-3. The number of patients treated in this way is, however, still too small to draw definite conclusions regarding the long-term outcome.

Methylprednisolone is the traditional drug for treatment of acute episodes of rejection of the pancreas or the kidney graft. Our present protocol is 0.5 g methylprednisolone as the first dose, followed by 0.25 g daily for another three days. If by the 5th day the rejection has not culminated (steroid resistent rejection), treatment is carried on with monoclonal (OKT-3) or polyclonal (ATG, or ALG) antibodies against T-lymphocytes, OKT-3, 5 mg/day is usually given for 10 days. ATG, 200 mg is given daily for three days, and then every second day until a total dose of 1000 – 1400 mg is reached or the rejection has been overcome.

A more detailed description of the most commonly used immunosuppressive agents is given below, with most emphasis on cyclosporine-A.

Cyclosporine-A (CyA)

Renal side effects of CyA: The most important side effect of CyA is the nephrotoxicity. Serum creatinine is usually increased by 10 – 40% and creatinine clearance and other GFR parameters are reduced in the majority of recipients of renal [8, 9] or cardiac grafts [10]. Although the nephrotoxicity is dose related, renal blood flow and GFR is usually somewhat reduced, also with the relatively low therapeutic doses which are now recommended in organ transplantation.

A reduction in renal blood flow secondary to an increased alpha-adrenergic stimulation of renal vessels has been demonstrated in early stages of CyA nephrotoxicity [11, 12]. Mean arterial blood pressure is increased from 5–15%, depending on the CyA dose. The increased blood pressure is probably also secondary to arteriolar vasoconstriction, but not correlated to the renal dysfunction. Serum potassium is usually moderately increased. This increase has been attributed to the reduced plasma renin activity which usually is seen on CyA treatment in man. Serum uric acid values are increased, often out of proportion to the creatinine values. At higher, toxic dose levels, CyA is also toxic to the renal tubular function [13].

The functional impairment of the kidney, which also is seen with therapeutic CyA dosages does not imply permanent renal damage as all pathological parameters usually are reversible after CyA withdrawal. With higher dosages, possibly also after long-term treatment at low dose levels, specific morphological changes can be seen in the kidney: toxic tubulopathy with giant mitochondria, isometric vacuolization and microcalcifications, arteriolopathy and ultimately striped interstital fibrosis with tubular atrophy [14]. Patients with other organ transplants, such as single pancreas transplants, seem to be at the same risk for kidney damage as renal transplant patients. Prospective trials are now in progress to evaluate if co-administration of calcium-antagonists, alpha blockers or prostaglandin analogs can reduce the renal toxicity of CyA.

Effects of CyA on pancreas function and carbohydrate metabolism: Distribution studies have documented the highest tissue concentrations of CyA in fat tissues and in the pancreas. Cytoplasmatic vacuolar lesions in pancreatic islet cells and a decrease in insulin positive cells have been demonstrated in rats after CyA 25 mg/kg, intraperitoneally for 3 weeks [15]. In another study in rats, therapeutic dosages of CyA induced reversible glucose intolerance due in part to inhibition of insulin secretion, and also possibly inhibition of synthesis [16].

Replacement of azathioprine with CyA 1–7 months after kidney transplantation in man was followed by a small rise in fasting blood glucose and plasma C-peptide levels suggesting that CyA induced insulin resistance, but did not affect beta-cells adversely [17]. In a European multicentre trial [8], fasting blood sugar was the same on CyA as in the azathioprine group. In a group of non-diabetic multiple sclerosis patients randomized to treatment with CyA or placebo for 2 years, no abnormalities were observed in basal levels of glucose, insulin, C-peptide or in glucose disappearance rates and pancreatic islet beta-cell function after stimulation [18]. In summary, the data from clinical studies indicate that the effects of CyA on glucose metabolism and endocrine pancreas function are of minor importance. As prednisolone dosages are generally lower when CyA is used, the tendency to steroid-induced insulin resistance should be reduced on CyA.

Effects of CyA on serum lipids: Complications of atherosclerosis have been reported to be several times more frequent in recipients of renal or cardiac transplants than in the normal population. Both hyperlipidemia and hypertension contribute to the accelerated atherosclerosis. A number of other known risk factors such as age, sex, diabetes, transplant rejection and prednisolone therapy are also independently associated with posttransplant vascular disease [19]. Vascular risk factors are common in diabetics, hence the effect of immunosuppressive treatment on serum lipids is important in kidney and/or pancreas allografted diabetes patients.

A survey of posttransplant hyperlipidemia in 566 CyA treated renal transplanted patients documented a 37,6% incidence of hypercholesterolemia within 6 months after transplantation [20]. There was a strong correlation between cholesterol levels and corticosteroid therapy. The cholesterol levels were reduced when the prednisone dose was lowered. Hypertriglyceridemia was more severe with CyA/prednisone than with azathioprine/prednisone treatment. The triglyceride levels were also strongly correlated to age, serum creatinine, diabetes and the use of beta-blockers.

In a prospective study of kidney allografted patients randomized either to CyA alone, CyA and prednisolone or to azathioprine and prednisolone, total cholesterol was unchanged in the latter group, but increased in both CyA groups, primarily due to an increase in LDL cholesterol [21]. On the other hand, CyA did not increase the incidence of coronary heart disease compared to azathioprine, at least in the 2 first years after heart transplantation [22]. In another study in heart transplant patients the prevalence of coronary heart disease was significantly lower 3 years after operation on double or triple treatment with CyA than with prednisolone and azathioprine [23].

It is reasonable to conclude that corticosteroids play a major pathogenetic role for hypercholesterolemia. The prednisolone dose is usually reduced in CyA treatment. Further studies will be required to assess if CyA has major adverse effects on serum lipids and on the pathogenesis of atherosclerosis.

CyA and drug interactions: CyA is extensively metabolized by the heterogenic cytochrome P 450 oxidase enzyme system. Inducers of this enzyme (like barriturates, phenytoin and other antiepileptic drugs, rifampicin and isoniazide) will reduce the blood concentration of CyA. Drugs which are metabolized by the same enzyme system will inhibit CyA metabolism by competitive binding to the enzyme (ketaconazole, erythromycin, some calcium channel blockers, cimetidine) and thereby increase CyA blood concentration, sometimes dramatically (for survey see Cockburn [24]). Secondarily to these pharmacokinetic interactions transplant rejection or increased CyA toxicity may be induced.

There are also many pharmacodynamic interactions. Drugs like amphothericin B, aminoglycosides, trimethoprim, antiinflammatory drugs (NSAIDs) and x-ray contrast media increase the nephrotoxicity. Calcium blockers have been claimed to reduce the nephrotoxicity, possibly also alpha blockers and postglandin analogs. Inhibitors of angiotensin converting enzyme have no documented interactions with CyA.

Interactions with lovastatin: Lipid lowering drugs are commonly used in diabetics, and lovastatin has been shown to have beneficial effects on plasma lipid levels in diabetics [25]. Lovastatin is extensively metabolized by liver and plasma lovastatin levels were increased 5-fold in one heart transplant patient on CyA. The patient suffered from severe muscle damage with myolysis and acute renal failure [26]. Later, other cases with rhabdomyoloysis with this drug combination were reported. Myopathia appears to have occurred in about 30% of 15 patients who had taken CyA together with lovastatin [27]. The interaction is dose dependent, and in most cases the daily dose was 40 mg or more.

At the present time the use of lovastatin and other inhibitors of HMG-CoA reductase are not recommended in diabetics or other patients treated with CyA. Prospective studies are in progress with 20 mg/day in selected patients groups.

Glucocorticoids

Synthetic glucocorticoids are regularly used as part of the immunosuppressive regimen following organ transplantation, most commonly prednisolone or prednisone. During acute rejection episodes the dose is either increased or soluble methylprednisolon is given in high dosages intravenously. Steroids are used for their cytostatic and cytolytic effects, particularly on the T-lymphocytes which are markedly inhibited in their functions. They also have a general stimulating effect on appetite and well-being, and cause a marked increase in the insulin need due to the catabolic and gluconeogenetic effects [28].

Most glucocorticoids are fully absorbed from the gastrointestinal tract. Cortisone and prednisone are inactive, but are quickly and completely metabolized in the liver to cortisol and prednisolone which are the active substances. Methylprednisolone is active directly. Half-lives vary and are shortest for cortisol and cortisone, longer for prednisone and prednisolone. Like cortisole, most synthetic glucocorticoids are bound to transcortine, albumin and other serum proteins, and are excreted as conjugated metabolites.

Long-term treatment causes more long-lasting suppression of the ACTH-cortisole axes, and sudden stopping of the drug may be dangerous and a slow reduction of dose is advised over 2–6 weeks. In any crises or other disease, extra cortisol substitution may be necessary.

The use of glucocorticoids causes development of Cushingoid features, increased tendency to gastritis, gastric ulcer, and also gastric and colonic perforation. Aseptic bone necroses, especially of the femur head, are common. All complications due to glucocorticoids are rarer since the introduction of cyclosporine A, which permits lower dosages to be used.

Azathioprine

Azathioprine is metabolized to the active drug mercaptopurine following its absorption. The absorption of azathioprine is, however, more reliable and complete. It is given orally, usually once daily in the morning with a meal. Too high dosages cause suppression of bone marrow, but rarely in the dosages given following transplantation. Liver toxicity, increase in serum transaminase levels, hepatitis and acute pancreatitis occasionally occur. Allopurinol slows azathioprine metabolism and the combination should be avoided. If it must be given, the dose of azathioprine should be reduced by 1/3 to 1/4 and white blood cell counts should be monitored closely. The dose usually given varies in different immunosuppressive regimens. The tolerance to the drug differs, common safety procedures include white blood cell counts, frequently during the first few weeks until the drug tolerance is ascertained.

The dangers of immunosuppression

The complications which the immunosuppressive treatment as such are increased susceptability to infections, increased tendency to neoplasms and side effects associated with the drugs themselves as described.

The infections in immunosuppressed patients are often unusually virulent; and severe infections are often caused by microorganisms, often not associated with clinical infections in an individual with normal immune systems; e.g. fungi, pneumocystis carinii, cytomegalovirus. Some centres use low dose prophylactic trimetoprim-sulfa for several months to prevent pneumocystis pneumonia. The patients have to be thoroughly informed about the danger of infections and how important it is to contact their doctor early in cases of fever and other symptoms indicating possible infection.

Malignant tumors of all types with long-term immunosuppressive therapy are associated with an excess of skin cancers and lymphomas.

Diabetes management

Following isolated kidney transplantations, insulin will of course have to be given. Many different regimens have been used. In hospital a mixture of soluble and medium acting insulin given twice daily is the simplest regimen. Insulin dosages have to be adjusted at least once, preferably twice daily based on blood glucose results obtained every fourth hour, what is known about the patient's food intake, infections and the dose of prednisolone to be given. It is important that when increased dosages of steroids are given as part of anti-rejection treatment, there should be no delay in the increase in insulin dose. It is also important to make the patients and all of the staff caring for them aware of the need for insulin during increases in glucocorticoid treatment, even though the patient may not be eating.

Complete normalization or near normalization of blood glucose is impossible in the early stages following kidney transplantation. The goal should be to keep the blood glucose levels below 12 mmol/l, gradually obtaining better normalization once the patients are able to take over the blood glucose measurements themselves, and perhaps also start on more physiological insulin delivery systems using multi-injection therapy or pumps. In the long-term, the total insulin dose will be higher than prior to transplantation, due to the long term prednisolone therapy required.

Conclusion

With modern immunosuppressive therapy using cyclosporine-A in combination with other immunosuppressive drugs (glucocorticoids, azathioprine, antilymphocyte sera) kidney transplantation may be performed in cases of diabetic uremia with remarkable success, using the same immunosuppressive regimen as with non-diabetics. Transplantation of the uremic diabetic is as successful as for the non-diabetic, even when a combined kidney and pancreas graft is given. A successful pancreatic transplantation increases life quality and may possibly improve long-term survival. The introduction of modern immunosuppressive therapy using cyclosporine-A in combination with prednisolone and/or azathioprine has much improved the results of transplantation in diabetic patients.

References

[1] Kelly WD, Lillehei RC, Merkel FK et al. Allotransplantation of the pancreas and duodenum along with the kidney in diabetic nephropathy. Surgery 1967; 61: 827–37.

[2] Melandri M, Dubernard MJ, Sanseverino R et al. Impact of immunosuppression on improvement of results of clinical pancreas transplantation. Diabetes 1989; 38 (suppl 1): 30–2.

[3] Merion RM, White DJG, Thiru S et al. Cyclosporine: five years' experience in cadaveric renal transplantation. N Eng J Med 1984; 310: 148–54.

[4] International Pancreas Transplant Registry. Personal communication.

[5] Brekke IB. Experience of the National Hospital, Oslo, Norway. In: Dubernard MJ, Sutherland DER, eds. International handbook of pancreas transplantation. Dordrecht: Kluwer Academic Publishers, 1989; 413–19.

[6] Sutherland DER, Moudry KC. Pancreas transplant registry. In: Dubernard JM, Sutherland DER, eds. International handbook of pancreas transplantation. Dordrecht: Kluwer Academic Publ, 1989; 291–322.

[7] Stratta RJ, Sollinger HW, Perlman SB et al. Early diagnosis and treatment of pancreas allograft rejection. Transplant Int 1988; 1: 6–12.

[8] European Multicentre Trial Group. Cyclosporin in cadaveric renal transplantation: one-year follow up of a multicentre trial. Lancet 1983; 2: 986–9.

[9] Canadian Multicentre Transplant Study Group. A randomized clinical trial of cyclosporine in cadaveric renal transplantation. N Engl J Med 1983; 309: 809–15.

[10] Myers BD, Sibley R, Newton L et al. The long-term course of cyclosporine-associated chronic nephropathy. Kidney Int 1988; 33: 590–600.

[11] Murray BM, Paller MS, Ferris TF. Effect of cyclosporine administration on renal hemodynamics in conscious rats. Kidney Int 1985; 28: 767–74.

[12] Dieperink H, Leyssac PP, Starklint H et al. Nephrotoxicity of cyclosporin A. A lithium clearance and micropuncture study in rats. Eur J Clin Invest 1986; 16: 69–77.

[13] Berg KJ, Førre Ø, Bjerkhoel F et al. Side effects of cyclosporin A treatment in patients with rheumatoid arthritis. Kidney Int 1986; 29: 1180–1187.

[14] Bergstrand A et al. Renal histopathology in kidney transplant recipients immunosuppressed with cyclosporin A: results of an international workshop. Clin Nephrol 1985; 24: 107–19.

[15] Teraoka S, Kawai T, Yamaguchi Y et al. Cyclosporine-associated toxicity in pancreatic islet cells and its prevention by K-MAP in cyclosporine-treated animals Transpl Proc 1989; 21: 2774–9.

[16] Yale JF, Roy RD, Grose M et al. Effect of cyclosporine on glucose tolerance in the rat. Diabetes 1985; 34: 1309–13.

[17] Gunnarsson R, Klintmalm G, Lundgren G et al. Deterioration in glucose metabolism in pancreatic transplant recipients given cyclosporin. Lancet 1983; 2: 571–2.

[18] Robertson RP, Franklin G, Nelson L. Intravenous glucose tolerance and pancreatic islet beta-cell function in patients with multiple sclerosis during 2-yr treatment with cyclosporin. Diabetes 1989; 38: 58–64.

[19] Kasiske BL. Risk factors for accelerated atherosclerosis in renal transplant recipients. Am J Med 1988; 84: 985–91.
[20] Vathsala A, Weinberg RB, Schoenberg L et al. Lipid abnormalities in cyclosporine-prednisone-treated renal transplant recipients. Transplantation 1989; 48: 37–43.
[21] Raine AEG, Carter R, Mann JI et al. Adverse Effects of cyclosporin on plasma cholesterol in renal transplant recipients. Nephrol Dial Transplant 1988; 3: 458–463.
[22] Hess ML, Hastillo A, Thompson JA et al. Lipid metabolism in organ transplantation: Does cyclosporine accelerate coronary atherosclerosis? Transpl Proc 1987; 19 (suppl 4); 71–3.
[23] Reid CJ, Banner N, O'Brien C et al. Prevalence and significance of coronary artery disease after cardiac transplantation in patients receiving cyclosporin and azathioprine. Brit Heart J 1988; 59: 116.
[24] Cockburn I. Cyclosporine A. A clinical evaluation of drug interactions. Transpl Proc 1986; 18 (suppl 5): 50–5.
[25] Garg A, Grundy SM. Lovastatin for lowering cholesterol levels in non-insulin-dependent diabetes mellitus. N Engl J Med 1988; 318: 81–6.
[26] Norman DJ, Illingworth DR, Munson J et al. Myolysis and acute renal failure in a heart-transplant recipient receiving lovastatin N Engl J Med 1988; 318: 46–47.
[27] Tobert JA. Rhabdomyolysis in patients receiving lovastin after cardiac transplantation. N Engl J Med 1988; 318: 48.
[28] Olefsky JM, Kummerling G. Effects of glucocorticoids on carbohydrate metabolism. Am J Med Sci 1976; 271: 202–10.

Subject index

Prevention and Treatment of Diabetic Late Complications

Edited by *C. E. Mogensen* and *E. Standl*

1989. 17 x 24 cm. X, 226 pages. With 44 illustrations.
Paperback **DM 86,–** ISBN 3 11 012297 9

International experts in diabetes mellitus review the latest knowledge of prevention and treatment of diabetic late complications. There are articles on epidemiology and clinical impact of diabetic late complications in IDDM and NIDDM. Separate papers deal with diabetic renal disease, retinopathy and neuropathy and, in addition, with heart diseases, cerebral, and peripheral vascular diseases in connection with diabetes. Special attention has been given to treatment in relation to risk factors in diabetes.

Elke Austenat / Tilman Stahl

Insulin pump therapy

Indication – Method – Technology

With the assistance of *Pia Magdalena Heinze, Erich Lange* and *Margrit Reinhold*

1990. 17 x 24 cm. XII, 187 pages. With 77 illustrations and 34 tables.
Paperback **DM 128,–** ISBN 3 11 012265 0

The insulin pump therapy is one of the latest methods in the therapeutic strategy of diabetes mellitus. The authors of this book are very experienced in application of the pump therapy and describe for example indications and contraindications of insulin pump therapy, prerequisites and techniques of these methods, education for pump patients, application procedures, special situations in insulin pump therapy (children during vacation, pregnancy and so on).

The insulin pump therapy is designed to prevent or at least to delay the diabetic late complications.

W DE G **de Gruyter**

Bei Fragen zur Produktsicherheit wenden Sie sich bitte an:
If you have any questions regarding product safety,
please contact:

Walter de Gruyter GmbH
Genthiner Straße 13
10785 Berlin
productsafety@degruyterbrill.com